Cannabis Pharmacy

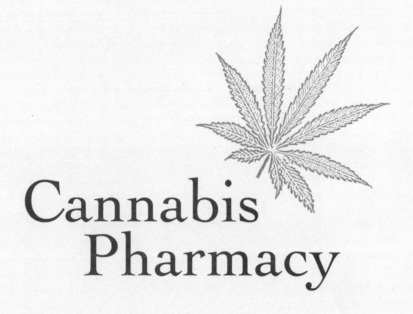

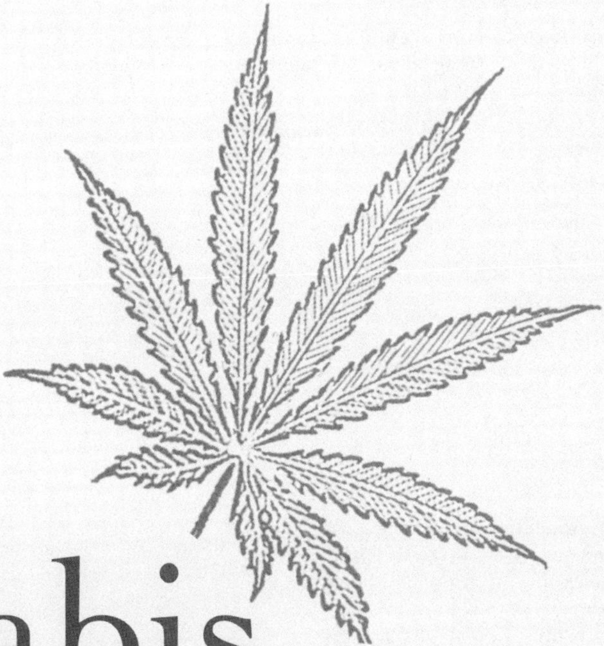

Cannabis Pharmacy

The Practical Guide to Medical Marijuana

Michael Backes

FOREWORD BY ANDREW WEIL, M.D.

BLACK DOG
& LEVENTHAL
PUBLISHERS
NEW YORK

This Black Dog & Leventhal Publishers, Inc. edition is published by arrangement with Elephant Book Company Limited and Michael Backes.

Black Dog & Leventhal Publishers, Inc.
151 West 19th Street
New York, NY 10011

Elephant Book Company Limited,
35, Fournier Street,
London E1 6QE
United Kingdom

Distributed by
Workman Publishing Company
225 Varick Street
New York, NY 10014

Manufactured in the
United States of America

Editorial Director: Will Steeds
Managing Editor: Laura Ward
Project Editor: Anna Southgate
Index: Christine Shuttleworth
Art Editor: Louise Turpin
Illustrations: Robert Littleford
Cover illustration: Louise Turpin

ISBN 13: 978-1-57912-951-4

hgfedeba

Library of Congress Cataloging-in-Publication Data available on file

DISCLAIMER
The cultivation, possession, use, and supply of cannabis are criminal offenses in most states, and in many countries, punishable by fine and/or imprisonment. This book is not intended to advocate or recommend the unlawful use of cannabis for any reason. It is based on the author's research into existing scientific and anecdotal information concerning the use of cannabis for medical purposes, and is not intended to provide guidance or prescription for self-medication or for any particular course of treatment incorporating cannabis, which should only be pursued under the care of a physician in states where such use is permitted by law.

Contents

Foreword by Andrew Weil, M.D.

From the perspective of someone who has studied traditional therapies as a career, it is surprising that cannabis ever left our medicine cabinets, since the plant has been used for millennia in cultures throughout the world as a curative for ailments of both mind and body. In 1942, the American Medical Association (AMA) fought to keep it as part of the U.S. Pharmacopeia. In spite of the long history of cannabis as a safe and effective treatment for many conditions, the AMA lost that battle, and cannabis was banned. Now, more than seventy years later, the American Herbal Pharmacopeia has begun publishing a two-part monograph on cannabis, returning the plant and its derivatives to their proper places as useful medicines.

During its long exile, cannabis was falsely characterized as a dangerous narcotic, though the reality of its medicinal value was known by many. Patients undergoing treatment for HIV shared that cannabis increased appetite. Multiple sclerosis patients reported that cannabis relieved stiffness and pain. And a few cancer patients for whom allopathic treatments failed, found that cannabis could occasionally help the body overcome drug-resistant tumors. The medical and research communities are only just beginning to discover and investigate what their patients have known for decades.

Michael Backes' excellent overview combines current research with real world observations from the patients utilizing cannabis dispensaries in California to present compelling evidence about the medical conditions for which the plant can often provide effective treatment. Intended as a guide for patients and their physicians, the book explains what has been recently learned and what has been rediscovered about the uses of the cannabis plant as a medicine. I have often said that Western medicine could benefit from using traditional plant remedies instead of, or in combination with, the synthetic drugs that dominate the modern pharmacopeia. I would also say that cannabis is one of the best examples of a safe and effective botanical remedy that is underutilized and still largely misunderstood by many conventional practitioners.

Owing to variations in their chemistry, different cultivated varieties of cannabis produce different physiologic effects, and sometimes widely different experiences, yet there is little evidence-based guidance about using particular cannabis varieties to address specific conditions or symptoms. This book helps fill that gap.

Clinical investigation is confirming that many common Western diseases such as diabetes and cancer may be closely linked to metabolic dysfunction caused by poor diet and inactivity. We are also beginning to see evidence that cannabis contains potent homeostatic regulators that can help balance and maintain metabolism. Its chemical constituents interact with the body's own endocannabinoid system, affecting every physiological process, including appetite, regulation of mood, and perception of pain.

My journey in developing integrative approaches to health and wellness began with a strong emphasis on mind-body interactions, and when I began studying cannabis in 1968, in my senior year at Harvard Medical School, I learned that it is capable of producing an extraordinary range of effects. This work was conducted two decades before the endocannabinoid system was discovered. Since that time, science has continued to confirm what experience has told us for centuries. With the evidence presented in this informative guide, the value and utility of cannabis as medicine becomes even clearer.

It is my strong hope that the work of Michael Backes and other like-minded professionals will inspire further rational and scientific approaches to cannabis, steer us away from the political agenda that has made it difficult for patients to access the benefits of this useful plant, and guide the medical community to use it intelligently.

Introduction

When we consider the arguments against the use of cannabis as a medicine, we must first look at the evidence. What we know is that cannabis is certainly not a panacea, but for specific individuals and circumstances, it is very useful and quite safe. Both advocates and detractors of medical cannabis continue to promote a somewhat shocking range of misconceptions about medical cannabis. Cannabis won't cure every cancer; it does produce side effects; and it is not right for everyone. Before the publication of this book, finding evidence-based information about herbal cannabis medicines often proved challenging. I wrote this book primarily because I needed information on the history of medical cannabis, how to use it appropriately, and the varieties and conditions it has successfully treated for my work in California with patients using cannabis under a physician's supervision. But with only 21 U.S. states permitting the medical use of cannabis in late 2013, I recognize that there are many seriously ill individuals who must rely on illicit sources for cannabis, and these patients have an acute need for accessible and informed guidance. This book is not intended to replace professional medical advice and supervision. Anyone comtemplating using cannabis as a medicine should seek advice from a doctor.

The prohibition of cannabis has unfortunately ensured that a spectacular amount of nonsense about cannabis and its medical uses is taken as fact. In my experience, opponents of medical cannabis remain opponents only until an illness strikes. Numerous times, politicians, judges, and law enforcement officials who suddenly find themselves in need of some cannabis advice have approached me for discreet consultations on behalf of themselves or their loved ones.

Since the 1980s, a small coterie of determined scientists and physicians have studied cannabis and its effects. Conducting that work has been arduous in a hostile regulatory environment in which the study of cannabis is severely restricted and often prohibited altogether. But these determined individuals have not only persevered, they have succeeded in greatly broadening our understanding of the plant.

Cannabis and cannabis medicine remains a moving target. Every month, new studies further our understanding as to how cannabis works and might be used as a medicine. And our understanding of both the benefits and risks of using cannabis also continues to deepen. Because cannabis does not exhibit the toxicity of drugs such as opioids, dosing cannabis as a medicine tends to be imprecise.

A brave group of activists choose to challenge the status quo and demand access to cannabis as a medicine. This book would not exist without the courageous precedent that these activists set. Organizations such as the Wo/Men's Alliance for Medical Marijuana, Americans for Safe Access, Marijuana Policy Project, Drug Policy Alliance, and NORML have fought hard to ensure that medical cannabis is available to those in need.

Far too many people have gone to prison for using or providing cannabis as a medicine. Laws that prohibit physician-supervised access to medical cannabis are fundamentally wrong and must be reformed. California was the first U.S. state to provide legal access to medical cannabis. Initially, California failed to create a regulatory system to provide storefront access to cannabis, and this created an uncertain climate in which some Californian cities tolerate dispensaries, very few permit them, and most ban them. Even laws that intend to enable storefront access to medical cannabis often create an oppressive bureaucracy that can be dauntingly difficult to navigate.

In this work, I attempt to provide a comprehensive overview of the uses of cannabis as medicine, even though the scientific and medical understanding of how cannabis works as a medicine continues to evolve. Cannabis is an extremely complex medicine, made more so because different varieties and forms of cannabis produce a range of medicinal effects. Part 1 provides a historical and scientific overview of cannabis as a medicine. Part 2 offers a guide to using medical cannabis. Part 3 focuses on 27 cultivated varieties of cannabis and how they produce different effects. And Part 4 provides information about using cannabis effectively with different ailments under a doctor's supervision. The research collected herein is drawn from hundreds of recent studies, but this book hopes to present this evidence in an accessible manner for the layperson. *Cannabis Pharmacy* is designed to encourage further inquiry, so I have attempted to avail myself of as many open and accessible sources as possible in its creation, so that patients and physicians wishing to dig deeper may do so easily and inexpensively. I hope that this book will encourage patients and physicians to discuss the advantages and limitations of cannabis as a medicine. It would be great if patients and physicians felt as comfortable discussing the potential use of cannabis as they do discussing an herbal medicine such as echinacea.

On the rear flap of the 1967 book, *Pot: A Handbook of Marijuana*, the author John Rosevear writes:

"The author does not pretend to impartiality in this controversial question but he does claim that this handbook is an objective statement of the truths about marihuana. Once the prejudice and hysteria surrounding this subject are put aside, these truths are quite simple."

Nearly a half-century later, the prejudice and hysteria may finally be fading, but the truth about cannabis as a medicine is more interesting and complex than anyone could have imagined.

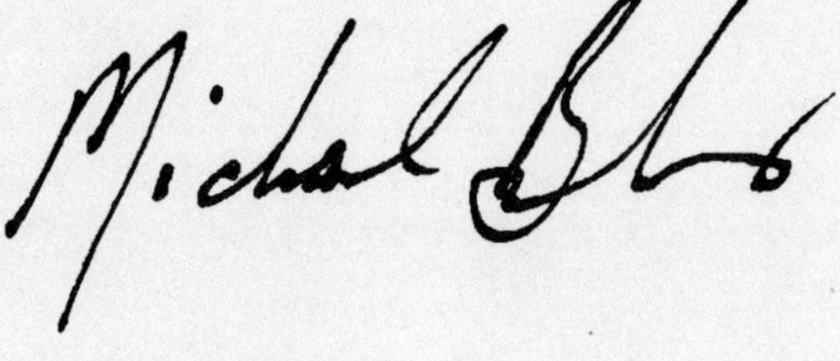

Cannabis as a Medicine

For over 12,000 years, the cannabis plant has provided humankind with food, fiber, inebriation, and medicine. Cannabinoids, medicinally active substances produced within the plant, interact with the protein receptor molecules of the body's own system. Different varieties of cannabis express different chemistries, which in turn produce a varying range of medicinal effects. Understanding the chemical ecology produced within cannabis allows both the patient and the recreational user to use cannabis medicines more predictably and effectively.

1

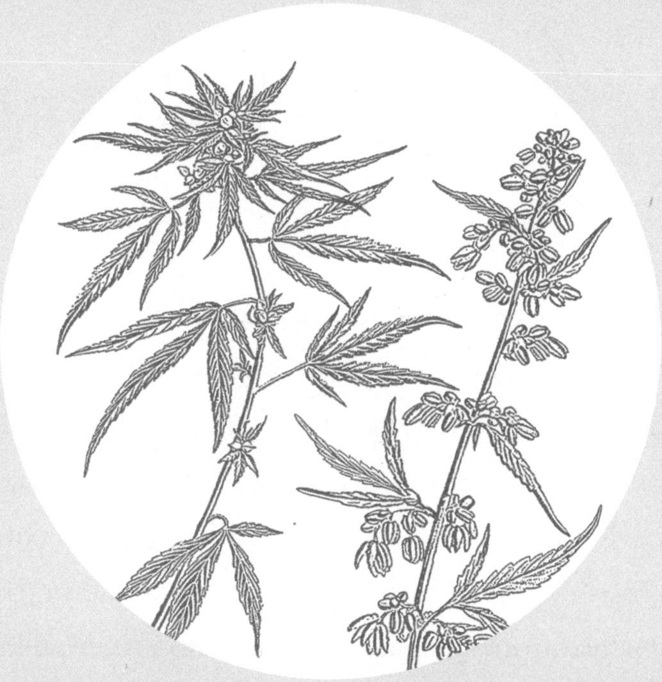

HISTORICAL CONTEXT

Humans may have cultivated cannabis for longer than any other plant. It has been grown for fiber, medicine, and inebriation for at least 12,000 years, since the end of the last Ice Age. The cannabis plant is believed to have first emerged around 36 million years ago in Central Asia, near the Altai Mountains, where Siberia, Mongolia, and Kazakhstan converge. Forty-thousand-year-old human remains have been found in the Altai region, so cannabis plants growing along the region's riverbanks may likely have first attracted human attention as a food source.

The earliest extant evidence for cannabis usage are 10,000-year-old dried cannabis flower specimens: they were found in a clay jar at a Jomon-era Japanese archaeological excavation. According to researcher Dave Olson, "A neolithic cave painting from coastal Kyushu in southwest Japan depicts tall stalks with hemp-shaped leaves. Strangely dressed people, horses and waves are also in the painting, perhaps depicting the Korean traders bringing hemp to Japan. The hemp plant figure itself reflects the sun/plant image, similar to the hieroglyphic likenesses used by Mediterranean cultures."[1]

The earliest written accounts of cannabis used as medicine originate in ancient China, where cannabis is part of the oral, generation-to-generation transmission of plant lore. This oral tradition extends back to the legendary Emperor Shen-Nung, who reigned 4,700 years ago. In his teachings, Shen-Nung cited cannabis as an important herbal remedy, along with ginseng and ephedra. Following Shen-Nung's reign, Chinese medical traditions were passed along orally for the next 2,000 years. And by the first century CE, Chinese oral traditions concerning medicinal cannabis had expanded to cover over 100 medical conditions. This knowledge was incorporated into the first Chinese pharmacopeia, *Pen-ts'ao Ching*.

A photograph of a neolithic cave painting discovered in southwest Japan. Between the two tall hemp leaves, it is just possible to discern human and horse figures above the swirling waves.

> *"Ma-fên (fruits of hemp)... if taken in excess will produce hallucinations... If taken over a long term, it lightens one's body."*[2]
> Pen-ts'ao Ching

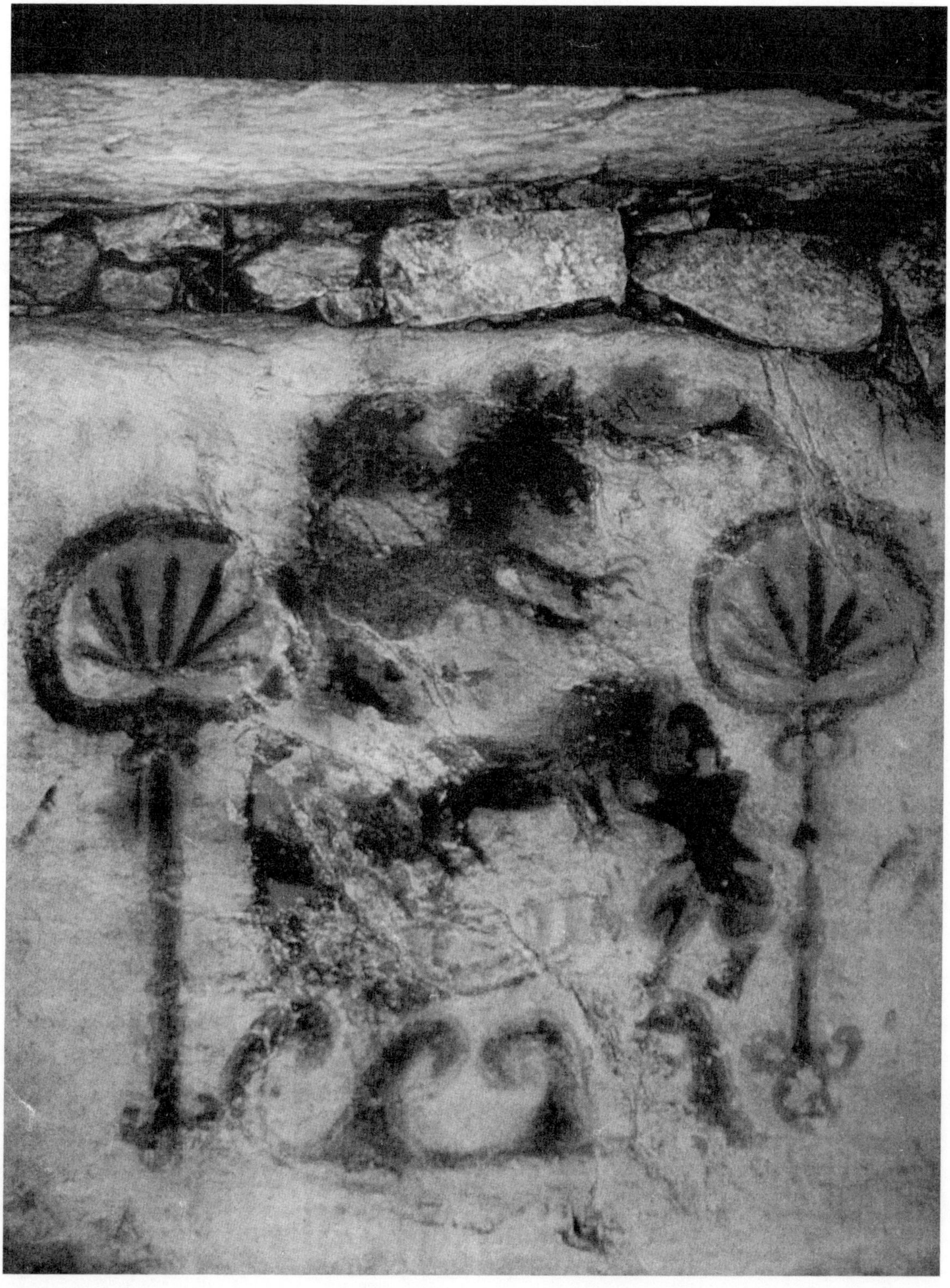

Cannabis on the Move

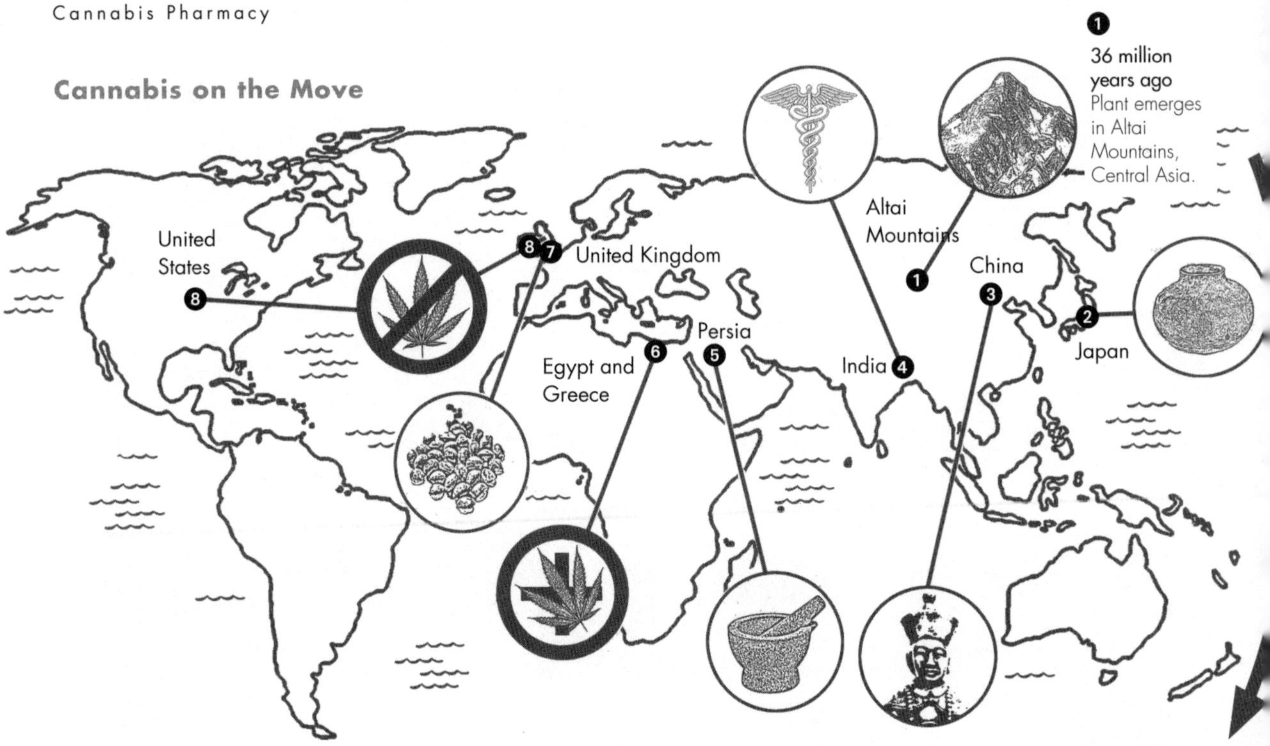

8	7	6	5	4	3	2	
1920s/1930s Cannabis banned in the U.K. and all 48 U.S. states.	1894 Hempseed considered beneficial in moderate doses in the U.K.	200 BCE Cannabis used as a medicine in Egypt and Greece.	500 BCE Cannabis ranks as the most important of all known medicinal plants in Persia.	1500 to 200 BCE Cannabis used as a medicine in India.	4,700 years ago Cannabis considered an important herbal remedy in China.	10,000 years ago Cannabis flowers stored in clay jars in Japan.	

From 1500 to 200 BCE, cannabis was used as a medicine in the Mediterranean region, in Egypt and Greece, and in India. In the *Avesta*, the religious text of Zoroastrianism of ancient Persia (now modern-day Iraq), cannabis was ranked as the most important of all known medicinal plants.[3] Further, Polish anthropologist Sula Benet has claimed, controversially, that cannabis provided a key ingredient—*q'neh bosm*—in the holy anointing oil recipe recounted in the Hebrew Old Testament's book of Exodus.[4]

In early Islamic medicine, cannabis is both lauded as widely useful and condemned as a poison. The great Persian physician Mohammad-e Zakariã-ye Rãzi (865–925 CE) cited a wide range of uses for cannabis as a medicine, while the tenth-century physician Ibn Wahshiyah, in his book *On Poisons*, claimed that the mere aroma of cannabis resin would kill within days of exposure.[5]

Cannabis Travels West

Until the seventeenth century, very little was written in the West about the medicinal uses of cannabis. In his oft-quoted *Anatomy of Melancholy*, the English scholar Robert Burton included "hemp-seed" in a laundry list of plant remedies for depression, and renowned herbalist Nicholas Culpeper included hemp as an anti-inflammatory

William O'Shaughnessy

Sir William Brooke O'Shaughnessy (1809–89) was an Irish physician working in Calcutta, India, who studied the medicinal uses of cannabis. O'Shaughnessy first experimented with animals to gauge cannabis' toxicity. While O'Shaughnessy's animal subjects ranged from dogs and pigs to fish and birds, he could only induce symptoms of inebriation in his human subjects, as the animals recovered regardless of the dose they received. O'Shaughnessy went on to experiment with alcoholic tinctures of *Cannabis indica*, working with people suffering from medical conditions including cholera, tetanus, rheumatism, and infant convulsions. He found cannabis to be uniformly effective at calming these patients. O'Shaughnessy even tried a cannabis tincture on a person suffering from rabies, and, although the patient died from the disease, O'Shaughnessy noted that he believed the medicine helped the individual pass much more peacefully. William O'Shaughnessy's work extended far beyond his interest in cannabis, however. He wrote a standard chemistry textbook, considered to be the first to stress the importance of biochemistry. O'Shaughnessy also developed the first intravenous fluid replacement treatment, which was used successfully to counter the fatal dehydration caused by many diseases, including cholera. Finally, he introduced the telegraph to India and even ran the county's telegraphic service, for which he was knighted by Queen Victoria, in 1856.[6,7]

Hemp in Moderate Doses

The nineteenth century's most noted study of cannabis came in the shape of the enormous "Indian Hemp Drugs Commission Report," conducted by the British government and published in 1894. The report consisted of seven volumes and 3,291 pages of testimony from 1,193 interviews conducted across India. The conclusion of the report? "The Commission have now examined all the evidence before them regarding the effects attributed to hemp drugs. It will be well to summarize briefly the conclusions to which they come. It has been clearly established that the occasional use of hemp in moderate doses may be beneficial; but this use may be regarded as medicinal in character."[8]

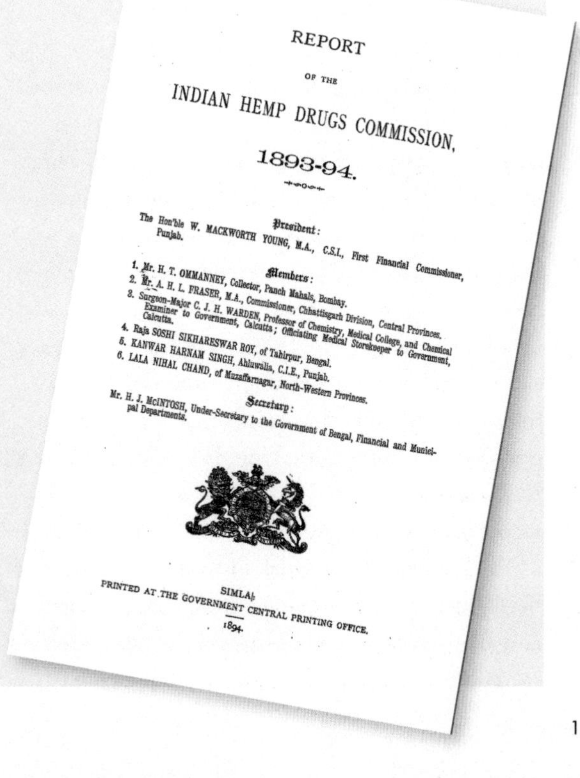

REPORT

OF THE

INDIAN HEMP DRUGS COMMISSION,

1893-94.

President:

The Hon'ble W. MACKWORTH YOUNG, M.A., C.S.I., First Financial Commissioner, Punjab.

Members:

1. Mr. H. T. OMMANNEY, Collector, Panch Mahals, Bombay.
2. Mr. A. H. L. FRASER, M.A., Commissioner, Chhattisgarh Division, Central Provinces.
3. Surgeon-Major C. J. H. WARDEN, Professor of Chemistry, Medical College, and Chemical Examiner to Government, Calcutta; Officiating Medical Storekeeper to Government, Calcutta.
4. Raja SOSHI SIKHARESWAR ROY, of Tahirpur, Bengal.
5. KANWAR HARNAM SINGH, Ahluwalia, C.I.E., Punjab.
6. LALA NIHAL CHAND, of Muzaffarnagar, North-Western Provinces.

Secretary:

Mr. H. J. McINTOSH, Under-Secretary to the Government of Bengal, Financial and Municipal Departments.

SIMLA:
PRINTED AT THE GOVERNMENT CENTRAL PRINTING OFFICE.
1894.

in *The English Physitian* [*sic*]. It is interesting to note that both of these uses would have relied on English fiber cannabis varieties constitutionally low in tetrahydrocannabinol (THC; the main psychoactive constituent in cannabis) and likely higher in cannabidiol (CBD), an excellent anti-inflammatory.

In 1838, *Cannabis indica* was reintroduced to Western medicine by William O'Shaughnessy, an Irish physician working and teaching in India, who published a noted account of his experiments with the plant.[9]

In its usage in O'Shaughnessy's India, cannabis—both as a medicine and an inebriant—was typically consumed orally, rather than smoked. The use of *bhang* (ground marijuana) in *bhang lassi*, a drink consisting of milk, spices, and cannabis, had been present in the Indian subcontinent for over 1,000 years. Interestingly, recipes for *bhang lassi* often call for up to an ounce of cannabis flowers and leaves. Such a recipe could easily deliver 200 milligrams of THC per cup of *bhang*—an enormous dose. So why doesn't a glass of *bhang lassi* deliver a huge effect? Simply because *bhang* is typically not heated above the temperature at which THC acid becomes psychoactive. Since *bhang lassi* recipes call for first making a cannabis water tea, before folding in the milk, this means that few of the non-water-soluble cannabinoids will be extracted. *Bhang lassi* is intended to be mild in its effect, and its preparation method supports that outcome.

O'Shaughnessy's work in India—then part of the British Empire—gained notice back in Britain, and British doctors would spend the next 50 years studying cannabis and its uses as a medicine.

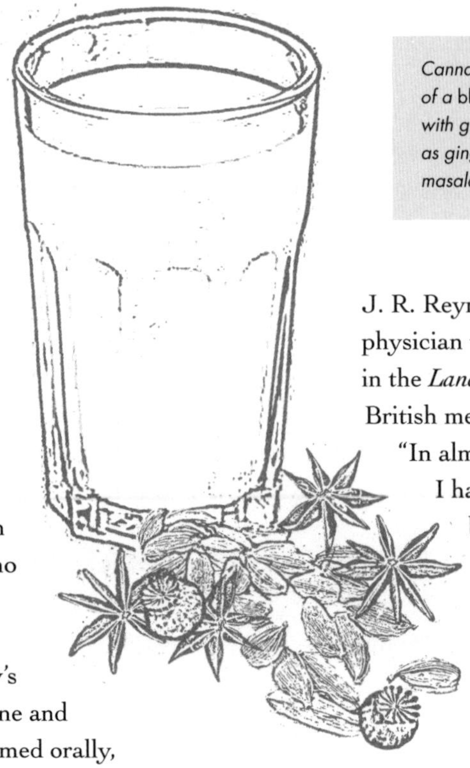

Cannabis-infused milk forms the basis of a bhang lassi, *which is thickened with ground almonds. Aromatics such as ginger, aniseed, cardamom, garam masala, and poppyseeds add spice.*

J. R. Reynolds, personal physician to Queen Victoria, wrote in the *Lancet* (a highly respected British medical journal) in 1890, "In almost all painful maladies I have found Indian hemp by far the most useful of drugs."[10] Despite rumors to the contrary, there is no evidence that Reynolds provided cannabis to Victoria for her menstrual cramps.

From Prohibition to Present

In 1925, the League of Nations endorsed and ratified the International Opium Convention, which included language banning cannabis and its derivatives except for medical and scientific use; this specific form of cannabis prohibition has continued internationally to this day. The U.K. banned cannabis a few years later, in 1928.

By the mid-1930s, cannabis had been banned in all 48 U.S. states, and though it remained listed in the U.S. Pharmacopeia (USP) as a medicine, access was virtually impossible.[11] The federal government subsequently banned cannabis with the Marihuana Tax Act of 1937. During the hearing on the Tax Act, the American Medical Association's legislative counsel, Dr. William C. Woodward, testified to the House Ways and Means Committee that "there are potentialities in the drug that should not be shut off by adverse

From Medicine to Narcotic and Back: Cannabis Scheduling and Reform

The Single Convention on Narcotic Drugs of 1961 is the principal international treaty prohibiting the production and supply of proscribed classes of drugs around the world, including cannabis, LSD, cocaine, and heroin. This treaty requires signatory nations to pass laws that align with the provisions of the Single Convention. Evolving from a series of treaties in the 1920s, which sought to control international trade in opium, cocaine, and certain derivatives, the Single Convention was the first time that cannabis had been included in such a document. It explicitly permits the production and supply of the scheduled drugs for medical or research purposes. Government officials often cite that reforming cannabis laws on a national or state level will require modifying this treaty. The reality is that nations often choose to shun provisions of treaties to which they are signatories, if doing so is considered politically acceptable and expedient within their home nations.

Raphael Mechoulam

Since the early 1960s, Dr. Raphael Mechoulam (b. 1930) has conducted cannabinoid research in Israel. The U.S. government, through the National Institutes of Health, has funded much of Mechoulam's research into cannabis chemistry. Even though cannabidiol (CBD) had first been isolated from Mexican cannabis and Indian hashish samples back in 1940, no further studies had been conducted into CBD for 25 years when Dr. Mechoulam started studying CBD and other cannabinoids in the early 1960s. Mechoulam and his colleagues built upon their 1963 research on the CBD cannabinoid molecule to help them isolate THC the following year. Mechoulam went on to identify the two "best candidate" molecules which were later proven to be the body's own cannabinoids, a group of substances called endocannabinoids.

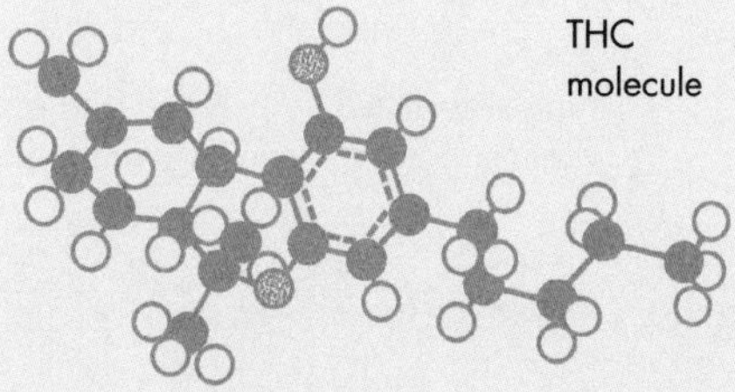
THC molecule

legislation. The medical profession and pharmacologists should be left to develop the use of this drug as they see fit."[12] Dr. Woodward and the AMA objections were ignored.

By the mid-twentieth century, the perception of cannabis and its extracts had devolved from being a safe and effective medicine to a dangerous narcotic. The American Medical Association continued to oppose the removal of cannabis medicines from the U.S. Pharmacopeia for five years after the passage of the Marihuana Tax Act, before it was finally excised in 1942. From World War II until the early 1960s, cannabis was only studied in the context of being a dangerous narcotic. The U.S. government discouraged any research into cannabis as a potential medicine.

The "modern" scientific era of cannabis research arrived in 1964, with the discovery of the major psychoactive ingredient in cannabis: delta-9-tetrahydrocannabinol, or THC. This clear, tasteless liquid was discovered by Raphael Mechoulam, an Israeli researcher in Jerusalem.

THE CANNABIS PLANT

Current genetic understanding places cannabis within the plant family Cannabaceae. This small family consists of flowering plants that originated within the temperate regions of the Northern Hemisphere. Besides cannabis, the Cannabaceae family includes two species of hops, whose female flowers are used for making beer. The leaves of hop plants share their palmate (finger-shaped) form with cannabis. More recently, the Cannabaceae family has broadened to include 70 species of hackberry trees, previously thought to be part of the related Ulmaceae family, which also includes elm trees.

In the genes: cannabis shares family traits with hops and hackberry trees.

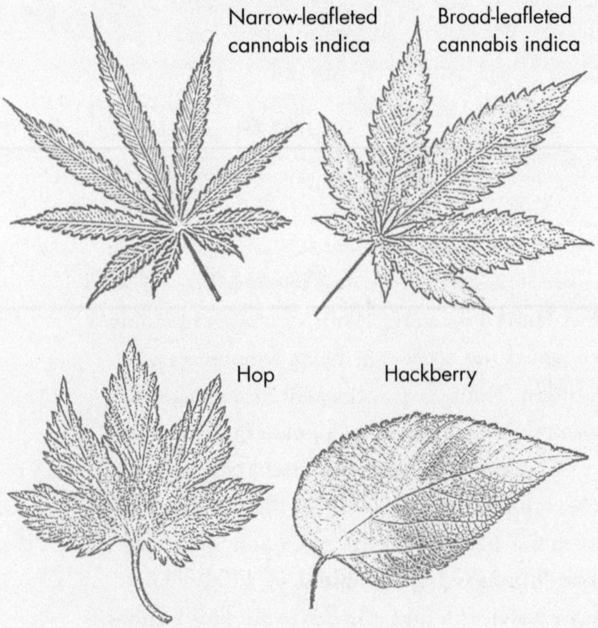

Genetic evidence supports the argument for cannabis appearing to have split into two species: *sativa* and *indica* (see page 52). *Sativa* is the fiber type of cannabis that produces more CBD and typically less than 1 percent THC. *Indica* is the drug-rich cannabis, whose THC content can reach 25 percent of the plant's dry weight. In common parlance, *sativa* is used to describe narrow-leafleted and taller drug varieties from more tropical climes, while *indica* is applied to the broad-leafleted and shorter drug varieties from Afghanistan and Pakistan. While the Afghan plants rarely grow to more than 6½ feet (2 meters) in height, their Southeast Asian counterparts, for example in Vietnam, have been reported to exceed 27 feet (7 meters) in height.

Cannabis for Everything

Cannabis is a truly multipurpose plant. Its extraordinarily strong fibers have been used to make hemp cloth and paper for thousands of years. The Vikings used hemp to make sails for

The relative heights of the two cannabis species when compared to an average human being. The narrow-leafleted sativa grows to as much as three times the height of the broad-leafleted indica. To some extent the ultimate height of a plant depends on cultivation methods and whether a plant is grown outdoors, indoors, or in a greenhouse.

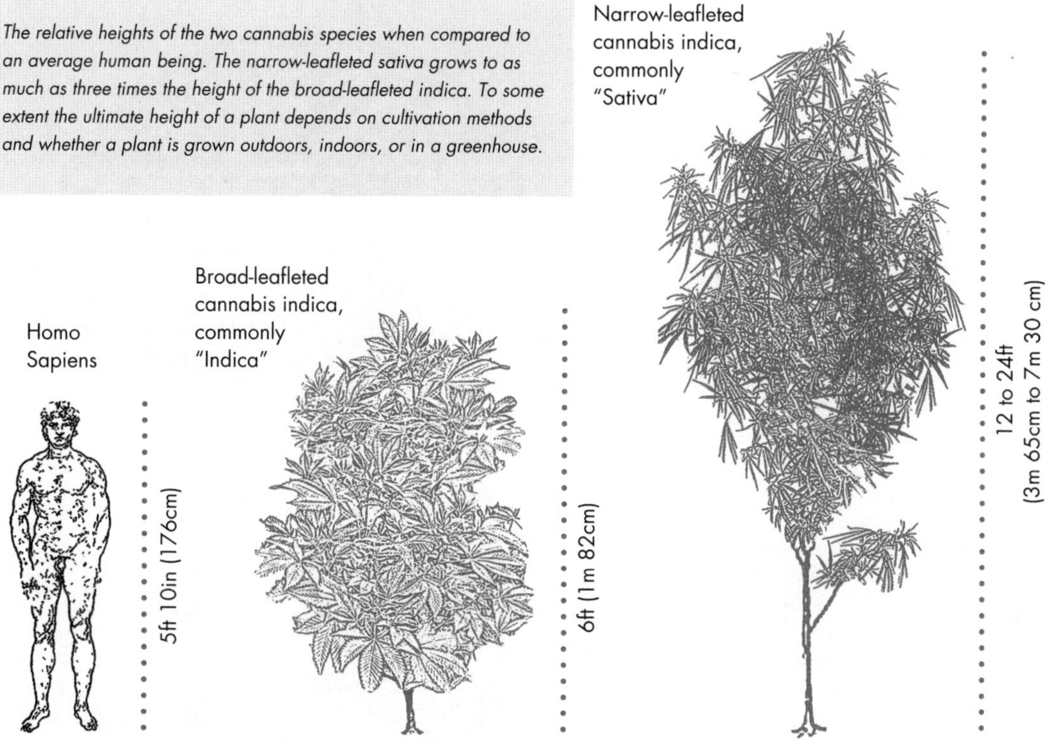

their ships to voyage from Scandinavia to Nova Scotia. Betsy Ross sewed the first United States flag from hempen cloth. The American Declaration of Independence was written on hemp paper, and deutsche marks—now obsolete German currency—were once printed on hemp paper. In the Netherlands, windmills were often built to crush hemp stalks.[13]

As already mentioned, cannabis' potential as a food source is likely what first drew early humans' attention. Cannabis seed (hempseed)—which is strictly speaking a nut rather than a seed—is exceptionally rich in polyunsaturated fats, essential fatty acids, and proteins (see page 20). This composition qualifies it as a functional food (that is, a food that can benefit a person's health in ways other than purely nutritional) and indeed hempseed has been used in Asian cultures as both a food and a medicine for three millennia. Despite the sweeping American prohibition of cannabis products, over the last two decades hempseed has been permitted in the U.S. for use in food.[14]

Cannabis resin's utility as a drug, both for medicinal and psychoactive use, has encouraged breeding favoring the plant's production of resin (see pages 24–25). Breeding for increased resin production has produced a range of cannabis drug chemotypes regionally around the globe, with some cultivars producing only THC, other cultivars producing THC and CBD, and a few cultivars expressing propyl THCV and/or CBDV (see pages 42–46).

The Sexes of Cannabis

Cannabis is dioecious, meaning that it produces male and female flowers on separate plants. By contrast, the majority of flowering plants exhibit both male and female reproductive organs on the same plant, developing mechanisms that are geared to reduce inbreeding and self-pollination. Cannabis likely evolved two sexes to encourage a wider genetic diversity.[15] Molecular genetic markers have been found within cannabis, meaning that the plant's sex can be determined before any visible signs are observed.[16]

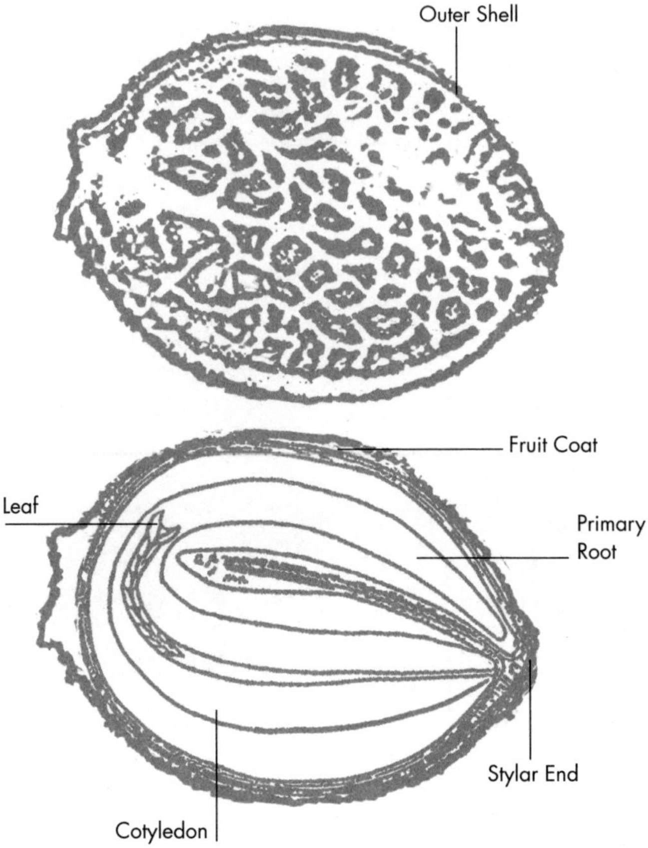

Hempseeds contain all of the essential amino acids, a good number of essential fatty acids, as well as high levels of magnesium, iron, and potassium. It is processed into various forms, including hemp flour, hemp milk, and hemp oil.

Outdoor vs. Indoor—Why Cannabis Is Not a Houseplant

Throughout the Western world, a debate rages over whether outdoor or indoor cultivation of medical cannabis produces better medicine. Indoor cultivation within a controlled environment can produce five crops per year of small, pristine plants with vast numbers of intact trichomes. Outdoor cultivation typically produces a single crop of very large plants, from which an individual can produce as much as 5 pounds (2.3 kilograms) or more of flowers. Outdoor cultivation requires good sun, water, well-drained soil, and reasonable maintenance. Indoor cultivation takes high-intensity lighting, hydroponics equipment or soil pots, environmental control, and constant maintenance. Pests (see pages 68–69) are more difficult to control indoors, therefore preventative measures to control them are crucial. The future of medical cannabis cultivation likely belongs to a hybrid of indoor and outdoor: the greenhouse. As with most flowering plants, cannabis thrives in a properly maintained greenhouse. Greenhouse cultivation is also much more environmentally friendly than conventional indoor cultivation (see also, page 75).

The dioecious nature of cannabis plants means that male and female cannabis plants produce their own types of flowers. The female (left) grows seed pods, while the male (right) develops sacs full of pollen for fertilization.

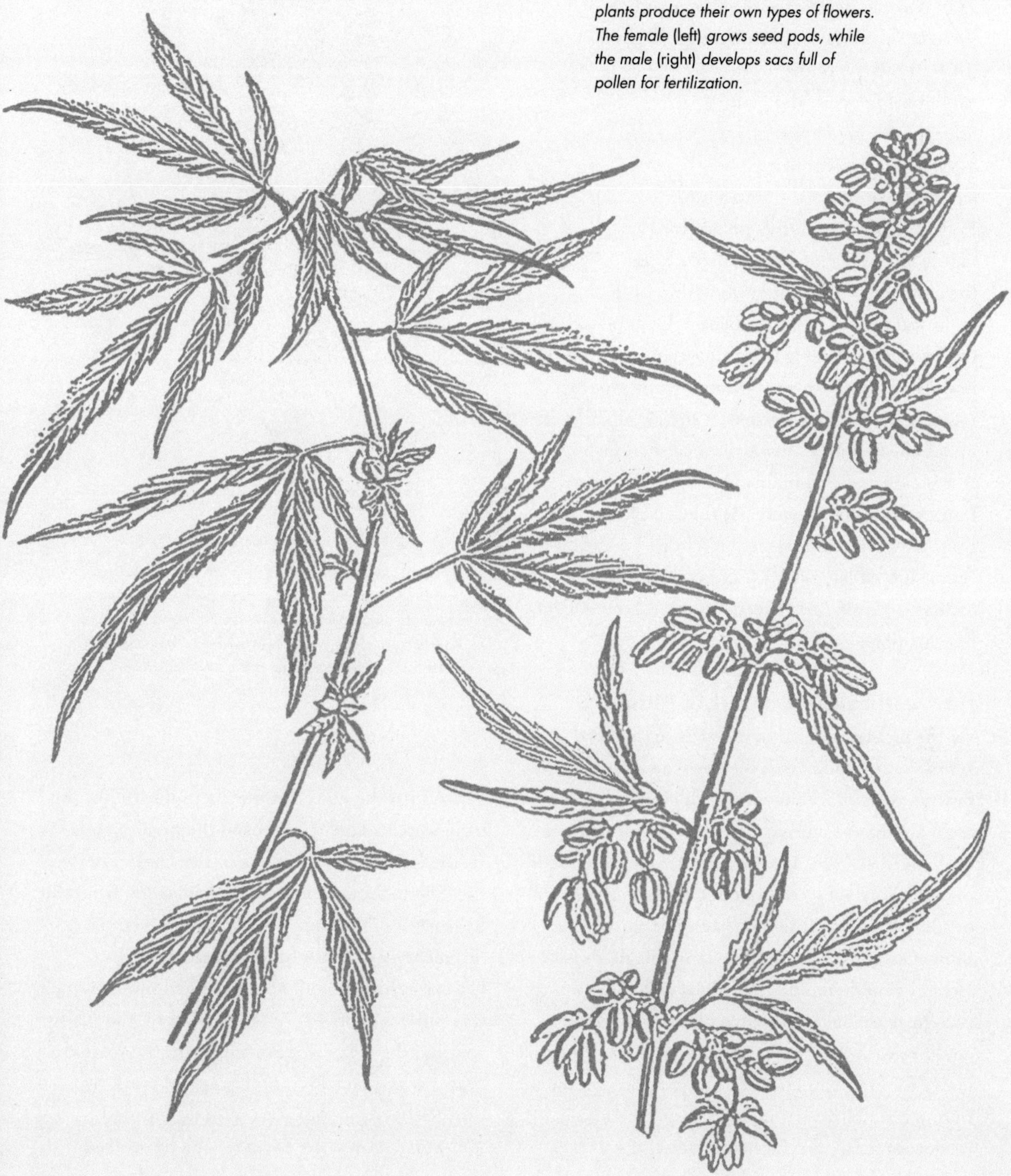

Cannabis is an annual plant, which means that it completes its life cycle within a single year. Most cannabis seeds will germinate three to seven days after planting. During the first three months of the cannabis life cycle, the plant undergoes a rapid vegetative growth phase, producing leaf mass for optimal photosynthesis. Following the vegetative phase, longer nights after the summer solstice trigger the cannabis flowering cycle within both male and female cannabis plants. Depending on the latitude, cannabis flowering requires 10 to 12 hours of night. Flowering cannabis produces fewer leaflets (small leaves) as the plant shifts its metabolic resources toward reproduction.[17] A typical female cannabis plant will produce hundreds of tiny flowers. At the top of the plant these flowers are clustered in a huge mass that in Spanish is called a "cola." Colas of outdoor female cannabis plants can exceed 4 feet (1.2 meters) at harvest time.

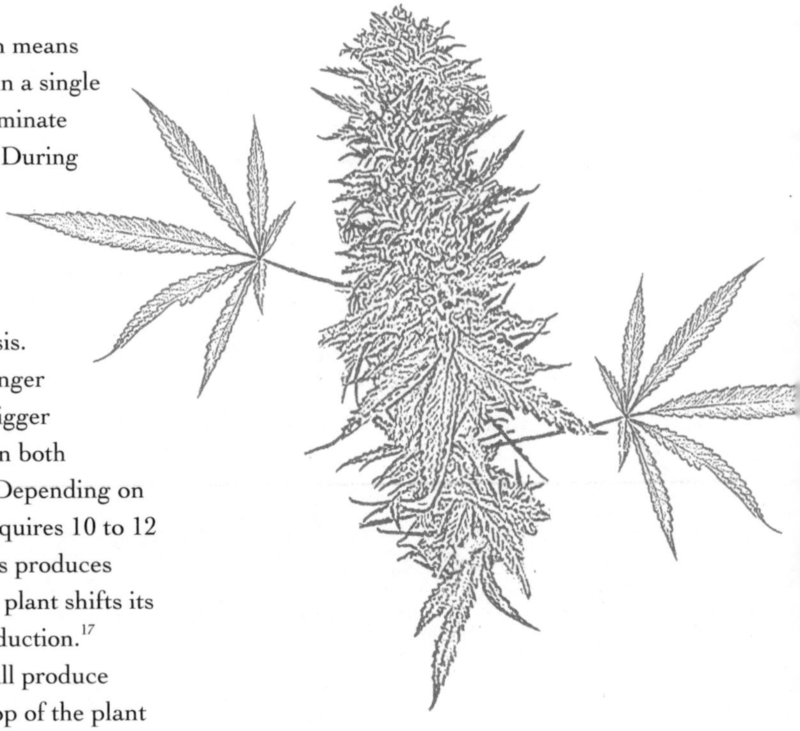

A cola at the top of a female cannabis plant. A cannabis plant will develop one large cola at the top of its main stem. There may be smaller colas on either side, too. There are several methods by which it is possible to train cannabis plants to grow several larger colas, and not just one.

Harvesting the Cannabis Plant

By the nineteenth century, it was discovered in India that unpollinated, seedless female cannabis flowers were more potent, producing more drug resin and hence more cannabinoids and terpenes (see pages 42–49). This technique of culling male plants before they could pollinate the females produced a form of female cannabis flowers known as ganja. The Indian cannabis fields in Bengal would employ specialists called *poddars* to recognize the male cannabis plants before they could release their pollen, and then mark these males for eradication.[18] The ganja approach meant that instead of diverting energy and metabolic resources to the production of seed, the unfertilized female cannabis plant would continue to produce resin while it awaited pollination.

When introduced to California in the 1960s, this technique radically increased the quality and aesthetics of drug cannabis in the United States.

The technique was called *sinsemilla*, from the Spanish for "without seed." Carolyn Garcia, former wife of Grateful Dead member Jerry Garcia, wrote a book about the technique, which was published in 1977.[19] But the book that truly sparked the *sinsemilla* movement in the United States was a lavishly photographed work by Jim Richardson and Arik Woods, entitled *Sinsemilla: Marijuana Flowers*, which received limited distribution in 1976. This work provides the best photographic reference of the different varieties of high-end drug cannabis being produced in the mid-1970s in the United States.[20]

The advantages of producing seedless drug cannabis come with a downside, however. Seedless crops are typically produced not from seeds, but from "clones," a term used to describe cuttings taken from vegetative "mother plants." While providing more uniformity in the crop, growing drug cannabis from clones nevertheless eliminates the opportunity for varietal improvement that accompanies propagating the crop from seed. Using the clones-and-mothers approach has kept certain lines of drug cannabis alive for decades, although accident, interdiction, and neglect have resulted in many early clone lines being lost.

Since the turn of the century, tissue culture techniques have been used with varying success in the United States, Israel, the United Kingdom, Austria, and Canada to propagate cannabis plants from tissue samples. This work was first pioneered using fiber cannabis varieties in China as early as the 1980s.[21] Tissue culture of cannabis can also be used to create "artificial seeds," a feat accomplished by a group led by Dr. Hemant Lata at the University of Mississippi.[22]

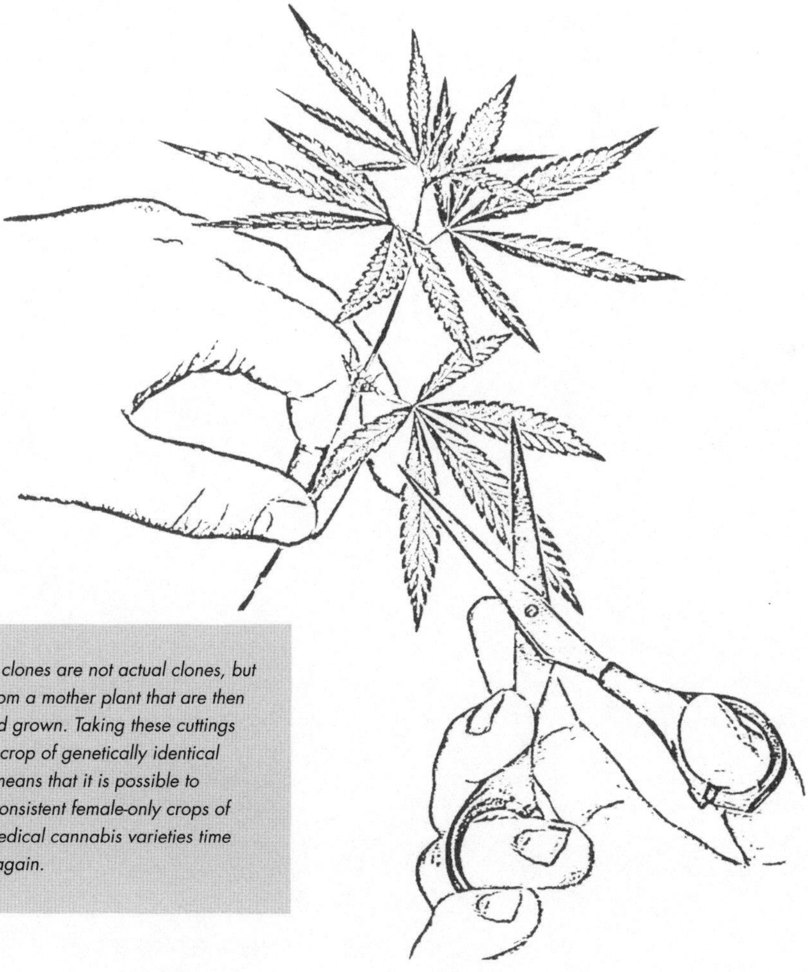

Cannabis clones are not actual clones, but cuttings from a mother plant that are then rooted and grown. Taking these cuttings ensures a crop of genetically identical plants. It means that it is possible to produce consistent female-only crops of desired medical cannabis varieties time and time again.

Medicine in the Resin

The cannabis plant produces a number of capitate-stalked glandular trichomes. The tips of these specialized plant hairs secrete the resin, a medicinal psychoactive substance, which consists of terpenoids, fats, and cannabinoids. The unpollinated female cannabis plant produces far greater concentrations of interesting medicinal substances in its resin than the male. This resin is primarily produced in the flowering tops of the female. Each tiny cannabis flower within these clusters consists of a single, curled leaf known as a bract. Each cannabis bract is covered with vast numbers of tiny hair-like gland cells called trichomes. Under magnification, a trichome resembles a golf ball sitting atop a tee. The golf ball is the trichome's resin head, a waxy pillow of oils secreted from cells at the tip of the trichome's stalk. When resin heads are ruptured, they release intense aromatic chemicals called terpenoids (see page 47), which are associated with the smell of cannabis. (Cannabinoids, pages 42–43, are themselves odorless.) These resin heads contain the most medically interesting chemicals produced

The Structure of the Female Plant

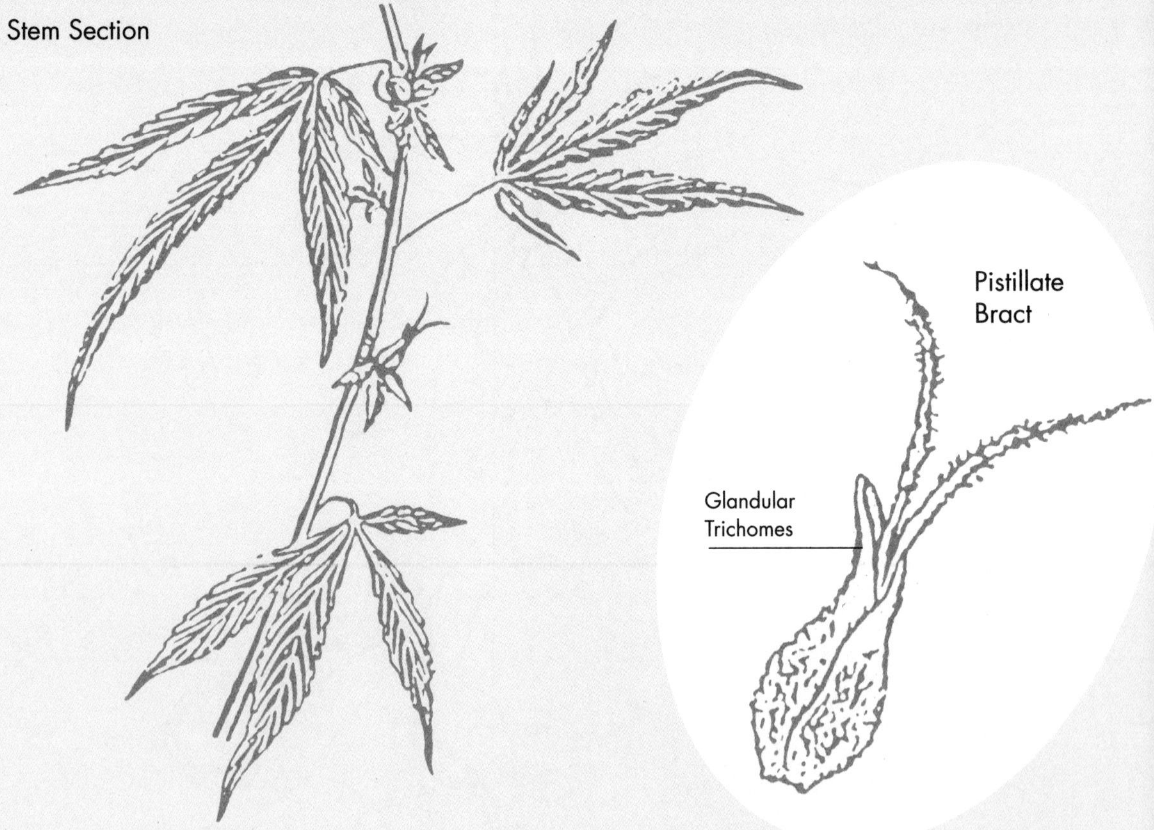

by the cannabis plant, including cannabinoids and terpenoids. They are also the plant's most delicate structure. And since they contain the majority of the medicine, trichome heads must be handled extremely gently to avoid rupture and subsequent oxidation.

Between the resin head and the trichome stalk is an abscission layer, which allows the resin head to be separated from the stalk. These little balls of cannabis resin can be collected by sifting dried cannabis over a fine mesh screen, which allows the tiny resin heads to pass through the screen (see page 81). Alternatively, agitating the cannabis in ice water makes the trichomes brittle and they shear off, allowing the resin heads to be sieved from the water with a mesh screen.

The reasons why the cannabis plant secretes its precious resin are somewhat disputed. Claims have been made that the cannabinoids act as ultraviolet (UV) filters to protect the plant's reproductive tissues from sunlight damage. A strong case has also been argued that the resin protects the plant from predation by insects and grazing animals.

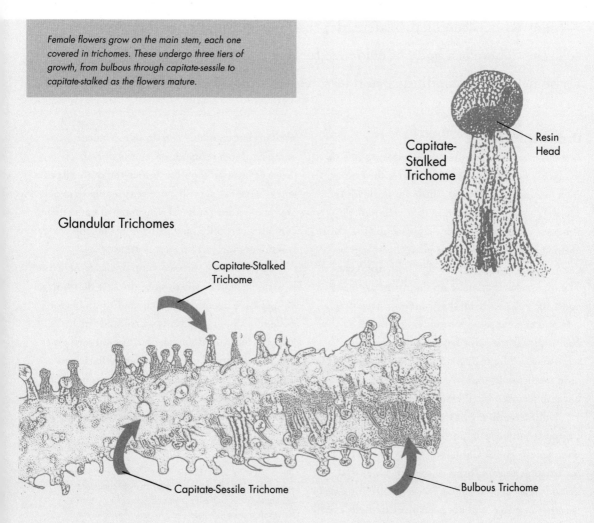

Female flowers grow on the main stem, each one covered in trichomes. These undergo three tiers of growth, from bulbous through capitate-sessile to capitate-stalked as the flowers mature.

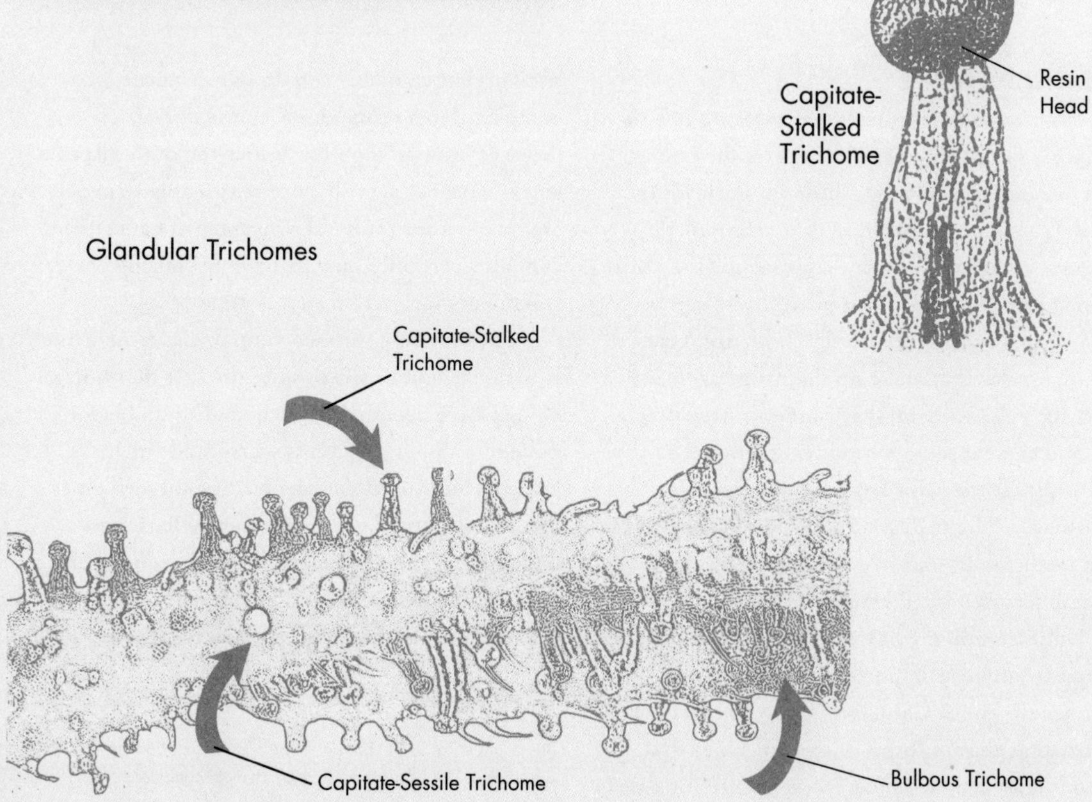

HOW MEDICAL CANNABIS DOES AND DOESN'T WORK

According to a recent survey by the International Association for Cannabinoid Medicines (IACM), most individuals who use cannabis for medical reasons are seeking symptomatic relief from pain or physical discomfort—for example, back pain, injury or accident, migraine, etc. —followed by sleeping disorders, depression, neuropathy, and multiple sclerosis. There is a body of evidence for using cannabis as a medicine for some of these conditions, and less evidence for others.

Use or Abuse?

Although cannabis is often cited as being one of the most commonly abused drugs on the planet, such a characterization is a little bit misleading. There is a common and false distinction made between the misuse of licit drugs versus the abuse of illicit ones. Both licit and illicit drugs can be used rationally and irrationally; both are misused. The molecules that make up the drugs are neither good nor evil. To claim that cannabis is completely safe and can cause no harm is as irrational as claiming that cannabis has no medicinal use whatsoever. The reality is that cannabis can be used medicinally, and that cannabis can cause harm if not used intelligently.

Understanding what we don't know about cannabis can be as important as making use of what we do know. Cannabis may well be effective for treating certain forms of cancer. Does that mean it is a cure for cancer? No. A cure for cancer is something that will keep a cancer patient free from cancer for at least five years. It has not been proven that cannabis can do that. Cancer is complex. It's not one disease; it is dozens of diseases lumped together under the umbrella of a single word: cancer. It's not reasonable to expect any one plant to solve the mystery of cancer. But cannabis certainly may provide promising treatments for certain cancer types.

The way to approach cannabis as a medicine is to do so cautiously, despite the fact that human beings have been using medicinal cannabis for millennia. Such caution is warranted since humans have used various traditional medicines incorrectly, and have inadvertently harmed ourselves in the process. It is worth remembering that arsenic was used as a medicine by nearly every doctor in the eighteenth century.

The results of an IACM survey on the uses of cannabis as a medicine. The tables reveal which medical conditions are treated most frequently (top) and types of symptoms for which patients are most likely to seek alleviation through the use of medicinal cannabis (bottom).[23]

SURVEY OF MEDICAL CONDITIONS AND THE NUMBER OF PEOPLE TREATING THEM

ADHD or hyperactivity	33
Allergy	7
Amyotrophic lateral sclerosis	1
Anxiety disease	38
Arthrosis or degenerative arthritis	35
Asthma	15
Autism	4
Back pain	113
Bechterew disease	6
Bipolar disorder	13
Cancer	14
Cancer chemotherapy	7
Chronic obstructive pulmonary disease	6
Crohn disease or ulcerative colitis	17
Dependency from alcohol, opiates, or other	14
Depression	64
Epilepsy	15
Fibromyalgia	33
Gastritis or gastric ulcer	5
Glaucoma	10
Head or brain injury	4
Hepatitis	23
HIV or AIDS	28
Irritable bowel syndrome	13
Lupus erythematosus	4
Menstrual pain	5
Migraine or headache	33
Multiple sclerosis	39
Neuralgia	9
Neurodermitis	2
Neuropathy	23
Obsessive compulsive disorder	7
Osteoporosis	2
Pain from injury or accident	59
Parkinson disease	2
Phantom limb pain	7
Postpolio syndrome	3
Posttraumatic stress disorder	31
Restless legs syndrom	3
Rheumatoid arthritis	19
Schizophrenia or psychosis	7
Scoliosis	7
Sleeping disorder	66
Spinal cord injury	22
Tinnitus	1
Tourette syndrome	3
Trigeminus neuralgia	1

SURVEY OF SYMPTOMS AND THE NUMBER OF PEOPLE SEEKING ALLEVIATION

Anxiety	174
Appetite loss or weight loss	102
Bladder problems	8
Breathing problems	14
Chronic inflammation	35
Chronic pain	278
Depression	50
Diarrhea	8
General malaise	17
Hyperactivity	22
Impotence or decreased sexual desire	3
Inner unrest	22
Irritability	22
Nausea or vomiting	22
Nightmares	6
Pruritus or itching	-
Seizures	7
Sleep disorders or insomnia	49
Spasms	28
Spasticity	10
Sweating at night	3
Tics	1
Tremor	1

The Chemical Ecology of Cannabis—A Question of Synergies

While much of this book focuses on THC, there is a lot more cannabis chemistry of increasing medicinal interest. Doctors and pharmacologists, including Ethan Russo, John McPartland, and Geoffrey Guy, have spent the last few decades examining the chemical ecology of the cannabis plant. McPartland and Guy have proposed a "coevolution hypothesis" which posits that humankind has been breeding selected cannabis varieties purposely so as to interact safely with the human body's endocannabinoid system. Perhaps the human body evolved to eliminate cannabinoid receptors from the brain stem. Were this not the case, a cannabinoid overdose would be fatal. What is known for certain, however, is that the cannabis plant produces a range of cannabinoids and terpenoids that modulate the effects of one another and often reduce the side effects of one constituent while enhancing the effects of another. Cannabidiol (CBD) reduces the anxiety that can be caused by tetrahydrocannabinol (THC) and also reduces the forgetfulness produced by moderate doses of THC. Pinene, a terpenoid produced by some varieties of cannabis, also reduces the short-term memory impairment that can be caused by THC. It is extraordinary that one plant can produce so many safe, pharmacologically active substances, and it is likely not an accident either. The number of potential chemical synergies of medicinal interest found within the cannabis plant boggles the mind and should keep researchers quite busy for at least the next decade.

Changing Practice

Cannabis is a remarkably nontoxic substance; but within our bodies it mimics some of the most fundamental regulatory molecules that we produce. The endocannabinoid system (with which cannabis interacts, see pages 39–41) appears to have a key role in regulating pain, appetite, immune function, and dozens of other internal processes. The study of the endocannabinoid system is so new and moving so quickly that there will almost certainly be additional discoveries, perhaps major ones, between the time that I type these words and this book ends up in your hands.

Most of the information that is available to medical cannabis patients in the United States comes from the marijuana underground, and not from medical research. That situation is changing perhaps, but not as quickly as cannabis science is advancing. Cannabis prohibition has opened up an immense gulf between the contemporary practice of medicine and the use of cannabis as a medicine. Today's physicians are not taught that cannabis can be an effective medicine; they are taught that cannabis is a dangerous drug open to all kinds of abuse.

Patients using cannabis as a medicine typically know more about cannabis than their doctors. The problem stems from the difficulty of conducting peer-reviewed medical research on the medical uses of cannabis when the primary U.S. government agency supervising that research is dedicated to the proposition that cannabis is a dangerous drug of abuse with no accepted medicinal use. This is the endgame of the politicization of science. However, this situation is changing. There is every chance that cannabis research will soon be unfettered, although there are those who have been saying the same thing since the 1960s.

Cannabis, Kids, and Pets

"What about the kids?" is the mantra of the War on Drugs. The kids and drugs combination is a minefield of good intentions and poor decisions. Which drugs are appropriate and safe for use with children is not easily answered. When neuroscientists are still unable to distinguish the difference between Ritalin and cocaine in patients undergoing state-of-the-art brain scans (because their mechanism of action appears almost identical), it underscores the challenge of making definitive statements about the risks or benefits of using cannabis with young patients. There is simply not enough evidence. So what about medical cannabis and children? Like all medicinal uses of cannabis, the answer requires a thoughtful physician. There is some evidence that the THC found in many varieties of cannabis could influence brain development and perhaps even harm genetically susceptible young people, though this evidence is far from conclusive. And yet there is also evidence that constituents in cannabis such as CBD and CBDV may be significant value in treating certain intractable forms of childhood epilepsy. What's the answer? There is no easy one, but even the difficult answers should rest with the parent and the child's healthcare professional.

As for pets, some folks think that everything they do to themselves is just fine for their companion animals. There's a phrase for that: anthropomorphic shortsightedness. The truth is that cannabis won't kill your dog or cat, but it can temporarily paralyze the animal, cause it to lose bladder control, and generally make the creature terribly disoriented.

Is there a use for medical cannabis with animals? Probably. A small number of veterinarians in the U.S. are currently researching the uses of medical cannabis with pets. Always consult a veterinarian before you dose Rover or Kitty, but dosage between species will vary considerably.

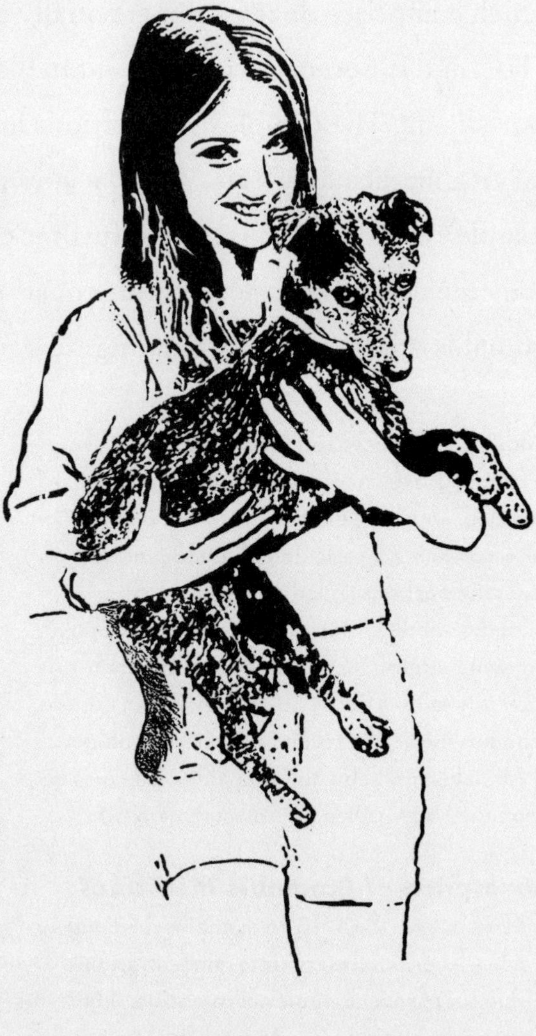

HOW CANNABIS WORKS WITHIN THE BODY

The cannabis plant produces more than 700 chemical compounds, of which the best known is THC, or tetrahydrocannabinol. Yet THC is just a single component of a remarkable chemical ecology produced within cannabis, which comprises dozens of medicinally active substances. Cannabis is not just THC, and different varieties of cannabis produce differing ratios of active ingredients. The complex interactions and ratios of these chemicals produce varying medicinal effects. This variation in potency and constituency, plus the complex chemical interactions, further combined with the way in which the body metabolizes these cannabis constituents, make consistent medicinal cannabis dosage very challenging.

Understanding how and where the constituents of cannabis medicines are absorbed, metabolized, excreted, and stored within the body is important for establishing a basic understanding of how cannabis works as a medicine. But such an understanding is, from a scientific standpoint, a moving target. There is only so much that is currently known about how the body acts upon cannabis medicines (called the pharmacokinetics of cannabis) and how the cannabis medicines act upon the body (called pharmacodynamics).

Absorption of Cannabis Medicines

When smoked, the THC in cannabis medicines reaches its peak blood plasma concentrations within six to seven minutes of ingestion. THC from smoking is actually detectable a few seconds after inhalation. The ability of a patient to absorb THC through smoking or vaporization appears to be a learned behavior, with experienced users more than twice as efficient in their rate of absorption as occasional users. The efficiency of inhaled cannabis is dependent on the size and duration of the inhalation, plus how long the breath is held. Holding one's breath only slightly increases absorption.[24]

Sublingual (under the tongue) or oromucosal (on the tissues of the mouth) administration of cannabis medicines is not as efficient as administration by inhalation, although absorption and onset of cannabis medicines placed beneath the tongue has been known to occur as quickly as five to 15 minutes after application. Peak blood concentrations for sublingual THC are reached within four hours, with other cannabinoids such as CBD taking slightly longer to peak.[25]

Oral absorption of THC (sublingual or oromucosal) in cannabis medicines is both slow and inconsistent. This inconsistency has often been cited as the reason why many oral cannabis preparations that were popular in the nineteenth century subsequently fell out of favor with both doctors and patients. Maximum blood plasma levels are often reached within two hours, but in some studies human subjects have needed up to seven hours to reach these levels. Furthermore, some THC is destroyed by stomach acid. Then, the liver grabs much of the THC before it can become bioavailable. This liver absorption of THC is called a first-pass effect.

Topical absorption of THC is difficult and not particularly efficient but can be accomplished by blending the THC into a fatty acid and propylene glycol. This approach has been used to treat skin conditions including psoriasis and inflammatory ailments including osteoarthritis.

Metabolism of Cannabis Medicines

Once absorbed, 90 percent of THC will be bound to proteins in the blood plasma. Because it's being moved by the blood, THC ends up being distributed to tissues that have lots of blood vessels, including the heart, liver, fat cells, etc. Only about 1 percent of the administered THC will find its way to the brain.

Certain organs in the body can break THC down into other molecules called metabolites. This metabolism takes place primarily within the liver, but also within the tissues of the heart and lungs. When the liver breaks down THC, the primary metabolite is 11-hydroxy-THC, twice as psychoactive and lasting twice as long as THC. Eventually, 11-hydroxy-THC undergoes further metabolic changes into an inert metabolite, before being excreted from the body.

Absorption, Metabolism, Excretion

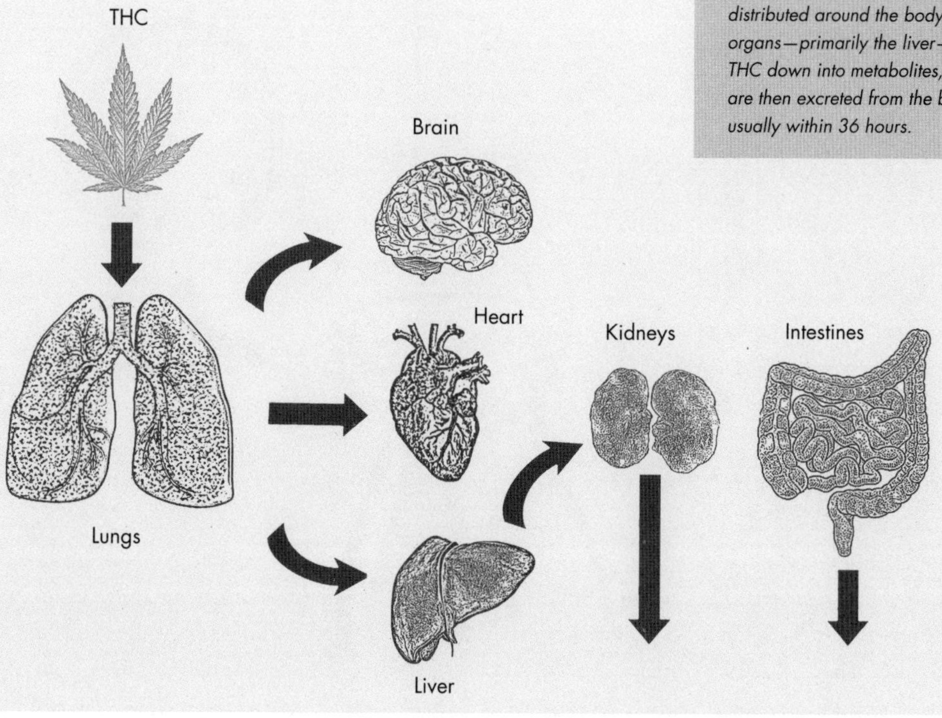

Once inside the body, THC is absorbed into the bloodstream and distributed around the body. Certain organs—primarily the liver—break THC down into metabolites, which are then excreted from the body, usually within 36 hours.

Cannabidiol is metabolized by the liver into 7-hydroxy-CBD. Very little is known about the pharmacology of this CBD metabolite.

Elimination of Cannabis from the Body

Within roughly 36 hours after ingestion, THC and its psychoactive metabolite will be eliminated from the bloodstream. THC's non-psychoactive metabolites can hang around for weeks in heavy users. Eventually, these metabolites will be excreted—around 30 percent excreted in urine and 70 percent in feces (5 percent of an oral dose will be excreted in the feces unchanged).[26]

Neutral vs. Acidic Cannabinoids and Bioavailability

Within the cannabis plant, THC and the other cannabinoids exist in the form of acids—for example, THCA. The human body does not easily absorb these cannabinoid acids. This ability of a drug to be absorbed is termed its bioavailability. When heated, however, cannabinoid acids give up a carbon dioxide molecule and transform into a neutral state—a process called decarboxylation—which makes them considerably more bioavailable. Cannabinoid acids are very delicate. Even room temperatures will slowly encourage

The conversion of THCA to THC in herbal cannabis medicines can be quickly accomplished at 310°F (154°C) maintained for a period of seven minutes. Great care should be exercised when handling this decarboxylated cannabis and especially cannabis concentrates, since their high bioavailability makes accidental overdosage by licking one's fingers painfully simple. There's even a colloquial phrase for this accidental ingestion: becoming a cookie casualty.

Conversion of THCA to THC

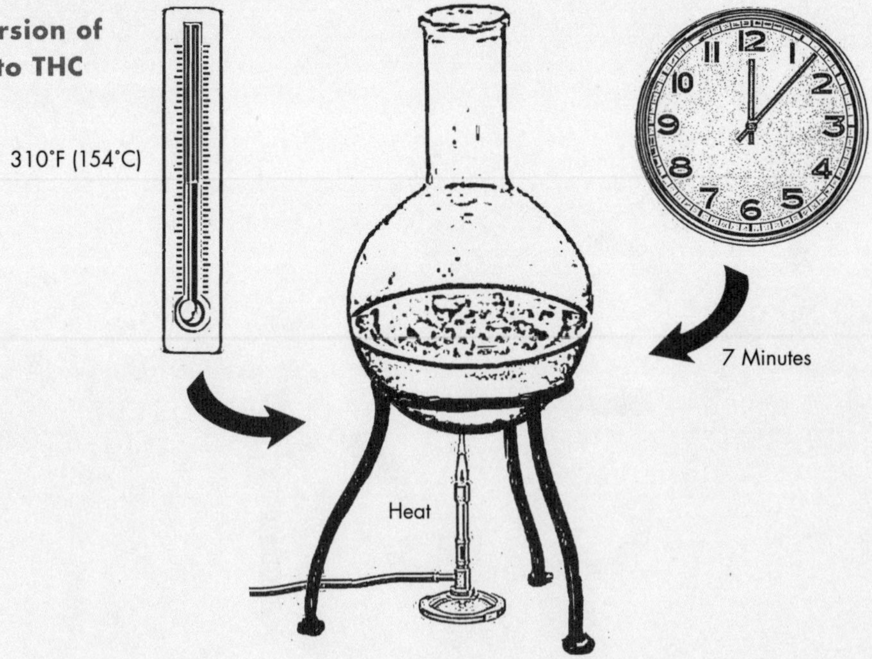

their conversion to their bioavailable neutral forms. The high heat used to smoke, vaporize, or cook cannabis quickly transforms cannabinoid acids into this neutral form (see opposite). It is also possible to convert the various cannabinoid acids into their neutral forms with the steady application of moderate heat at a temperature that is below boiling or combustion points of the cannabis constituents.

Are Cannabinoid Acids Effective Medicines?

Recently a small study was published that controversially claimed that decarboxylated THC was more bioavailable than THC acid, but that CBD acid was *more* bioavailable than decarboxylated CBD. Dutch scientist Arno Hazekamp noted in his work on cannabis tea that even though the water used was not hot enough to decarboxylate the THC, patients were still noting medicinal effects—just not getting very "high." It may be that cannabinoid acids have been overlooked as a form of medicine until now. Just because these cannabinoid acids do not produce psychoactive effects, it certainly does not mean that they cannot be medicinally effective. However, the assertion remains unproven that raw cannabis and its cannabinoid acids might be more effective medicinally, or better absorbed, than the neutral cannabinoids produced by the application of heat.

When It Comes to Cannabis Dose: *Less* Likely Leads to *More* Effect

Studies have recently shown that consistently high doses of cannabis cause the brain to reduce the density of cannabinoid receptors in the body, apparently in response to these high doses. This result makes sense in the context of the overall purpose of the endocannabinoid system, which is to regulate and balance signaling throughout the body. High doses can cause an imbalance of the endocannabinoid system, and the body therefore adjusts by reducing cannabinoid receptor density. So, if there is a rule of thumb for cannabis dosage, it should be: use the smallest possible dose required to meet the medicinal need, then set the shortest possible treatment course at that dosage in order to reduce the chance of a patient developing dose-tolerance issues.

Variance in Cannabis Effects among Patients

Numerous studies have shown the enormous range of effects occurring when cannabis medicines are administered to different patients. This variance depends on several factors, some genetic. With orally administered cannabis medicines, there is a large observed range of delivered doses, from 4 to 12 percent. This means that one patient could absorb three times the dose that another patient absorbs.

Additionally, the target can be sized differently among different patients. In the case of THC, one of its targets is the CB1 receptor. The density of the target CB1 receptors in the brain can vary with an individual's level of tolerance to cannabis medicines. A patient with an extremely high tolerance to the effects of cannabis may be able to withstand a dose of cannabis 100 times greater than a novice patient.

Among some users of cannabis, a high tolerance is sometimes viewed as an accomplishment, when actually it's simply the body's attempt to establish an equilibrium after consistent overmedication. A high tolerance to the effects of cannabis is typically the result of needless overmedication.

ADVERSE EFFECTS OF MEDICAL CANNABIS

While this may not be the most pleasant topic, understanding the side effects and contraindications of using herbal cannabis as a medicine can make the experience both safer and better informed. It is important to speak with a physician or healthcare professional if a user feels that he or she is experiencing *any* side effects from *any* medication, including cannabis.

Cannabis can produce adverse effects and also interact negatively with other medicines. A commonly held belief among certain circles is that cannabis is completely safe, but the reality is that cannabis is a potent drug capable of producing significant side effects. The side effects of cannabis medicines can be frightening to novice users, who may be unaccustomed to its psychoactive results. Elderly patients without prior experience can become very uncomfortable indeed. Dosage of medical cannabis to older and inexperienced patients must be approached with close supervision and considerable caution.

The important factor when dealing with common cannabis side effects is simply to remain calm, breathe slowly, and relax. Most of the cannabis side effects noted opposite are associated with THC, the primary psychoactive ingredient. By using cannabis medicines that also contain CBD, a non-psychoactive cannabinoid, some of the following THC side effects might be reduced or eliminated altogether.

Patients who are either new to cannabis medicines or who have accidently overmedicated can occasionally experience a condition called postural or orthostatic hypotension. After using cannabis, especially at high doses, this can result in sudden lightheadedness or loss of consciousness upon standing from a seated or reclining position. It can be particularly dangerous if the person topples onto a hard surface. Suddenly passing out upon standing up has become increasingly common among users of highly concentrated cannabis oils. It has also been observed that, while reclining, novice cannabis users tend to experience an upward spike in their blood pressure. This spike should be noted with particular caution if elevated blood pressure is potentially an issue.

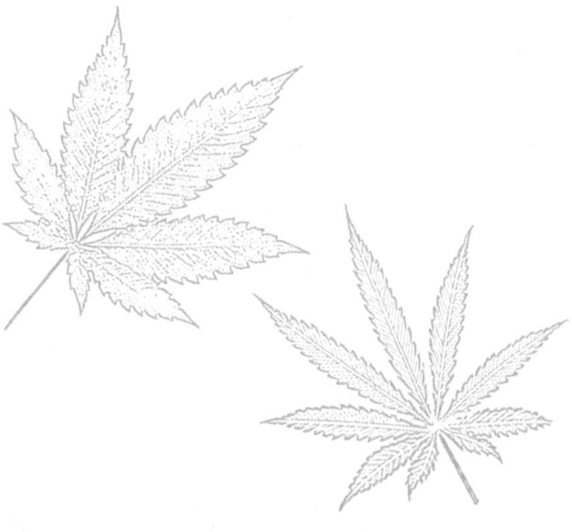

Before Using Cannabis

CONSULT YOUR PHYSICIAN if you have been diagnosed with, or believe that you may suffer from:

- Schizophrenia, bipolar disorder, or severe depression
- Heart disease, high blood pressure, angina, or irregular heartbeat
- Chronic obstructive pulmonary disease
- An immune disorder

You must speak with your physician or healthcare professional before using medical cannabis, as the use of cannabis may not be safe for you, or special precautions may be advised. Additionally, if you are under 22 years of age, speak with your doctor about the safety of using high-THC cannabis medicines. There is certain conflicting evidence that exposure to THC may interfere with some specific aspects of brain development and may possibly encourage the development of schizophrenia in a very small, but susceptible, group of young people, especially those with a family history of the disorder. A number of studies are currently underway that should help to provide more evidence to support or disprove this concern. Until then, younger patients should exercise significant caution before using THC-dominant cannabis medicines and consider using cannabis medicines with higher CBD to THC ratios.

THE MOST COMMONLY REPORTED MILD ADVERSE EFFECTS AMONG USERS OF MEDICAL CANNABIS

- Rapid heartbeat, technically referred to as tachycardia. Rapid heartbeat typically subsides within 15 to 20 minutes. Slow, steady breathing for a few minutes can help while the racing heartbeat gradually begins to subside.

- Dry mouth, informally called "cottonmouth." Dry mouth can be addressed with water or, even better, lemonade. Lemonade with added lemon peel is a popular local remedy in North Africa to reduce the mild side effects of cannabis use.

- Dizziness or lightheadedness can seem less pronounced when the eyes are kept open and focused on something, such as watching television.

- Red, irritated eyes can be treated using mild eyedrops, such as VISINE, which quickly relieve any itchy or burning eyes.

- Coughing caused by inhaled cannabis smoke or vapor is rarely dangerous and usually subsides quickly. It is most easily avoided by simply reducing the amount inhaled. A glass of water can also help. Care must be taken when inhaling concentrated forms of cannabis, such as cannabis resin (hashish) or oil (hash oil, butter, wax, or dabs), since too much can result in a brutal coughing fit that can damage the lungs. If airway irritation becomes an issue with inhaled cannabis, then oral or sublingual cannabis administration methods should be explored.

None of the listed side effects is immediate cause for alarm, but calming someone who is experiencing any one of them for the first time can be quite a challenge.

Pregnancy and Breast-Feeding

The use of cannabis during pregnancy and breast-feeding cannot be recommended. There are some indications that women who smoke cannabis produce babies with lower birth weights. While the cognitive tests given to children of cannabis-using mothers are contradictory, caution should be observed. The most recent research on endocannabinoids indicates that they are involved in several aspects of fetal and childhood development, which alone should encourage caution. Cannabinoids from cannabis medicines are passed along in the mother's breast milk.

Short-Term Psychological Adverse Effects

By far the most commonly experienced, acute psychological side effects of cannabis medicines are confusion, anxiety, and feelings of panic. All of these are dose-dependent side effects. If these feelings or psychological symptoms escalate, it is vital that the patient sees a healthcare professional as soon as possible. Typically, a doctor will prescribe an antianxiety medication, such as Xanax (alprazolam), and bed rest. These sensations may be avoided in the future by monitoring the cannabis dose until a comfortable baseline has been established. Such a baseline is easier to establish with smoked and vaporized cannabis medicines than with oral and sublingual preparations. Using herbal cannabis medicines rich in CBD, limonene, and pinene may reduce some of these effects.

Long-Term Adverse Effects

There can be long-term adverse effects from using cannabis medicines, which is why responsible physicians recommend a defined course of treatment for their patients. Heavy, long-term smokers of cannabis can develop severe and chronic bronchitis. A range of cognitive deficits (that is, affecting the ability to think) has been noted in long-term cannabis users. On the plus side, evidence indicates that most of these deficits are likely reversible. A recent brain scanning study of heavy cannabis users has shown that the density of their cannabinoid receptors had declined considerably. This receptor density was completely restored in all the study participants after 28 days of abstinence from cannabis.[27] Decline in receptor density is called "receptor down-regulation." It is likely responsible for the

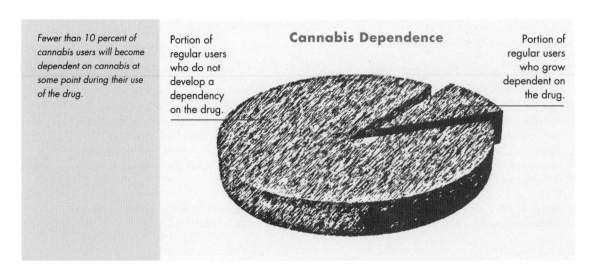

Fewer than 10 percent of cannabis users will become dependent on cannabis at some point during their use of the drug.

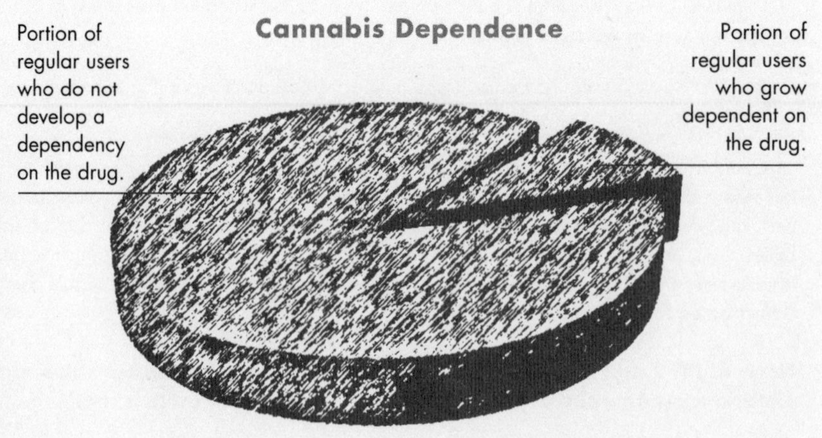

DRUGS THAT CAN *INCREASE* THE EFFECTS OF ORALLY ADMINISTERED CANNABIS
Amiodarone (Cordarone): treating cardiac arrhythmias
Clarithromycin (Biaxin): antibiotic
Diltiazem (Tiazac, Cardizem, Dilacor): treating high blood pressure, angina
Erythromycin (Robimycin, Ilosone, Acnasol): antibiotic
Fluconazole (Diflucan, Trican): antifungal
Isoniazid (Nydrazid, Rifamate): treating tuberculosis
Itraconazole (Sporanox): antifungal
Ketoconazole: antifungal
Miconazole (Monistat): over-the-counter antifungal
Ritonavir (Norvir): HIV protease inhibitor
Verapamil (Calan, Veralan, Isoptin): treating cardiac arrhythmias

DRUGS CAN *DECREASE* OR INTERFERE WITH THE EFFECTS OF ORAL CANNABIS
Carbamazepine (Tegretol, Equetro, Carbetrol): anticonvulsant
Phenobarbital: sedative, anticonvulsant
Phenytoin (Dilantin): anticonvulsant
Primodone (Mylosine): anticonvulsant
Rifabutin (Mycobutin): Mycobacterium avium complex (MAC) disease
Rifampicin (Rifampin, Rifadin, Rifater, Rimactane): antibiotic
St. John's Wort: herbal antidepressant
Additionally, cannabis medicines (smoked, oral, sublingual, or vaporized) increase the effects of alcohol, benzodiazepines (Ativan, Halcion, Librium Restoril, Valium, Xanax, etc.), and opiates (codeine, fentanyl, morphine, etc.).

development of "tolerance" over time to the effects of cannabis. Cannabis tolerance can be controlled through a measured approach to cannabis dosage.

Drug interactions When taken orally, the active ingredients in cannabis medicines interact with enzymes as part of the body's process in metabolizing the cannabis medicine. This drug interaction can increase or decrease the effect of cannabis or other medications. Special caution should be used when taking oral cannabis with the drugs listed above. The interaction of smoked or vaporized cannabis with these other drugs is unknown, but caution is nonetheless advised.

Cannabis Hyperemesis: A Newly Described Adverse Effect

Recently, a new condition related to the use of medical cannabis has been described both in Australia and the United States. This condition, known as cannabis hyperemesis, is characterized by vomiting and abdominal pain associated with the use of cannabis. A recent study at the Mayo Clinic, based in Rochester, Minnesota, looked at 98 case reports.[28] In many of the sufferers, the symptoms seemed to be relieved by taking either a hot bath or shower. The syndrome is also reported to resolve itself completely upon cessation of cannabis use.

Because THC in cannabis medicines is strongly bound to blood plasma proteins, caution is advised when taking any other medications that are also strongly bound to plasma proteins.

Can Cannabis Cause Heart Attack or Stroke?

The short answer: yes, cannabis can likely increase the chances of stroke or heart attack in certain populations.[29] The latest research indicates an increased risk of stroke in young people who use cannabis, primarily smoked cannabis, recreationally. This risk is still extremely small, but considered significant by the researchers. Additional research shows higher rates of heart attacks among older patients who use or have used cannabis.[30]

In Case of Overmedication with Cannabis

Accidental overmedication with cannabis is not life threatening. It can be an extremely unpleasant experience for three to eight hours, but it will not be a fatal one. No human being has ever died from an overdose of cannabis.

If a child accidently consumes medical cannabis, call 911 and your doctor.

The most common form of cannabis overdose is by oral administration. Hallucinations, paranoia, panic, rapid heartbeat, and nausea can all manifest in a cannabis overdose. The best approach is reassurance and trying to make the person as comfortable as possible. The bottom line is that the patient is going to have to rest until the symptoms subside. Plenty of water is recommended, but don't force it. If the victim is a child, call the nearest poison control center. If the adult victim needs to be transported to the hospital, he or she will typically be given an antianxiety medication and sent home to rest. New treatments for severe cannabis overdose may be developed from pregnenolone, one of the body's own steroid precursors, which can prevent intoxication. The bottom line for those wishing to use cannabis as a medicine is that 99 percent of all adverse effects can be controlled through careful and informed dosage. That is, provided that no underlying conditions preclude the use of cannabis by the patient (see page 35).

Is Stoned a Side Effect?

It might sound absurd, but there are more and more patients looking to reduce the level of psychoactivity of cannabis medicines. Most hashish cultivars around the world, including the oldest cannabis medicinal crops, are so high in CBD that they produce reduced levels of psychoactivity when compared to today's cannabis varieties. Some older patients that used cannabis in the 1960s and 1970s remember these low-THC varieties fondly, and often claim that today's cannabis, while stronger, does not produce as interesting an effect. What if there were a cannabis variety that relieved the symptoms of pain and anxiety, elevated mood, and even relaxed muscles, but didn't impair its user in any fashion? Some cannabis breeders think that this could be the cannabis of the future.

It may be that prohibition spiked THC content, but also upset the balance of the plant's chemistry. Writers in the late 1970s and early 1980s complained when "*indica*" genetics were introduced. Those critics claimed that the cerebral clarity of the best *sativa* cannabis was replaced with a dull, "stoned" lethargy of the *indica* varieties. Perhaps the clock will be turned backward over the next few years, as some of these earlier approaches to cannabis breeding and taste are revisited.

THE ENDOCANNABINOID SYSTEM: A BRIEF PRIMER

Humans have used cannabis for centuries, but only in the last 50 years or so has any scientific understanding emerged as to how cannabis works within the human body. While the discovery of the first plant cannabinoids took place in the 1940s, it was not until 1964 that THC produced by the cannabis plant was first characterized and synthesized.

The discovery of THC in 1964 (see page 17) led to a long search for a receptor in the body with which THC might be interacting. The first cannabinoid receptors in the body were not characterized until the late 1980s. These receptors turned out to comprise a new series of regulatory mechanisms within the body, called the endocannabinoid system. Many of the physiological effects of cannabis occur due to the interaction of cannabinoids with the endocannabinoid receptor molecules.

The endocannabinoid system consists of this network of endocannabinoid receptors, which are distributed throughout the body. The system is a very complex regulatory system, broad in its function, and found within all complex animals, from fish to humans. The endocannabinoid system supports such diverse functions as memory, digestion, motor function, immune response, appetite, pain, blood pressure, bone growth, and the protection of neural tissues. Many researchers believe that there are even more physiological processes with which the endocannabinoid system is involved, still yet to be discovered.

Cannabinoid Receptors

The two primary subtypes of cannabinoid receptor in the endocannabinoid system are CB_1 and CB_2. These receptors are distributed throughout the central nervous and immune systems, and within many other tissues, including the brain, gastrointestinal system, reproductive and urinary tracts, spleen, endocrine system, heart, and circulatory system. Furthermore, researchers have uncovered new evidence that points to at least three other cannabinoid receptors throughout the body, in addition to CB_1 and CB_2.

Following the discovery of the cannabinoid receptors, the hunt was launched for the substances produced within the body that were binding to them. This led to the discovery of the first endocannabinoids, anandamide and 2-AG, in the early 1990s. So far, five endocannabinoids have been isolated. All of them are derivatives of polyunsaturated fatty acids, closely related to the popular omega-3 fatty acids (which are often purchased as supplements from health stores). Since they are fats, endocannabinoids are not water-soluble and have difficulty moving efficiently through the body; thus, they are designed to work locally.

One local activity occurs when endocannabinoids serve as the primary messenger across synapses (the gaps between nerve cells): they signal neurons to communicate with each other through the release of neurotransmitters. In recent years, it has become increasingly clear that the role of endocannabinoids in this synaptic function is both more important and far more complex than previously thought. Endocannabinoids modulate the flow of neurotransmitters, keeping our nervous system running smoothly.

Endocannabinoids are produced on demand, released back across the synapse, then taken up into the cells and rapidly metabolized. Endocannabinoids appear to be profoundly connected with the concept of homeostasis (maintaining physiological stability), helping redress specific imbalances presented by disease or by injury. Endocannabinoids' role in pain signaling has led to the hypothesis that endocannabinoid levels may be responsible for the baseline of pain throughout the body, which is why cannabinoid-based medicines may be useful in treating conditions such as fibromyalgia (a condition marked by muscular pain and stiffness). This could also mean that the constant release of the body's own endocannabinoids could have a "tonic" effect on muscle tightness (spasticity) in multiple sclerosis, neuropathic pain, inflammation, and even baseline appetite. The value of proper

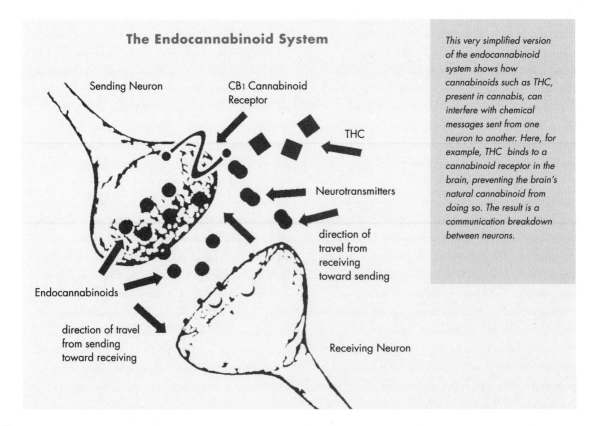

The Endocannabinoid System

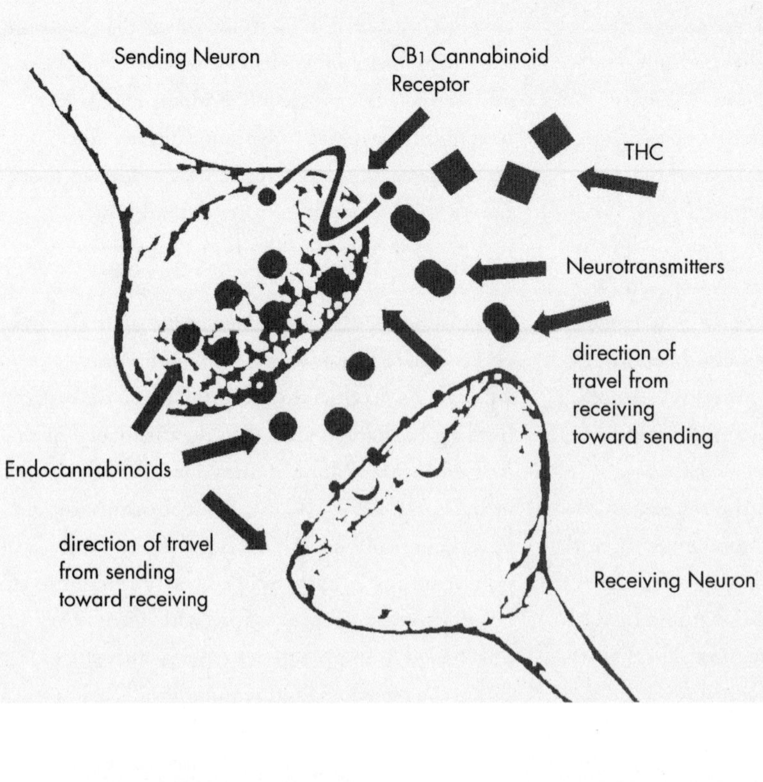

This very simplified version of the endocannabinoid system shows how cannabinoids such as THC, present in cannabis, can interfere with chemical messages sent from one neuron to another. Here, for example, THC binds to a cannabinoid receptor in the brain, preventing the brain's natural cannabinoid from doing so. The result is a communication breakdown between neurons.

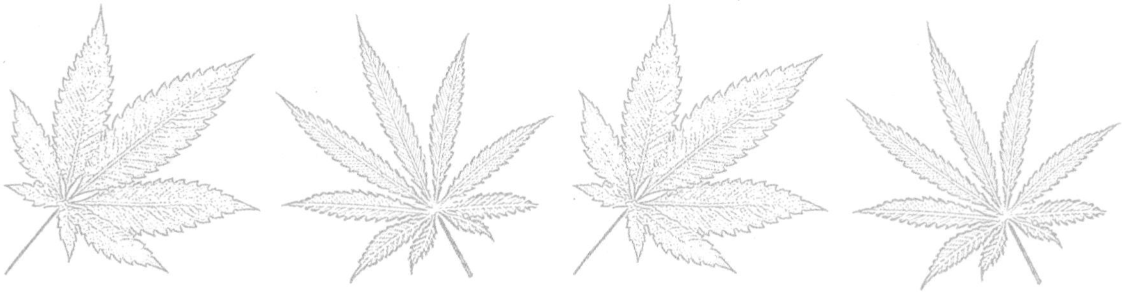

"endocannabinoid tone" throughout the body could be very significant to general well-being.

The CB_1 receptor is expressed throughout the brain, where endocannabinoids and CB_1 combine to form a "circuit breaker," which modulates the release of neurotransmitters. The list of brain functions that are affected by the endocannabinoid system is enormous: decision-making, cognition, emotions, learning, and memory, as well as regulation of bodily movement, anxiety, stress, fear, pain, body temperature, appetite, sense of reinforcement or reward, motor control, and much more. One brain region that does not have many CB_1 receptors is the brain stem, responsible for respiration and circulation, which is a primary reason why cannabis overdoses are not fatal. It is activation of this CB_1 receptor that is responsible for the psychoactive effects of cannabis.

While CB_1 activation results in the psychological and physical effects commonly associated with cannabis ingestion, CB_2 receptor activation does not. The CB_2 receptors are primarily found in blood cells, tonsils, and the spleen. From these sites, CB_2 receptors control the release of cytokines (immunoregulatory proteins) linked to inflammation and general immune function throughout the body.

The endocannabinoid system as a target for drug delivery goes well beyond the use of cannabis. Cannabinoid-based medicines can either enhance or interfere with the endocannabinoid system's balancing act. But designing drugs that interact safely with the endocannabinoid system is difficult, and drugs that antagonize or interfere with the function of cannabinoid receptors have met with decidedly mixed success. Rimonabant, a CB_1 antagonist, was approved for sale in Europe in 2006 as an obesity treatment. However, the Food and Drug Administration refused to approve it in the U.S., citing concerns that the drug was linked to episodes of depression and suicidal behaviors. Because the cannabinoid receptors are dispersed so widely throughout the body, activating or suppressing them for a single medical purpose can unleash a host of unwanted activity elsewhere.

Recent research has started to focus on developing drugs that can interact with cannabinoid receptors, but that do not cross the blood/brain barrier, in hopes of preventing some serious side effects. As mentioned above, Rimonabant, which blocked the effects of the CB_1 receptor in hopes of reducing appetite as a diet drug, was removed from the market because of psychiatric side effects. However, it is believed that these types of side effects might be reduced by limiting the ability of these new drugs to block or interact with these receptors. Other drug candidates seek to slow down how quickly anandamide—one of the key endocannabinoids—is metabolized. These proposed drugs show promise as treatments for conditions ranging from cancer to colitis.

PHYTOCANNABINOIDS AND TERPENOIDS—THE PRINCIPAL ACTIVE INGREDIENTS OF MEDICINAL CANNABIS

More than 700 chemical constituents are produced within the cannabis plant.[31] Of these, the cannabinoids, a group of over 80 molecules with chemical structures called terpenophenolics, have attracted the most interest from medical researchers. Cannabinoids are molecules that interact with cannabinoid receptors; receptor protein molecules are found throughout the bodies of plants and animals.

The body produces its own cannabinoids in the form of endocannabinoids. By contrast, phytocannabinoids are cannabinoids produced by the cannabis plant in the form of carboxylic acids: THCA, CBDA, and so on. Upon heating, or gradually warming up to room temperature over time, these cannabinoid acids are converted to their chemically neutral and more widely known form: THC, CBD, etc. It is this neutral form of THC that is psychoactive in humans. Cannabinoids have extremely high lethal dose requirements in humans, which is why no fatal overdose has ever been directly attributable to cannabinoids.

Until very recently, phytocannabinoids referred solely to those cannabinoids that are produced by the cannabis plant. More recently, however, it has been discovered that compounds produced by other plants, including lichens and even black pepper, can interact with cannabinoid receptors as well; therefore the definition of phytocannabinoids has been expanded to include any natural plant compounds that interact with cannabinoid receptors.

For much of the last 100 years, a small handful of cannabinoids were thought to be the only active pharmacological constituents of cannabis. But over the last decade, researchers have tried to get to the bottom of why different varieties of herbal cannabis appear to produce differing medicinal or psychoactive effects. One explanation for the variation is a synergy between cannabinoids and other components of cannabis' essential oil, called terpenoids or terpenes. It is now believed that both cannabinoids and terpenes, acting in concert, are responsible for the differences in both medicinal and psychoactive effects produced by cannabis varieties.

Cannabinoids

While there are over 100 cannabinoids produced by cannabis, only a few are produced in any significant quantity. They can be categorized into 10 structural types, of which four are primary:

- THC (tetrahydrocannabinol)
- CBD (cannabidiol)
- CBG (cannabigerol)
- CBC (cannabichromene)

A fifth type, CBN (cannabinol), is not produced by the plant but results from the oxidation of THC as it breaks down.

THC Delta-9-tetrahydrocannabinolic acid or THCA is the most common phytocannabinoid produced by drug cannabis varieties. Certain varieties of drug cannabis can produce up to 25 percent of the plant's dry weight in THC acid —an extraordinary amount for a single secondary metabolite in any plant species. The production of THC within the plant is controlled by a small group of genes. These genes controlling THC production are dominant in most drug forms of cannabis. THC is produced by an enzyme reaction within the plant using CBG as its precursor (see page 44).

THC is the primary psychoactive constituent of cannabis, although in its raw acidic form within the plant, it is not at all psychoactive. Upon heating through smoking, vaporization, or cooking, THCA is converted (decarboxylated) into THC (see page 32) and becomes highly psychoactive. Besides its psychoactivity, THC is a potent anti-inflammatory and analgesic,[32] is neuroprotective,[33] and reduces intraocular pressure, spasticity, and muscle tension.[34]

THC interacts with both the CB_1 and CB_2 endocannabinoid receptors. While THC is nontoxic, some physicians have characterized the unpleasant effects of THC overdoses as "psychotoxic." For example, THC can produce anxiety, sedation, and rapid heartbeat in novice users—although some of these adverse effects can decline over a course of treatment. High doses of THC over time are linked to receptor downregulation and tolerance to its effects.

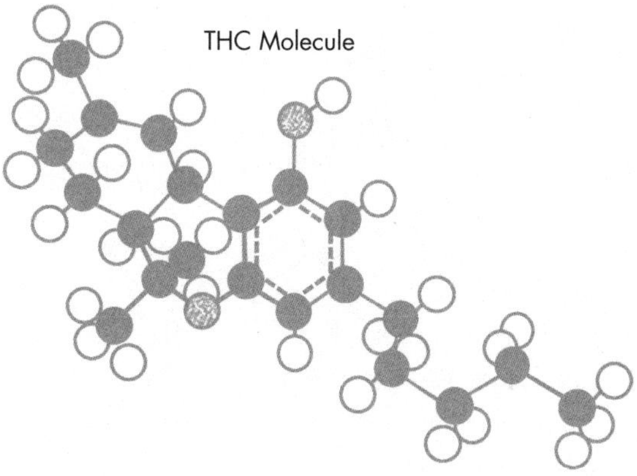

CBD Cannabidiolic acid or CBDA is the most common phytocannabinoid produced by fiber cannabis (hemp) varieties, and the second most common in some drug cannabis varieties. CBDA can be converted to CBD by heat over time, like THC. However, there are preliminary indications that CBD blood plasma levels are more easily achieved by using CBDA, rather than decarboxylated CBD. This study contradicts our current understanding of how cannabinoids work and more research needs to be conducted to confirm this assertion.[35]

CBD is produced from CBG, like THC, but employs a different set of genes and a different enzymatic reaction. Until recently, high-CBD cannabis varieties were unavailable in medical cannabis outlets in the United States. But with the advent of advocacy groups such as Project CBD, high-CBD cannabis varieties have reemerged in California and Colorado after testing laboratories began to screen for them. For example, a cannabis variety from Spain named Cannatonic has recently become available in California; it has a 20 to one CBDA to THCA ratio and peak dry weight concentrations approaching 17 percent CBDA. Varieties such as Cannatonic should dramatically increase the availability of CBD-dominant cannabis within the medical cannabis community. While CBD is not classically psychoactive, patients using high-CBD herbal cannabis have noted some effects akin to mild psychoactivity, though subjectively very different from THC-dominant cannabis.

In cannabis medicine formulations that combine THC and CBD, such as Sativex, CBD has been shown to eliminate some of THC's unpleasant adverse effects, modulating its psychoactivity and reducing the incidence of THC-induced sedation, anxiety, and rapid heartbeat.[36] Sativex appears to demonstrate the strong synergy between CBD and THC. For example, in a Sativex study conducted with cancer patients suffering from intractable pain, CBD and THC in combination reduced this pain significantly, while THC alone did not. CBD exhibits analgesic and anti-inflammatory effects across a wide range of symptoms and conditions. Cell studies have shown that CBD is also effective in vitro against lines of human brain, breast, and other tumor cells, while simultaneously protecting normal cells. CBD, along with its propyl cousin CBDV, is an effective anticonvulsant.[37]

CBD interacts with a wide range of receptors—more than THC—which may explain its broad effects. While CBD dosen't interact with CB_1 and CB_2, it does interact with a host of other signaling systems.[38] These interactions may lead to CBD-based treatments for conditions ranging from strokes to acne. CBD is even effective in inhibiting methicillin-resistant *Staphylococcus aureus* (MRSA; an infection-causing bacterium strain), more so than the antibiotic vancomycin.

The last 10 years have seen an explosion of interest in the medicinal value of CBD, which appears to act as a broad homeostatic regulator throughout the body.

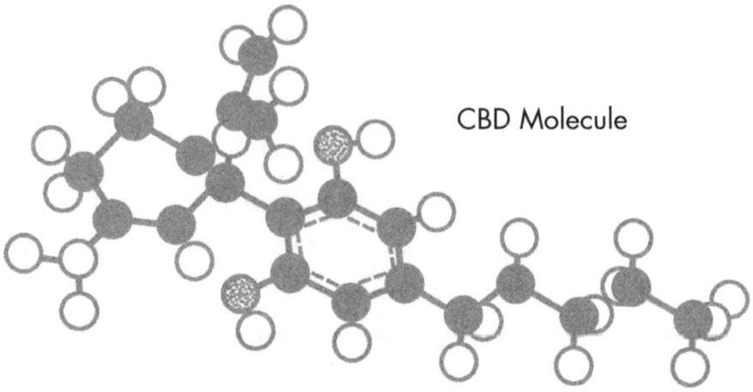

CBG Cannabigerol or CBG is an analgesic non-psychoactive cannabinoid that is the third most prevalent cannabinoid produced by the cannabis plant after tetrahydrocannabinol (THC) and cannabidiol (CBD). Cannabigerol is the precursor cannabinoid used by the cannabis plant to produce both THC and CBD. The propyl variation of CBG, cannabigerovarin is the precursor for THCV and CBDV. Only a few varieties of cannabis still have significant amounts of CBG remaining at maturity, and it is often produced more by fiber hemp than drug cannabis varieties.

Until recently, CBG had not been studied to the same degree as THC and CBD. A recent Italian study showed, however, that CBG was effective in treating the mouse model of inflammatory bowel disease (IBD).[39] In humans, IBD is an incurable disease that affects millions. CBG is unique among the primary cannabinoids, since it appears to interact predominantly with a range of receptors other than those of the endocannabinoid system.[40] CBG is also of potential interest as an antiseptic and antibiotic, since it is an extremely potent antibacterial agent against pathogens such as MRSA, a particularly virulent form of *Staphylococcus aureus* (commonly known as staph).[41] CBG may also prove of interest for its anti-tumor properties, especially for some forms of prostate and oral cancer.[42]

CBC Molecule

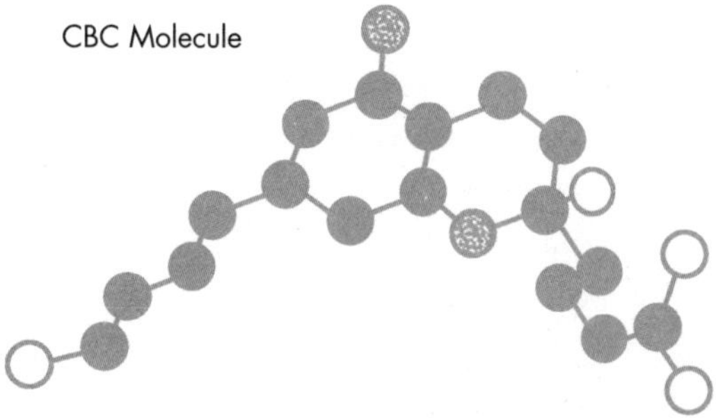

CBG Molecule

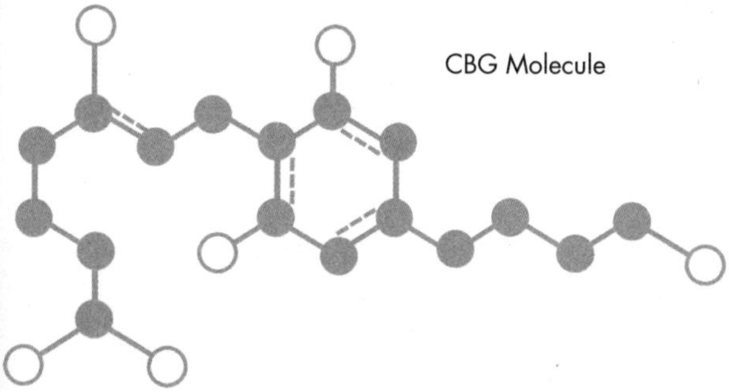

CBC CBCA or cannabichromenic acid is a rare phytocannabinoid produced very early in the flowering cycle of the cannabis plant. To date, CBC has been isolated from a few Central Asian cannabis cultivars, but it may exist in other varieties that have not been tested for CBC content during early flowering. Growing cannabis for its cannabichromene content currently entails collecting the immature flowers six weeks before floral maturity. It also appears that CBC may be concentrated in plant parts other than trichome heads.[43] CBC does not appear to interact with cannabinoid receptors, and it differs from THC in that it does not reduce intraocular pressure (fluid pressure within the eye).[44] However, CBC does exhibit a range of effects, including antibiotic and antifungal, which may help defend the cannabis plant in its early flowering phase.[45] Like many cannabinoids, CBC is anti-inflammatory and analgesic. It has also shown antidepressant effects in animal testing.[46]

CBN CBN is the oxidation byproduct of THC. It is not produced by the cannabis plant, but is readily detected in old samples of cannabis, cannabis resin, or oil. CBN is often an indication of poor storage of cannabis products. CBN is not psychoactive alone, but synergistically sedative with THC. Patients using herbal cannabis medicines high in CBN (greater than 0.5 percent by dry weight) subjectively describe the resulting interactivity as "thick" or "dull." Like CBD, CBN is effective against MRSA infections. Further, a recent study indicated that CBN might be useful in treating burns because it reduces perceived thermal sensitivity.[47] These potential uses of CBN demonstrate that even the most poorly handled and stored cannabis may retain some limited medicinal value.

CBN Molecule

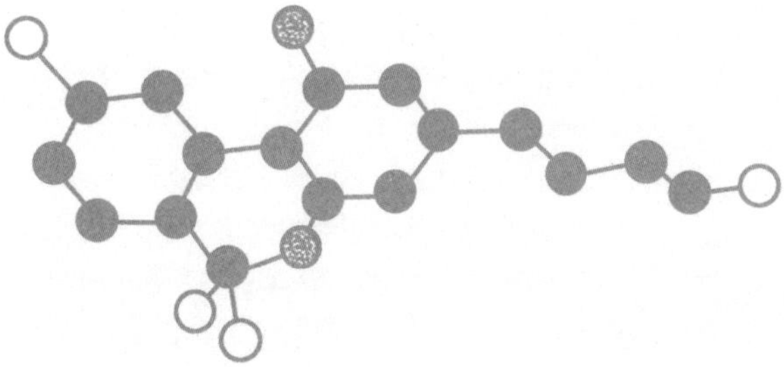

Pentyl vs. Propyl Cannabinoids

Common cannabinoids such as THC have "tails" of five carbon atoms. This feature defines this class of cannabinoids as pentyl cannabinoids. The precursor to pentyl cannabinoids is called olivetolic acid, which is used by the cannabis plant to make CBG. The CBG is then used to make THC, CBD, and/or CBC. But there is another class of cannabinoids that have three-carbon atom tails. These are the propyl cannabinoids. In some cannabis plants in southern Africa, cannabis evolved a different precursor to CBG called divarinic acid. When divarinic acid is used by the plant to make a variation on CBG acid called CBGV acid, CBGV can then be used by the plant to create the propyl cannabinoids: THCV, CBDV, or CBCV.

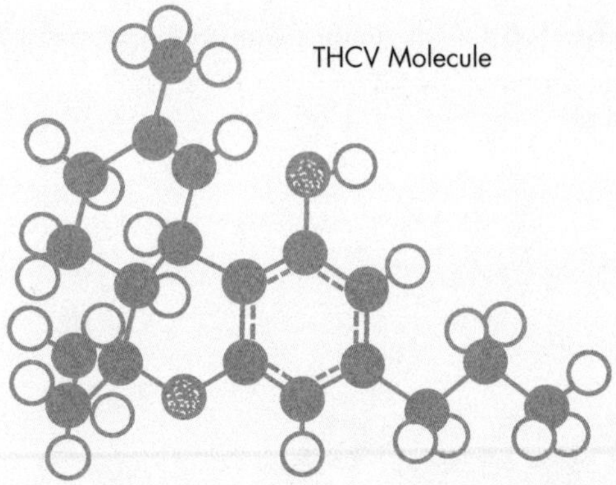

THCV Molecule

Tetrahydrocannabivarinic Acid

Tetrahydrocannabivarinic acid or THCVA is a scarcer propyl form of THCA produced by Afghan or Pakistani and southern African cannabis cultivars. THCVA, like all acidic cannabinoids, is converted to its bioactive neutral form, THCV, by heat or time. In these cultivars, the percentage of tetrahydrocannabivarinic acid (THCVA) rarely exceeds 2 percent by dry weight. GW Pharmaceuticals in the U.K. is believed to have bred THCV varieties approaching 10 percent THCVA and several Californian cultivars have tested with levels of up to 6 percent THCVA.

There appears to be some controversy about whether THCV is psychoactive or merely modulates the psychoactivity of THC, primarily since THCV's psychoactive effects have not been studied since the early 1970s.[48] Historically, THCV was considered to exhibit around 25 percent of the potency of THC, although more contemporary accounts claim that THCV produces no psychoactivity on its own. This contradiction may stem from the dosage employed, since THCV antagonizes the CB_1 receptor at low doses, but interacts with it at higher doses.[49] THCV is commonly considered to exhibit a range of effects diametrically opposed to those of THC. There is interest in molecules similar to THCV as potential diet drugs since they may encourage weight loss and increased energy expenditure in animal testing.[50] THCV is similar to THC as an analgesic and anti-inflammatory, and similar to CBD in its anticonvulsant effects.

Cannabidivarin (CBDVA) CBDVA is the propyl form of CBD. It has recently captured the attention of the cannabinoid medicine community for its potential value as an anticonvulsant, alone and in combination with CBD.[51] GW Pharmaceuticals has been working with cultivars that produce CBDV, but little information is known about these varieties, except that they originate from Central Asia.

CBDV Molecule

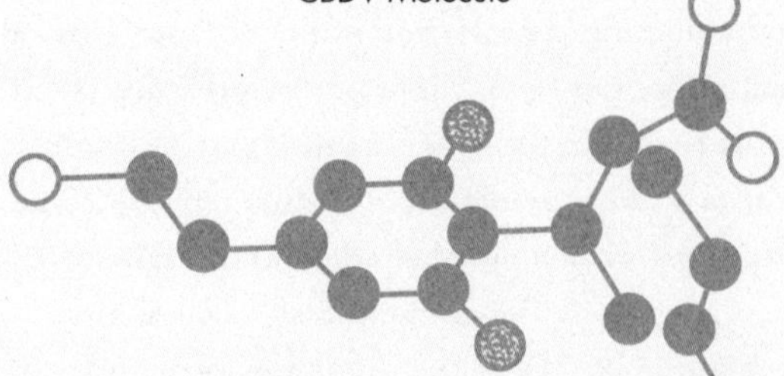

Terpenoids

When you smell perfume, you smell terpenoids, or terpenes as they are often called. And when you smell cannabis, you also smell terpenes, since cannabinoids themselves have no aroma. Cannabis produces more than 200 terpenes.[52] Terpenes are the most common plant chemicals in nature—30,000 of them have been identified. They are the aromatic constituents of all essential plant oils and are found in all spices, fruits, and vegetables.They are recognized as safe food additives by the FDA and are pharmacologically active and synergistic with cannabinoids.

In 2001, the paper "Cannabis and Cannabis Extracts: Greater than the Sum of Their Parts?" by John McPartland and Ethan Russo brought wider attention to the role of terpenes in the pharmacology of cannabis.[53] Cannabis users had long noticed subtle variations in the psychoactive effects among different cannabis varieties. Research on these terpenes and their synergies with cannabinoids is beginning to explain how different varieties of cannabis can produce a range of effects, even though they may share nearly identical cannabinoid profiles.[54]

Some significant terpenes found in cannabis include pinene, limonene, myrcene, ocimene, terpinolene, linalool, and beta-caryophyllene. They are primarily found in the plant's trichomes, as anyone touching cannabis flowers can attest. Terpenes are quite volatile, especially the fragrant monoterpenes, and are quickly lost from dried cannabis without proper storage measures. In the Netherlands, where the Jack Herer cannabis strain has been gamma-irradiated in pharmacies to reduce microbial counts, terpenes may be destroyed from such treatment. Similarly, orange juice that is gamma-irradiated has been shown to lose some terpenes in the process.[55]Terpenes are pharmacologically active, even at miniscule levels or concentrations, as low as 0.05 percent by weight. Interestingly, cannabinoids may increase the ability of terpenes to cross the blood/brain barrier, by increasing membrane permeability. Terpenes are lipophilic (fat-loving) and hydrophobic (water-hating), like cannabinoids, and they can interact with a wide variety of receptors throughout the brain and body.

Pinenes —Alpha-pinene and beta-pinene are monoterpenes found in many conifers. Pinene is responsible for much of the aroma of Christmas trees. It is also the principal ingredient in turpentine. The solvent activity of pinene is one reason that soft plastic bags are a poor choice for storing cannabis, since light terpenes can dissolve the plastic. Pinene inhibits enzyme activity in the brain and this inhibition aids short-term memory, which could explain why high-pinene cannabis varieties don't cause the memory issues associated with other high-THC varieties.[56] This terpene is associated with cannabis varieties such as Kona Gold.

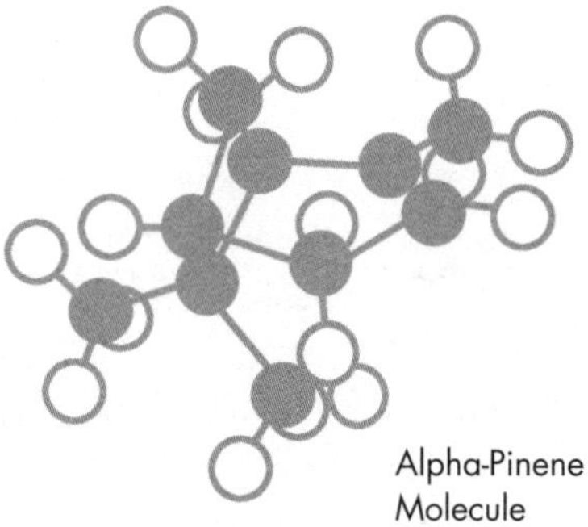

Alpha-Pinene Molecule

Limonene —Limonene is common in citrus fruits, especially their peels. Limonene and terpinolene are the terpenes responsible for the citrusy scent of some

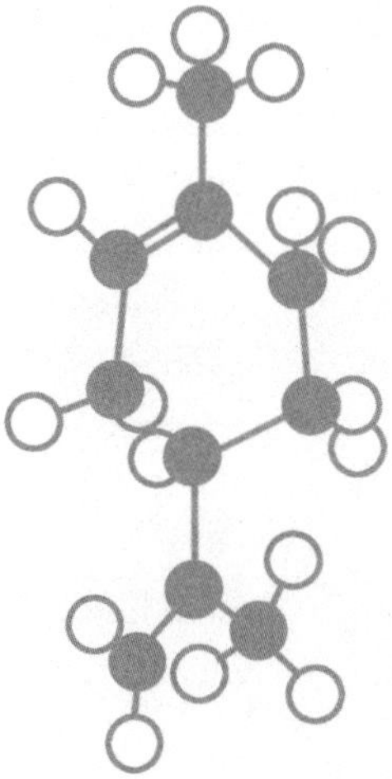

Limonene Molecule

cannabis varieties. Varieties such as Tangerine Dream are high in limonene, while Lemon Jack Herer is high in terpinolene, but both feature a pronounced citrus aroma. In cannabis, this aroma is associated with stimulating, mood-elevating, and quick-onset effects. Clinical studies with limonene and citrus oil have also demonstrated a significant antidepressive effect.[57]

Myrcene —Myrcene has reached the highest concentration of any terpene found in a cannabis variety, composing more than 30 percent of the total essential oil. Myrcene is the primary terpene produced by cannabis' closest relative in the plant kingdom: hop (see page 18). Bedrocan in the Netherlands produces a herbal cannabis medicine high in myrcene, specifically to deliver a sedative effect. Myrcene is typically associated with an "*indica*" or "couchlock" effect in cannabis. Myrcene relaxes muscles in animal models and also increases the effects of sedative drugs.[58]

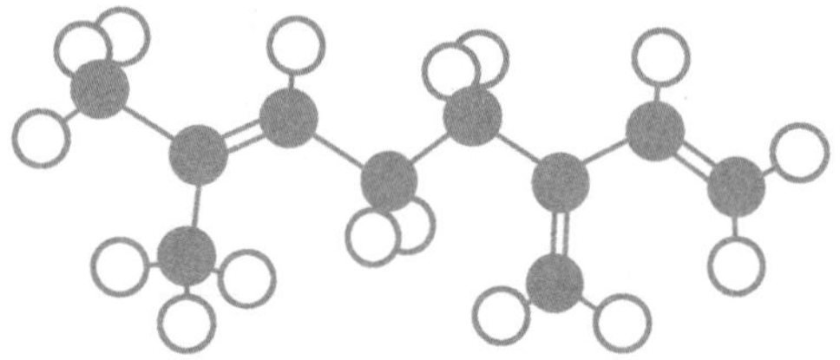

Myrcene Molecule

Beta-Caryophyllene —Beta-caryophyllene is the most common of the heavier sesquiterpenes found in cannabis and responsible for its more stimulating effects.[59] Beta-caryophyllene is also the most common terpene in decarboxylated extracts, since it typically survives extraction temperatures that the monoterpenes will not.[60] Beta-caryophyllene interacts with the CB_2 receptor and is found in black pepper and hops. This interaction makes beta-caryophyllene a "dietary cannabinoid." Black pepper could even be considered illegal in the United States under federal and state laws that strictly prohibit the distribution of cannabinoids and their analogs. Beta-caryophyllene was the first phytocannabinoid isolated outside of the *Cannabis* genus. It is an effective anti-inflammatory, both internally and topically. It may also be effective for relieving some of the hangover effects of THC overmedication.[61] The oxidation product of beta-caryophyllene is caryophyllene oxide. Drug detection dogs are trained to smell the caryophyllene oxide in cannabis.

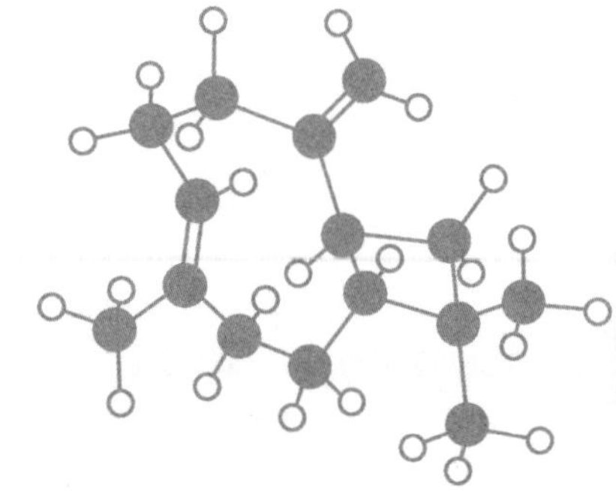

Beta-Caryophyllene Molecule

Linalool —Linalool is found in lavender and is mildly psychoactive. This naturally occurring chemical is associated with calming, antianxiety effects. It is found in varieties including Bubba Kush and several purple indica strains. Medicinally, linalool is sedative, analgesic, and anesthetic.

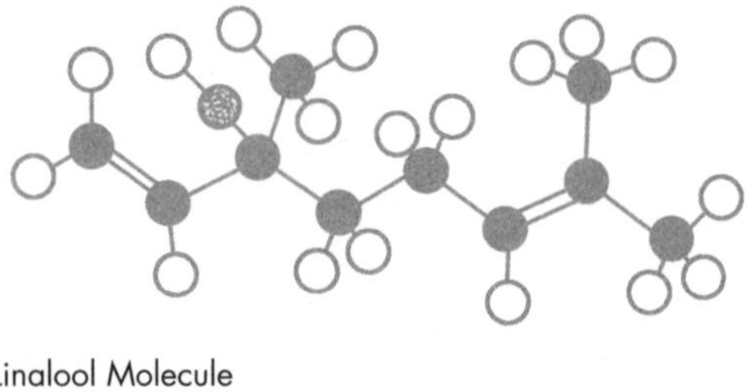

Linalool Molecule

TERPENOIDS AND THEIR PHARMACOLOGICAL ACTIVITIES

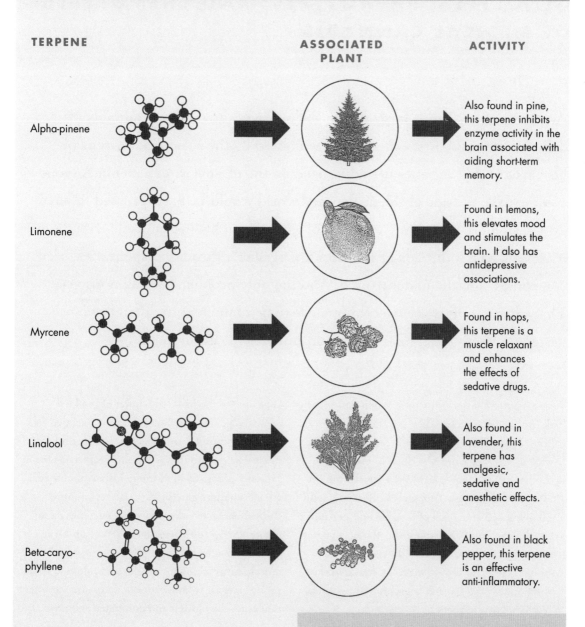

TERPENE		ASSOCIATED PLANT	ACTIVITY
Alpha-pinene	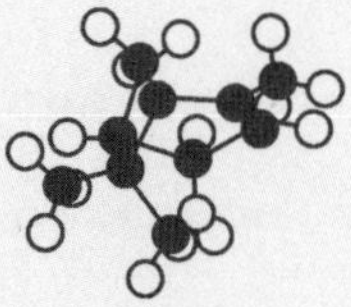		Also found in pine, this terpene inhibits enzyme activity in the brain associated with aiding short-term memory.
Limonene	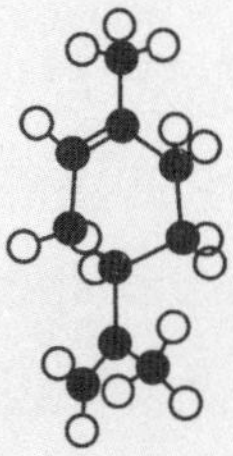	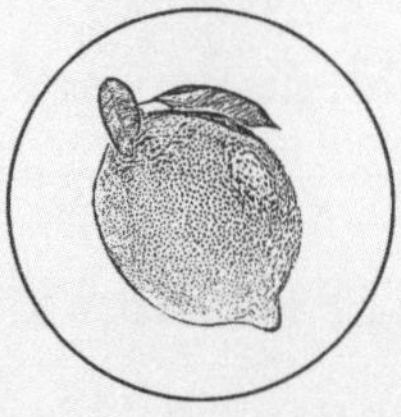	Found in lemons, this elevates mood and stimulates the brain. It also has antidepressive associations.
Myrcene	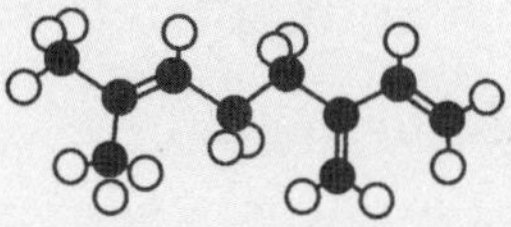	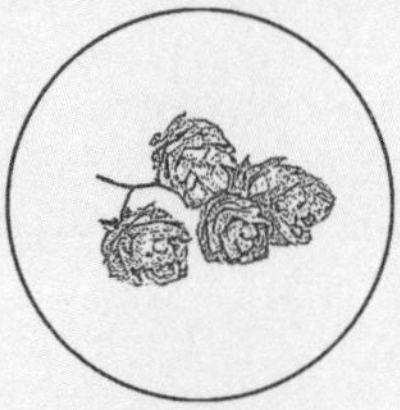	Found in hops, this terpene is a muscle relaxant and enhances the effects of sedative drugs.
Linalool	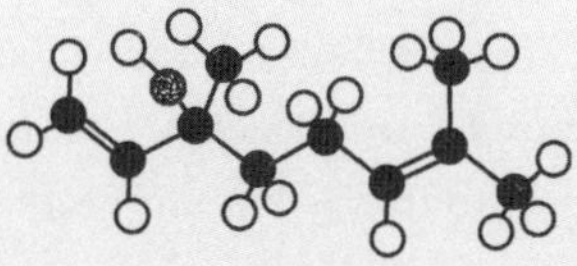	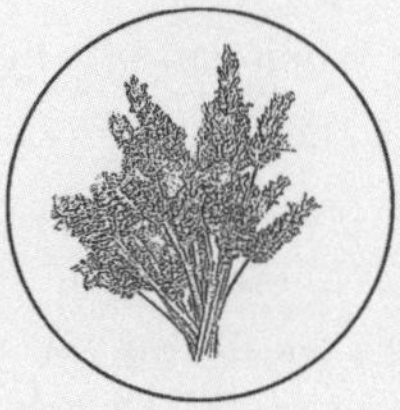	Also found in lavender, this terpene has analgesic, sedative and anesthetic effects.
Beta-caryophyllene	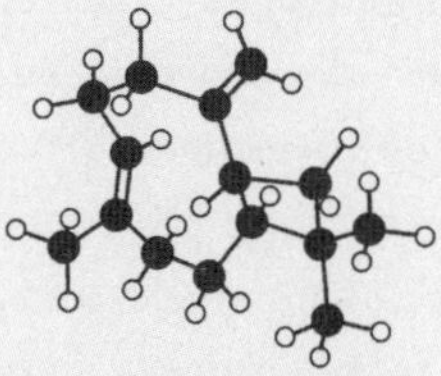	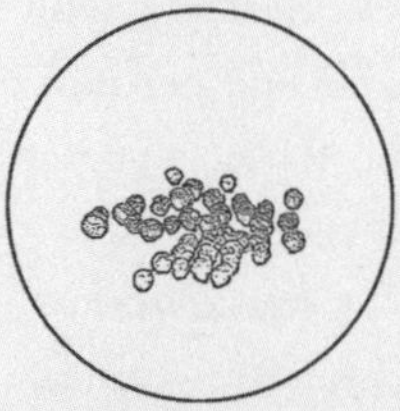	Also found in black pepper, this terpene is an effective anti-inflammatory.

This table offers a summary of five predominant terpenoids produced by cannabis, together with other plants that also produce the same terpenoid, and the pharmacological activities associated with each. The cannabis plant produces over 200 terpenoids, though most in trace amounts.

GENOTYPES, PHENOTYPES, AND CHEMOTYPES OF MEDICAL CANNABIS

Anyone walking into a large California or Colorado medical cannabis dispensary for the first time would be floored by the selection. Dozens of herbal cannabis varieties are advertised on the plasma screen menu. Anyone coming from outside of the dispensary world would be hard-pressed to have ever seen more than a few varieties of cannabis in his/her entire life. And now it appears as if hundreds of varieties are available through dispensaries, seed companies, and the underground. And the only problem? It's all nonsense. This apparent diversity is nothing more than a bunch of highly inbred varieties, where the similarities far outnumber the differences.

Take a visit to a large cultivation facility and really look for the differences. They are there, just tough to spot. Most of the leaflets are wide, even on the so-called *sativa* varieties like Sour Diesel. There is almost nothing that resembles a *sativa* from the 1970s, except perhaps Trainwreck. Basically, you are looking at a room full of cousins and perhaps even siblings. And what about the classic varieties from the past? Colombian Gold, Maui Wowie, Acapulco Gold, or Thai? Not to be found in the United States, and haven't been seen in decades. What happened to them?

Welcome to the isolated hamlet of modern cannabis genetics, where a bunch of related folk have intermarried and produced some odd offspring. Add to that a current preference for growing plants from cuttings rather than seeds, which hampers genetic diversity even more. Remember that today's medical varieties came of age during the government's War on Drugs. They were selected for THC content, ease of indoor cultivation, high yield, and minimal space requirements. In other words, to create varieties that could be hidden and cultivated with the

All this inbreeding has made for high-yielding and potent plants, just not always medicinally interesting ones.

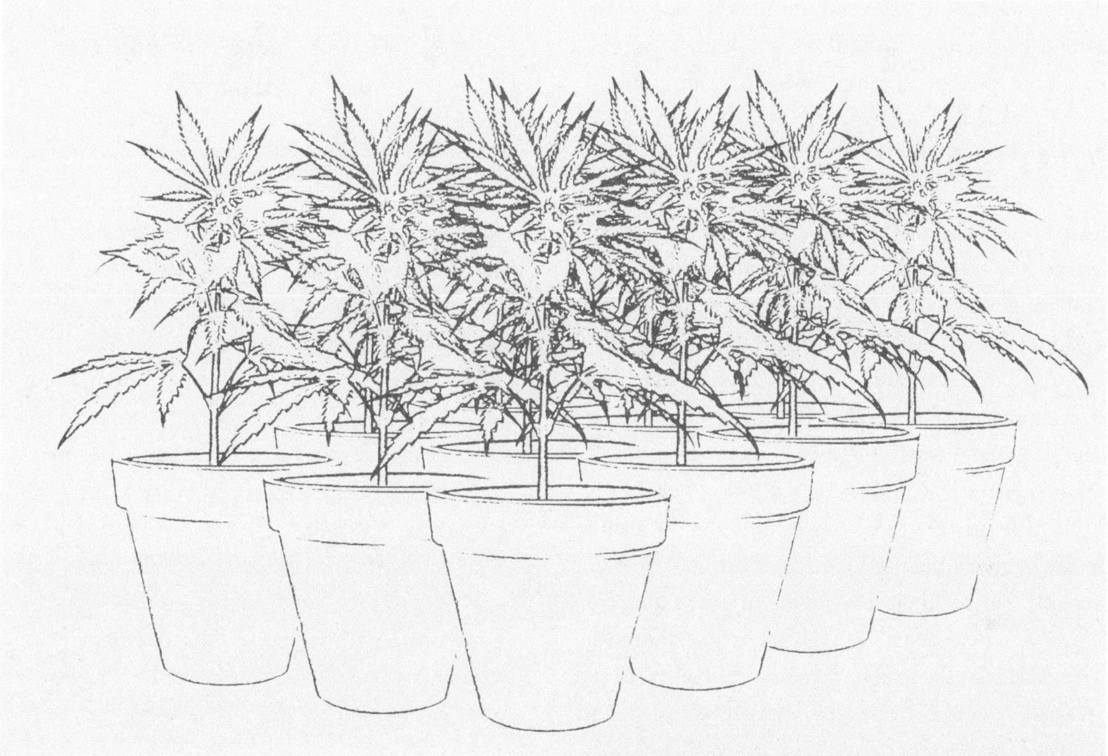

Cloning cannabis plants allows growers to focus on varieties that fulfill a certain number of criteria, be it THC content, rapid growth, or the size of plants and flowers, for example.

smallest footprint possible within the shortest period of time. And that's what we've got. Those Santa Cruz Hazes that weren't ready for harvest until Christmas? That tall wispy Kona Gold? Both dead as disco. Although the traits that made these varieties different in the sixties and seventies are still there, they've just shrunk into recessive traits, awaiting an iconoclastic breeder to coax them from hiding among the more popular genes.

The very first Afghan genetics to come to the U.S. in the late 1970s had a reasonable chance of being representative of the "Af-Pak" hashish genetics that filled the region before the Soviet invasion of Afghanistan. But they weren't. Instead, the plants that were selected were ones that expressed extremely high levels of THC, unlike the more common THC/CBD genetics found in the region. One of these selected plants became the legendary Afghan #1 (see pages 118–119). The irony was that it would be tough to find another plant in Afghanistan or Pakistan that resembles it, today or even back in 1975. Afghan #1 was selected for its high resin content, its compact shape, and its short harvest time, but also its high THC content. Was it the most medicinally interesting plant in Afghanistan? No. In fact, it probably wasn't the most medicinally interesting cannabis plant in the village.

But there is good news here. There are many places around the world where unique cannabis genetics still survive. Perhaps not as many as there were 40 years ago, but plenty, nonetheless.

The better news? Today we understand a lot more about the plant, and about what can make cannabis interesting from a medical standpoint.

Indica vs. *Sativa*

Let's explode a myth right now: the myth of *indica* and *sativa*. Ask most cannabis patients about *sativas* and they say: stimulating, mood-elevating, and good for daytime use. Ask them about *indicas* and you'll hear: body high, relaxing, stony, sedative, and more potent than *sativas*. The descriptors are correct, but the names are wrong. Ten years ago, Karl Hillig was working on his doctoral degree at Indiana University. Part of Hillig's dissertation was to examine the difference in the genetics between cannabis varieties from around the world, and he made an interesting discovery.[62] All drug strains of cannabis shared a relatively narrow range of genes. And all fiber strains of cannabis, the ones we call hemp, shared another small set of genes. And there was not as much crossover between them as might have been expected. So, Hillig decided to clean up the nomenclature. He decided that all fiber varieties, hemp, should be classified as *Cannabis sativa*. He classified all drug varieties as *Cannabis indica*, but noted some crucial distinctions. He divided drug *indica* cannabis into broad-leafleted drug (BLD) and narrow-leafleted drug (NLD) varieties. Most of today's drug cannabis varieties are a hybrid of these two biotypes, leaning toward the BLD side in appearance, but possessing characteristics from both cultivars. Most NLD-dominant hybrids are somewhat stimulating and cerebral when compared to pure BLDs such as Bubba Kush.

What about *Cannabis sativa*? It turns out that *sativas* are much more than just fiber and rope. They carry the gene to make the enzyme that converts CBG into CBD, rather than THC. All CBD genetics appear to trace their origins to hemp varieties of cannabis. And the CBD to THC hashish cultivars of the Middle East are likely true *indica/sativa* crosses. The classic early drug strains, such as Haze, contained some CBD along with THC. Eventually, the distinction between *indica* and *sativa* effects will be based on a variety's terpene, rather than its cannabinoid, content.

Primary Chemotypes of Cannabis

The simplest distinction between cannabis chemotypes is whether THC or CBD is dominant. The next distinction is which terpenes are dominant. Surprisingly, there are fewer terpene classes than expected, with the following being predominant in most drug cannabis: myrcene, limonene, beta-caryophyllene, terpinolene, pinene, linalool, or ocimene. Most cannabis varieties, because of *indica* heritage, tend to be myrcene dominant. Combinations of terpenoids will change the aroma of cannabis varieties, but terpenes also significantly influence the psychoactive and medicinal effects. A few varieties produce many different terpenes in quantity, for example OG Kush or Pincher's Creek, and these "entourages" are both rare and popular with patients.

So What Is Kush?

Kush takes its name from the Hindu Kush mountains of Central Asia centered in modern-day Afghanistan and Pakistan. These highlands are home to traditional hashish gathering cultures, whose denizens sift the cannabis to collect resin glands, which are then pressed into hashish (see pages 79–82). True kush cannabis genetics are squat, broad-leafleted plants with a spicy aroma and acrid smoke. A good example of today's problem in distinguishing cannabis varieties arises when discussing the popular OG Kush strain (see pages 152–55), which exhibits characteristics of a hybrid, but has little but potency in common with true kush varieties.

Have Cannabis, Will Travel

As drug cannabis was carried from Asia, where it originated, to Africa and then to the Americas, its chemistry changed. Local varieties, called landraces, became acclimated to the local conditions (see page 114). Thai, Acapulco Gold, and Durban Poison are examples of this. Such varieties began to exhibit new or different characteristics. Certain terpenes would repel molds, while others would repel insect pests or discourage some grazing animals. The plant was forced to adapt to survive. Narcotic myrcene varieties flourished in the mountains of Afghanistan, while stimulating pinene varieties were selected in India and Africa to help deal with tropical heat. By the time cannabis reached the highlands of Central Mexico, the effects took on what has been described as an almost spiritual intensity. Many consider these highland Mexican genetics to be the finest cannabis on Earth.

Medicinally interesting cannabis is cultivated from Vietnam to Lebanon, from Egypt to South Africa, from Argentina to Colombia, and from Panama to Russia. Only a handful of varieties among these landrace genetics have been characterized for their potential medicinal value. As cannabis prohibition is dismantled, many types of cannabis from around the world will reemerge or perhaps even be discovered. A golden age of cannabis varieties could be right around the corner.

In Search of the Lost Origins

When old cannabis cultivators sit around swapping tales, legendary strains are often discussed; Kona Gold, Panama Red, and Lemon Thai are just a few. As prohibition appears to be crumbling in the United States, and perhaps around the world, the opportunity looms to visit countries that once grew the landrace varieties that formed the foundation of modern cannabis genetics. Another approach is through tissue culture techniques. Scattered around the United States are a number of jars filled with vintage cannabis seeds. Conventional propagation is unlikely to germinate these ancient seeds, but tissue culture techniques can occasionally revive them. Eventually we may have access to our grandpa's cannabis medicine chest. The other advantage of rescuing these genetics is that they may contain compounds that have completely disappeared from modern cannabis varieties—compounds that have yet to be studied for their medicinal value.

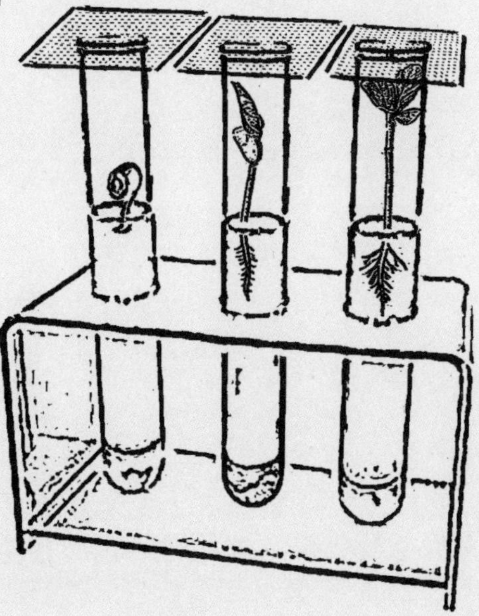

Using Medical Cannabis

As a plant medicine, cannabis can be eaten, smoked, vaporized, and applied as a topical cream or under the tongue. When most people consider using cannabis as a medicine, they think of smoked cannabis, even though for most of its history as medicine, cannabis was taken orally. Today, vaporization technologies provide a non-smoked alternative with similar speed of onset and dose control to smoking. There are also cannabinoid medicines, such as Sativex, which contains cannabidiol and terpenes to balance the effects of THC. Sativex can be considered the first modern prescription cannabis medicine, although the Golden Age of cannabis medicines is yet to come.

2

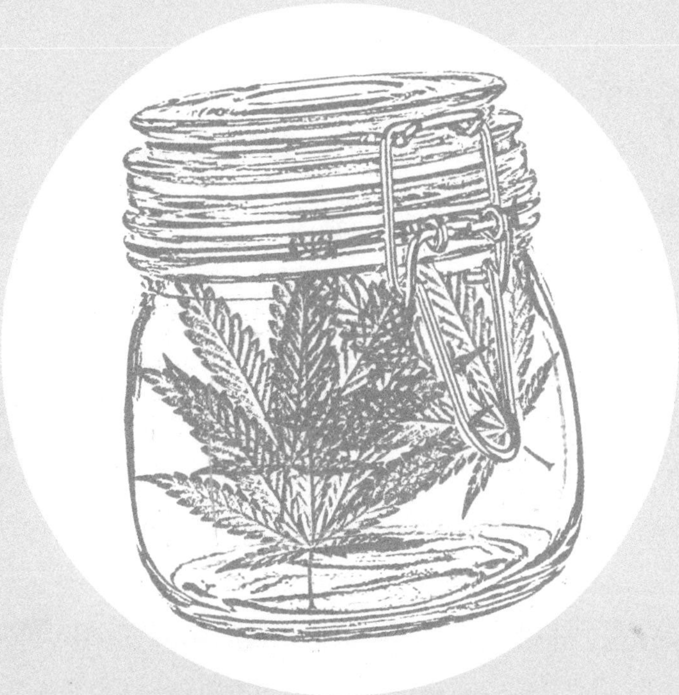

METABOLIZING MEDICAL CANNABIS

The form of cannabis and the method of its consumption profoundly affect how it works as a medicine. Different forms of cannabis have unique chemistries and the body metabolizes them differently. Various delivery methods impact the speed and efficiency with which a cannabis medicine works—and how long its effects will last. Due to cannabis prohibition and portrayals of cannabis use originating in the marijuana underground, there are not many popular models for using cannabis medicinally that are actually effective. For example, a bong is not the ideal way to take one's medicine.

As a natural product, cannabis has a shelf life, and knowing how to store it properly will extend its storage life. Occasionally, there is more in a sample of medical cannabis than should rightfully be there. Learning how to spot the various contaminants, and knowing which of them require a laboratory to detect, is a key skill for patients. Above all, learning how to master cannabis delivery methods and dosage can be of significant help in finding the best way to treat your specific medical condition.

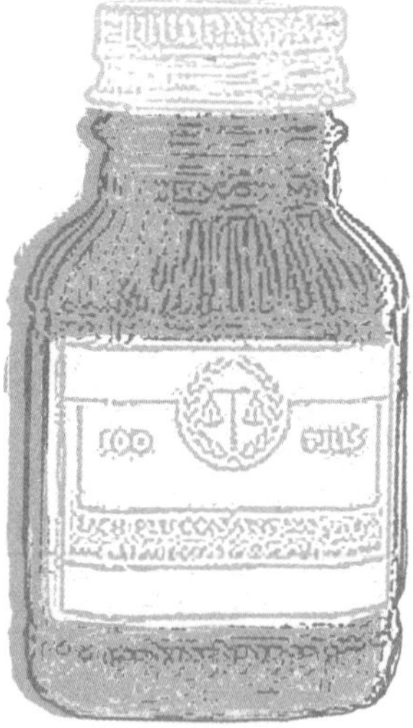

The Issue of Solubility

One of the trickiest issues when using cannabis medicines is that cannabinoids hate water and love fat. In technical talk, cannabinoids are hydrophobic and lipophilic. Since most medicines are taken orally, this insolubility in water poses some real issues. Cannabinoids are poorly and erratically absorbed when taken orally. This inconsistency is such a problem that cannabinoid medicines fell out of favor in the 1940s. However in the last 20 years, researchers have learned much more about how cannabis and cannabinoids can be absorbed effectively, from sublingual delivery to vaporization technologies. Many of these techniques are intended to detour around the gut and deliver the medicine into the bloodstream as quickly as possible.

DOSAGE: A SHORT INTRODUCTION

Many patients and even a few physicians have little idea of how to dose and deliver herbal cannabis medicines. Our only media models for cannabis use are stoner comedies, such as the Cheech and Chong movies or *Pineapple Express*. The model of cannabis dosage portrayed in these films is as inaccurate as learning how to drive an automobile by watching the chase sequences in *Fast & Furious*.

A more rational approach to medical cannabis dosage is to use the smallest effective amount of cannabis that delivers the desired symptomatic relief. This minimum effective dose is summarized quite simply by the phrase, "just a little bit."

"Just a little bit" emphasizes the small, controlled, and measured dosage approach to herbal cannabis. It can be challenging for patients new to cannabis to avoid overmedication, since many of the tools—such as bongs (water pipes) and vaporizers—don't come with detailed instructions encouraging informed, controlled dosage. Consistent overmedication with herbal cannabis can lead to tolerance to cannabis' medicinal effects, requiring increased dosage in order to relieve symptoms that were previously relieved with smaller doses.

Dose guidance is especially useful with THC-dominant cannabis medicines, which can be highly psychoactive. But what's a dose? The best-studied cannabis medicine is Marinol, the prescription synthetic form of THC. Clear dosage guidelines are well understood for

Media portrayals of cannabis use encourage patients to develop a skewed sense of the size and frequency of appropriate cannabis dosage.

Synthetic forms of THC, such as Marinol, can be taken in 2.5-mg, 5-mg, and 10-mg capsules, depending on the medical condition being treated.

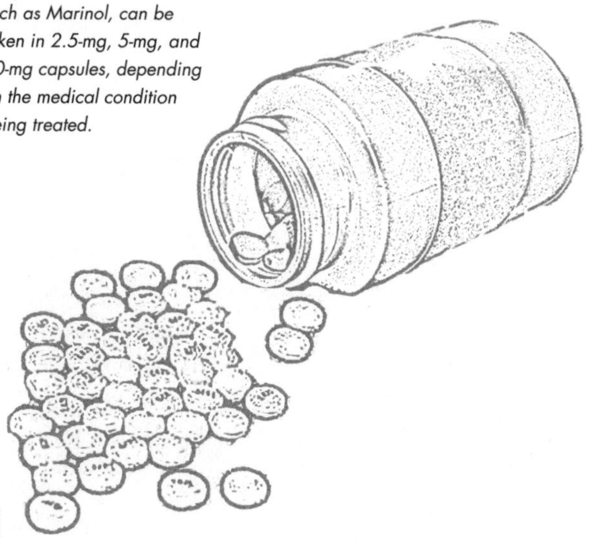

Marinol and can provide a starting point for developing dosage guidelines for herbal cannabis. A Marinol dose begins at 2.5 milligrams of THC for appetite stimulation. For chemo-induced nausea an effective Marinol dose can exceed 15 milligrams, depending on patient's height and weight. Psychoactivity is typically noticed by most patients at a dose of 5 milligrams of THC, so a 15-milligram THC dose can produce high high levels of psychoactivity that may be very unpleasant. Recent studies have shown that cannabis doses that deliver between 2.5 and 10 milligrams of THC can address a wide range of symptoms with tolerable levels of psychoactivity. There is increasing evidence that the other primary cannabinoid, CBD, found in some varieties of cannabis, can in fact reduce THC's psychoactivity levels.

When correctly dosed, cannabis can also be effective both orally and sublingually. However it can take 45 to 180 minutes for oral cannabis to take effect. When taken sublingually, delta-9-THC is absorbed directly into the bloodstream and the effects can be felt in five minutes. An oral cannabis dose is effective for two to three times longer than smoked or vaporized herbal cannabis, reducing the need for repeated administration.

What Cannabis Potency Means and How It's Changed

The media often cites studies indicating that cannabis potency has dramatically increased over the last 30 years. This trend is supposed to indicate that cannabis today is more dangerous than cannabis was in the 1960s. But is that true? Studies with smoked cannabis have demonstrated that patients quickly become adept at adjusting their dose, regardless of the potency of the cannabis they are using. The advantage to higher-potency cannabis is that less cannabis is needed to reach the desired dose. Cannabis in the 1960s would have averaged around 2 to 4 percent THC, while today cannabis in California dispensaries averages closer to 16 percent THC. If a patient is smoking cannabis, this could mean that the patient requires over 87 percent less cannabis to receive the desired dose. With certain cannabis concentrates, extremely high potency can make low doses nearly impossible. Most high-potency cannabis flowers can be easily and effectively dosed with simple guidance.

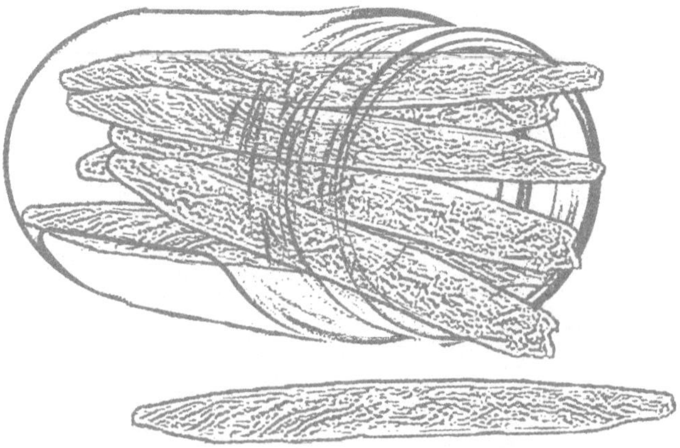

A "joint" is not a dosage guidance. A joint typically contains anywhere from 0.25g to 1g of cannabis. The levels of THC available in cannabis vary widely, and the ultimate dose depends on what percentage of the joint is smoked.

STORING CANNABIS

Whether you have dried flowers, pressed hash, tinctures, oils, waxes, or creams, there are a number of effective methods for storing cannabis, all of which serve to protect and preserve it for the longest possible time. As with all natural products, cannabis is susceptible to damage from exposure to heat, air, moisture, and light, so it pays to make the right choices for the longer term. Depending on the form being stored—particularly in the case of flowers—cannabis may also suffer from bruising and cross-contamination.

Cannabis is Perishable

To keep cannabis flowers and extracts in good condition, store them in a dark and cool place in an airtight, rigid container. For storage of fewer than 90 days, temperatures around 50°F (10°C) will maintain quality. At this temperature, 55 percent humidity should keep the cannabis from deteriorating. For long-term storage of flowers, however, a temperature below freezing is recommended—and the colder the better, though frozen flowers should not be thawed and refrozen. Cannabis should never be kept in temperatures over 80°F (27°C), neither should it be transported in a hot and confined space—such as a glove box or truck—except when stored in a chilled, well-insulated container. A lot of cannabis gets ruined by relatively short exposure to high heat in automobiles.

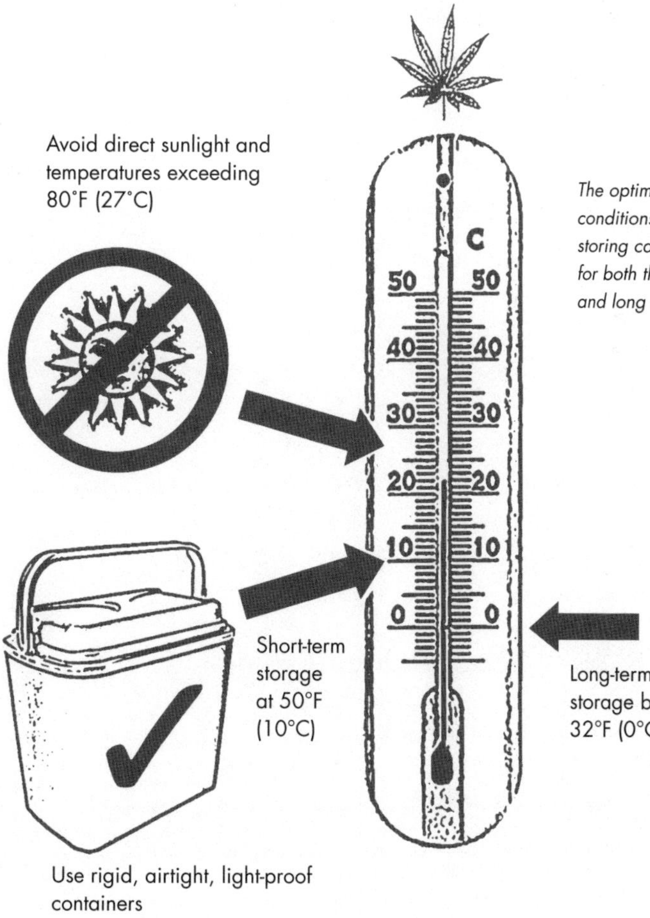
Avoid direct sunlight and temperatures exceeding 80°F (27°C)
C
50
40
30
20
10
0
Short-term storage at 50°F (10°C)
Long-term storage below 32°F (0°C)
Use rigid, airtight, light-proof containers

The optimum conditions for storing cannabis for both the short and long term.

Chemical-Resistant Plastic or Glass

Plastic sandwich bags are often used by drug dealers to package cannabis for selling. This leads to rapid bruising and deterioration of the cannabis. Keeping medical cannabis in good condition for a longer time requires a more robust approach to packaging.

Plastics such as polyethylene and polypropylene are good choices for containers storing cannabis. The key to choosing a good storage medium for cannabis is its chemical resistance. Anything that is considered safe for food storage and marked with NSF (certification from NSF International as being certified for food storage) is a safe bet.

You can reuse containers to hold cannabis flowers and extractions, but always clean them out between uses. To avoid the possibility

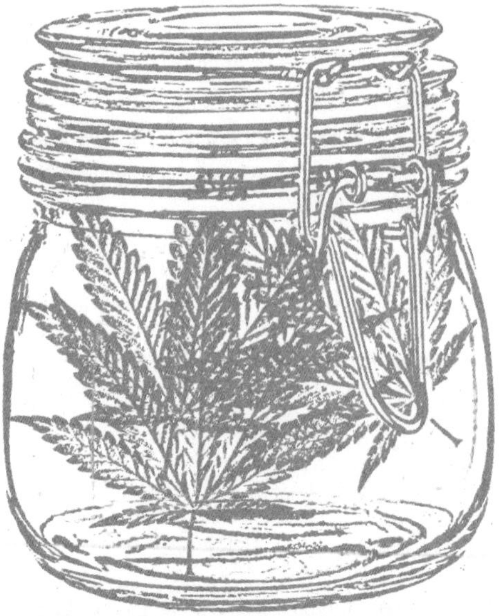

Glass jars offer one of the best methods for storing dried cannabis. They must be perfectly clean with airtight lids.

What Is Actually Being Stored and Protected?

The objective of correctly storing cannabis is not to protect the dried flowers as much as its millions of tiny "pillows." Microscopic, waxy pillows of oily resin are exuded from the tips of tiny gland hairs called trichomes. These incredibly delicate structures are where cannabis produces and stores its medicine. Anything brushing against these trichome resin heads will rupture them. When resin heads are ruptured, their terpenes evaporate and their cannabinoids break down. The waxy outer layer of the trichome head additionally keeps the highly polyunsaturated fats in cannabis oil from turning rancid. The reality is that dried cannabis flowers simply serve as a scaffolding to protect cannabis resin heads.

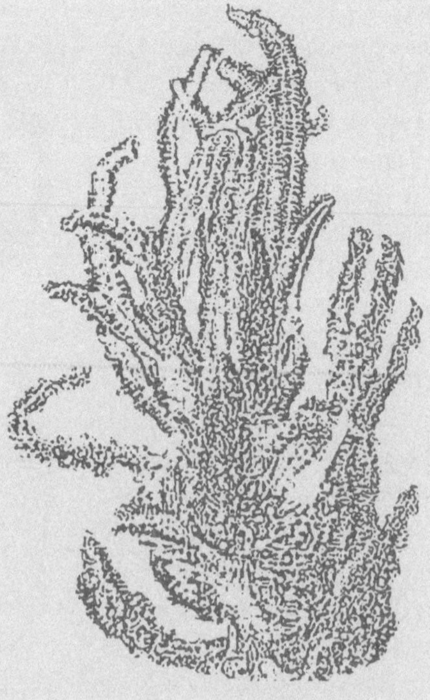

of cross-contamination, wash previously used containers thoroughly with soap and hot water. Never store cannabis in a dirty container. Remove cannabis resin buildup on used containers with 91 percent isopropyl alcohol, then rinse with hot water and allow to dry completely before use. If the used container is still even slightly sticky with resin, it's not clean.

A solid polypropylene, polycarbonate, or polyethylene jar with an airtight lid is an effective container for storing medical cannabis. The firmness of the jar's seal is crucial to maintaining freshness. Glass jars are also great for storing cannabis. However, neither glass nor plastic can protect cannabis trichomes if the container is violently shaken or otherwise disturbed. Whether it is plastic or glass, make sure that the container is not too large for the amount being stored in order to minimize exposure to air. Squeeze-top hinged plastic jars, while popular in California cannabis dispensaries, keep a poor seal and the cannabis stored inside them tends to dry out too quickly.

Sandwich and Turkey Bags Some medical cannabis dispensaries in California use soft plastic bags to package dried flowers and some extractions. The issue with this soft type of plastic is that a few of the oils produced by the cannabis plant, such as limonene, can dissolve the plastic and deposit its residue on the remaining cannabis. You really don't want to consume plastic-soaked cannabis. Oven-safe bags are a much better choice for soft packaging of cannabis. Cannabis cultivators often choose turkey-sized oven bags to store up to a few pounds of dried cannabis.

The Myth of Rehydration

Most containers used to store cannabis are not airtight, which means that the dried cannabis will continue to dehydrate. When dried cannabis drops below 7 percent water content, the cannabis loses its volatile terpene oils very quickly, and its aroma and some of its effect are lost. It is mistakenly thought that cannabis can be rehydrated back to original condition once it has dried out. This is not true; once the terpenes on cannabis have evaporated, they are gone. Water cannot bring back the aromatic constituents of cannabis that have evaporated.

People do dumb things thinking they are maintaining the freshness of cannabis. They spray the cannabis with water or throw bread/tortillas/orange peels in the container. Spraying cannabis with water returns the surface of the cannabis to the high-moisture condition in which opportunistic molds and bacteria can flourish. Putting organic material like bread or fruit into contact with dried cannabis is a surefire way to encourage rapid spoilage. Some folks recommend using fresh cannabis leaves to rehydrate dried-out cannabis. While the cannabis leaf technique may appear promising, its "like-to-help-like" approach means that the fresh cannabis will dry too slowly to be safe and may actually decay, providing fodder for all kinds of microbes and molds in the process.

Intended to withstand high temperatures, oven bags are quite inert and a safe storage choice. The primary drawback of turkey bags is they cannot protect flowers and trichomes from being crushed.

Heat Sealing and Vacuum Packing Heat-sealable bags are good for maintaining cannabis freshness, since they are truly airtight. They can also be resealed to minimize excess air in the package. This airtight feature is great for travel and general discretion since the aroma of cannabis is minimized; however drug-sniffing dogs can still detect the scent. However, traveling with medical cannabis continues to be a very risky proposition, since most jurisdictions often have very different laws concerning medical cannabis and few places extend reciprocity to patients from other regions.

Vacuum packing cannabis in soft bags is a bad idea since it crushes the trichomes and will lead to rapid spoilage of the cannabis when removed. Vacuum packing cannabis in hard containers is a much better way to store cannabis, provided that the packed cannabis has a safe anaerobic bacteria level.

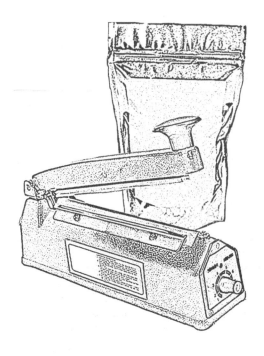

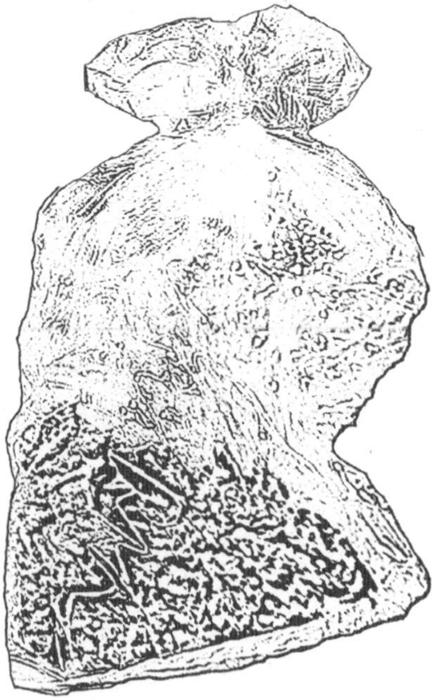

Cannabis stored in plastic bags (left) loses its potency more rapidly than cannabis stored in a heat-sealed or vacuum-packed bag (above). Trichome heads are easily crushed, increasing the oxidation rate of both cannabinoids and terpenoids. Rigid containers provide more protection to delicate, dried cannabis flowers.

Nitrogen Packing Recently, in Colorado and California, medical cannabis cultivators have begun storing their crops in nitrogen-filled bags. Nitrogen is an inert gas and prevents oxidation of cannabis constituents, and nitrogen packing is, therefore, an effective method for preserving medical cannabis. However, if the nitrogen-packed cannabis is allowed to become warm, some of its constituents can still break down. This modified atmosphere packing approach has not been shown to reduce microbial growth on fresh plants, but may have some advantages for dried cannabis and cannabis extractions.

Humidors and Moisture Packs Since they are used to keep tobacco fresh, wooden humidors and humidity packs are occasionally employed to maintain freshness in cannabis. Humidors are not intended to be airtight, so their moisture must be constantly monitored and replenished. Also, cigars and tobacco require more humidity than cannabis. Seasoning a humidor for cannabis will mean that the humidor must be slightly drier, around 60 percent humidity. The cannabis must have no direct contact with the humidor's moisture source, since this can trigger mold growth. If using humidifying packs, such as Boveda, it is also better to avoid prolonged contact between the surface of the pack and the cannabis. Never heat-seal a humidifying pack into a bag of cannabis, since the moisture pack may rupture if pressure is applied to the heat-sealed bag.

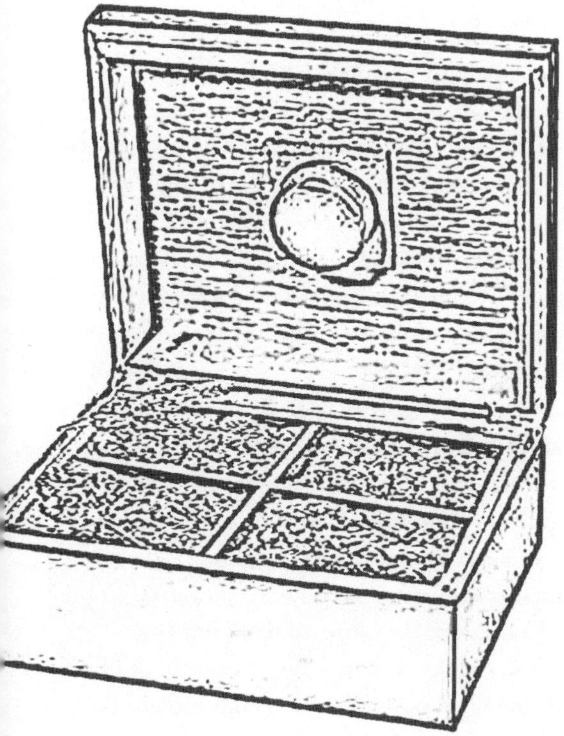

Packaged Cannabis

If you are acquiring sealed, prepackaged medical cannabis from a dispensary or shop, you are relying on the skill of the shopkeepers to maintain its freshness. Typically, a dispensary will provide a sample for patients to examine and smell. More sophisticated dispensaries may package their cannabis daily or weekly to ensure freshness. The best medical cannabis shops know how to store their medicines to protect the volatile constituents. Airtight containers are a good sign. Transparent plastic bags designed as food containers are typically not an indication of high-quality storage.

Storing Hashish and *Kif*

Pressing cannabis resin into hashish attempts to preserve the active ingredients from spoilage. Actually, the ideal method for resin preservation is to keep the fragile gland heads intact, unpressed, and very cold. Pressed hashish can also be stored for years in a conventional freezer at -4°F (-20°C), vacuum-sealed in a food-safe bag. The higher the pressure at which the hashish is compressed, the longer the hash may be stored. High-quality hashish is pressed with over 12 tons of pressure, using a hydraulic jack.

Unpressed, water-extracted hash or dry-sifted *kif* is more delicate, since the extracted resin glands have no protection from being ruptured

One of the most frequent problems encountered when using a humidor for storing cannabis is the development of mold. Moisture levels should be monitored regularly and kept at a constant rate to avoid disappointment. Any cannabis that shows signs of mold must be discarded.

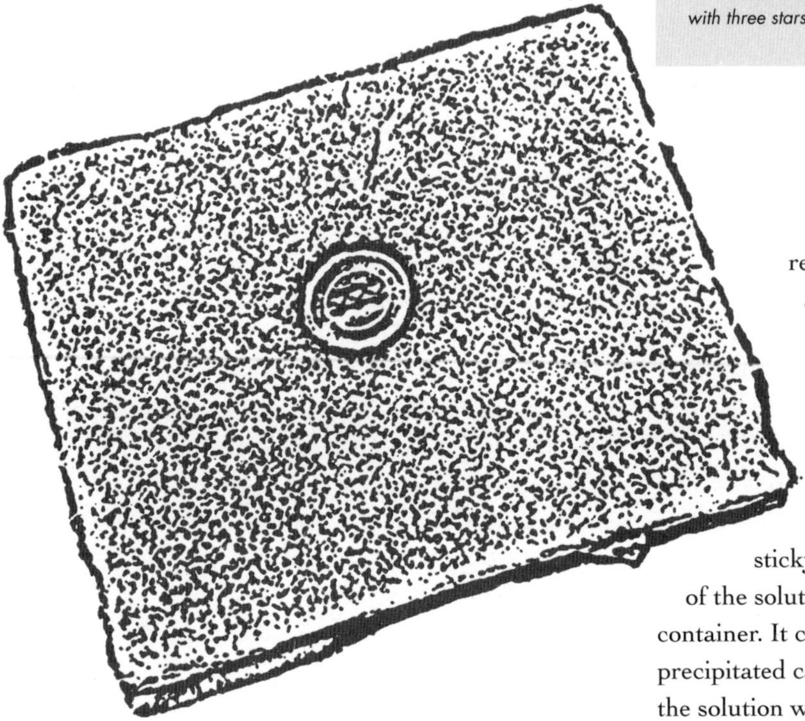

Afghan "primo" hash from the early 1970s, with a characteristic seal—a gold leaf disk embossed with three stars.

and oxidizing. The key to preserving water-extracted hashish is to first ensure that no residual water remains, since this will encourage mold and bacteria growth. Once the water is gone, the water hashish may be placed in a dark, cool, airtight storage container, where it should be left undisturbed until it is used. Always check stored water hashish for visible mold as it is highly susceptible to mold growth during the drying process. Compressing water-extracted hashish or dry-sifted *kif* reduces oxidation.

Storing Cannabis Tinctures

Tinctures are simple extractions of cannabis made by soaking the plant in ethanol (ethyl alcohol) or glycerin for a given length of time, then filtering out the plant matter from the resulting tincture. Storing ethanol and glycerin tinctures is best achieved with conventional refrigeration. Long-term storage of tinctures can be challenging. It is difficult to keep cannabinoids dissolved in the ethanol or glycerin, because the sticky cannabinoids will precipitate out of the solution and onto the walls of the container. It can be difficult to get these precipitated cannabinoids completely back into the solution within the tincture, but vigorous shaking of the container for a minute before each use will help. A handheld lab homogenizer, basically an ultra-high speed blender, can mechanically emulsify cannabinoids into glycerin for longer term stability. Also the addition of an emulsifier to the tincture can make it easier to keep the cannabinoids in ethanol or glycerin solution. Cannabis tinctures can be stored in the refrigerator and this will slow the breakdown of THC and CBD.

Storing Cannabis Edibles

Many patients take their cannabis medicines infused into everyday food items such as cookies or candies, commonly called "edibles." Medical cannabis edibles are perishable depending on the food item into which the cannabis has been infused, so long-term storage of cannabis edibles at room temperature is not recommended.

Baked goods, such as cookies, containing cannabis can be frozen, then thawed for use. Simple refrigeration of cannabis baked goods is not recommended, since normal refrigeration temperatures can encourage mold growth on baked edibles. Cannabis hard candies have a long shelf life, provided they are protected from moisture. These infused hard candies can be stored with small desiccant packs, like those used for potato chips.

Cannabis chocolates can be stored in the cool, dark conditions preferred by its constituent ingredient, cocoa.

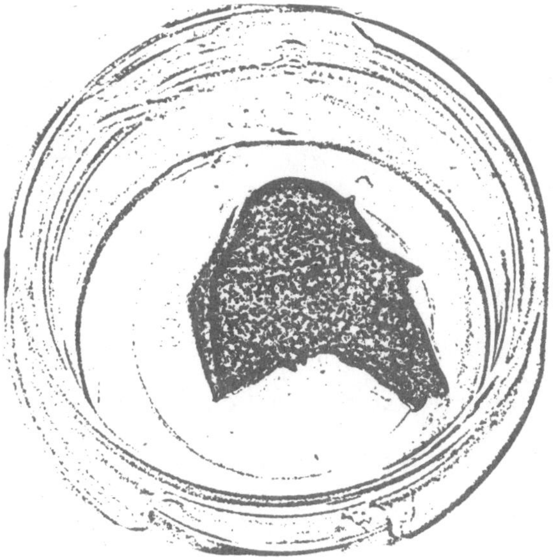

Cannabis oils and waxes are best stored in the freezer. Avoid freezing, thawing, and refreezing, however, as this will speed up deterioration.

Storing Cannabis Oils and Waxes

Cannabis oils and "waxes" are typically the most concentrated forms of medical cannabis available to patients, containing THC levels sometimes as high as 80 percent. The term "cannabis wax" refers to the consistency of the final product, which resembles a sticky wax. There are two basic approaches to making cannabis oils and waxes, either extraction with solvents such as butane or by using compressed liquid gases such as carbon dioxide. Both methods are effective for stripping cannabinoids from the raw cannabis. However, these methods strip more than just cannabinoids, and often will extract any fats produced by the plant. Extracted cannabis oils and waxes are extremely perishable if these extraneous plant fats and waxes have not been removed. These polyunsaturated plant fats oxidize within hours and turn rancid.

The rule of thumb is that all cannabis oils and waxes should be refrigerated to reduce spoilage and oxidation. Even better, divide the cannabis oil or wax into two or three dose portions and freeze them. Thaw one portion as needed in the refrigerator, and continue to store it there until it's finished.

The active cannabinoids and terpenoids in ethanol and glycerin tinctures may be diminished through direct exposure to light and heat. They are best stored, therefore, in small, dark bottles, preferably in a refrigerator.

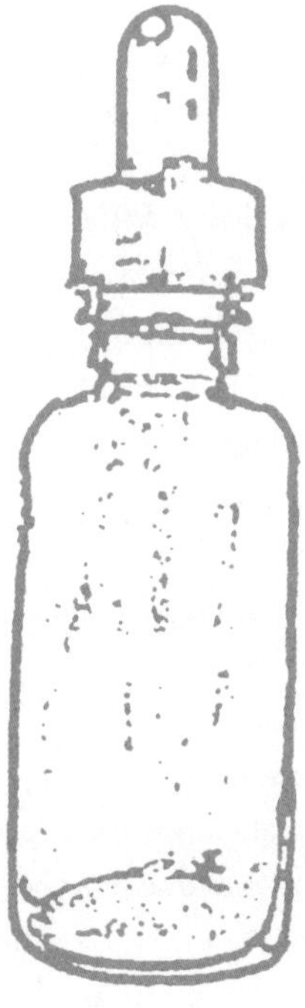

CANNABIS CONTAMINANTS, PATHOGENS, PESTICIDES, AND ADULTERANTS

Medical cannabis needs to be clean to protect patients from needless and occasionally dangerous exposure to pathogens, pesticides, and adulterants. The best way to avoid contaminated cannabis is to insist that it has been tested by a professional laboratory, qualified to detect microbiological and chemical contamination.

Just because a lab can test for cannabinoid content does not always mean the laboratory has the equipment or skills needed to detect the necessary range of contaminants, as many laboratories do not. Patients need to quiz their medical cannabis suppliers about the testing regimen to which their cannabis products are subjected. Testing and quality control measures are crucial to patient safety.

The vast majority of contaminated cannabis is the product of neglect during cultivation or processing, not malice.

Powdery Mildew and Gray Mold

Powdery mildew and gray mold are the most frequently reported fungal diseases of cannabis plants. Indoor cultivation sites commonly develop powdery mildew problems unless strict preventive measures are followed and adhered to. Crops cultivated outdoors in cool to moderate climates with rain during flowering season are often plagued by gray mold.

Gray mold loves big cannabis buds and can devastate a flowering crop in a matter of days. It typically appears as gray fuzz inside of cannabis buds, which can appear to have rotted the flower from the inside. Neither powdery mildew nor gray mold represent any health risk to the patient—just to the cannabis plant itself. A person could smoke a bowl of gray mold, and besides its unpleasant taste would suffer no ill effects.

Powdery mildew is actually caused by two varieties of fungus, one that develops from the plant's respiratory pores and another that grows upon the plant's surfaces. Powdery mildew often infests indoor cultivation facilities, where the plants tend to be crowded and stressed. The mildew appears as bright white threads on the smaller "water leaves" that surround the bracts (the collective term for the sepals, the tiny leaves that envelop the flowers of cannabis). While nontoxic, powdery mildew is a sign of poor cultivation technique and infested medicine should always be rejected.

Pesticides

Informal polling of several safety screening laboratories indicates that 1 to 2 percent of medical cannabis submitted by California dispensaries tests positive for pesticide residues. For an unregulated industry, as of late 2012, that is both encouraging and slightly ominous. It is heartening that pesticide residues appear to be scarce on California cannabis, but only a very few conscientious dispensaries even test for these residues. There is concern that the actual percentage of medications with unacceptable levels of pesticide residues might be higher. As medical cannabis laws are enacted and refined, then more pesticide screening will be mandated. Cultivator education and certification programs, such as Clean Green in California, can encourage and authenticate better practices among medical cannabis cultivators. And patients should demand clean and screened medicines. The pesticide residues that are detected on contaminated cannabis are rarely toxic to mammals, but they can be devastatingly toxic to honeybees or fish. Organic pesticides such as some pyrethrins can be used on medical cannabis plants, but only if the cultivator truly understands the amount of time required for the active pesticide to clear the plant. Often a positive pesticide test results from a cultivator using an otherwise safe substance too close to harvest.

Synthetic Plant Growth Regulators

Plant growth regulators (PGRs) such as daminozide and paclobutrazol have been used on cannabis to force the plant to flower more quickly, and to produce bigger and tighter buds. These chemicals are banned in the U.S. for any plants intended for human consumption; daminozide is considered a probable carcinogen in humans by the U.S. government. A few unscrupulous manufacturers of cannabis fertilizers have slipped

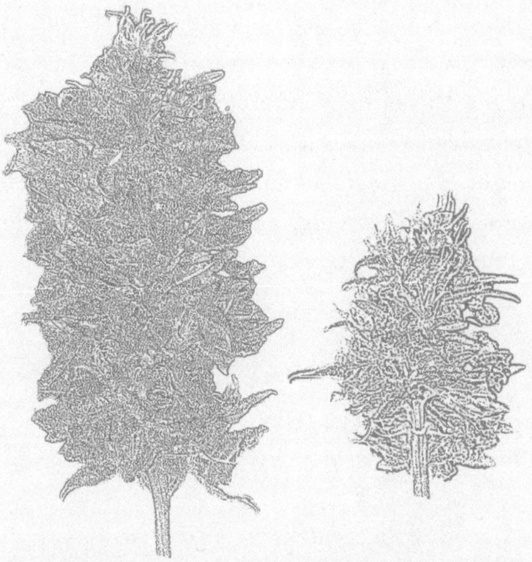

Plant growth regulators: A regular King Kush indoor-cultivated bud grows to around 1½in (4cm) while a King Kush bud grown indoors with the addition of PGRs could exceed 4in (10cm).

these PGRs into products without mentioning their inclusion on the products' labels. Always be somewhat suspicious of huge, indoor cultivated cannabis buds since they are often the result of using these illegal "plant steroids." If an indoor cultivated bud just looks too big to be normal, the flowers may actually be toxic.

Pathogenic Molds and Bacteria

Unlike powdery mildew or gray mold, the dangerous molds that can infest cannabis are difficult to detect with the naked eye. To find *Aspergillus*, *Fusarium*, or *Penicillium* molds requires laboratory tests. All of these dangerous molds are due to poor curing technique, not poor cultivation. These hazardous, pathogenic molds attack wet, freshly harvested cannabis. They are called opportunistic fungi because they attack rotting plant material. Specifically, they infest cannabis that stays too wet for too long during the curing process. These pathogenic fungi typically attack cannabis that is between 15 and 22 percent water weight. By contrast, correctly cured cannabis typically has between 8 and 12 percent water weight. The key to avoiding infestation by these storage molds is to dry harvested cannabis quickly enough so that it spends as little time as possible in the moisture "danger zone"—the time it takes for the plant to reach 15 percent water content. The biggest threat posed by pathogenic molds is aflatoxin, a poison produced by certain varieties of *Aspergillus* mold. Aflatoxins are not only toxic, but very carcinogenic. They are very rare on cannabis and can easily be prevented by careful drying and storage.

Dangerous bacteria such as *staphylococcus* and *E. coli* can also occasionally be found on cannabis. These bacteria end up on cannabis from human contact. Simple but thorough hand washing is all that is required to keep these dangerous bacteria in check.

Anaerobic bacteria are very rare on cannabis, as the plant is rarely exposed to the low-oxygen environments in which these bacteria can thrive. There are exceptions, however. Olive oil that is infused with whole, raw cannabis buds may provide an anaerobic environment that could result in botulism poisoning.

Conventional vs. Organic Production of Medical Cannabis

Conventional cannabis production employs chemical fertilizers and synthetic insecticides. The organic production of cannabis, on the other hand, uses manures and composts for fertilizing, as well as botanical extracts and beneficial insects to control pest species. Conventional agriculture relies heavily on synthetic herbicides to kill weeds, while organic farming controls weeds by crop rotation, tilling and mulching, and the judicious application of plant-derived herbicides. It is a commonly held belief that organic production of herbal medicines, including cannabis, is the superior approach.

Recently, other approaches to organic agriculture have gained credence vis-à-vis cultivating medical cannabis. Veganics is an organic approach whereby only plant-derived nutrients and pest control are used. Nontoxic cultivation is where no toxins, whether synthetic or organic in origin, are used in the cultivation of cannabis. The ideal method of producing medical cannabis is one by which the final product contains no trace of anything except cannabis… no residual nutrients, no additives, and no residues whatsoever.

Pests

Visible evidence of infestations on dried cannabis flowers is indicative of poor cultivation technique and lower-quality medicine. These attacking pests often weaken and kill cannabis plants, lowering the potency of the resulting product. Eradicating spider mites, the most common cannabis pest found indoors, can be extremely difficult once they are established. Most indoor and greenhouse cannabis cultivation sites will have to tackle a spider mite infestation at some point. Such a plague will lower the quality of medicine that the cannabis plant can produce because these pests weaken the plant, interfering with its ability to produce medicinal resin. Spider mites reproduce so quickly that their population can explode in a just a matter of weeks, resulting in thousands of mites feeding on every plant.

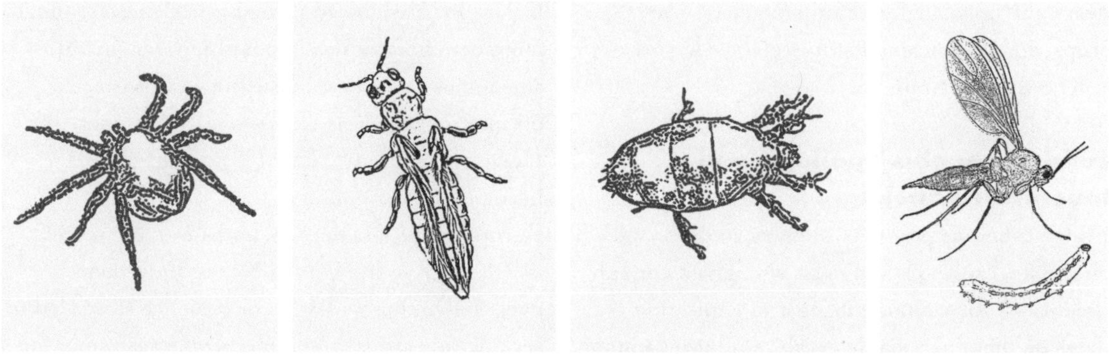

LEFT TO RIGHT *The four main pests that cause problems for cannabis growers: spider mite, thrip, broad mite, and fungus gnat with its larva. All indoor- and greenhouse-cultivated plants run the risk of being infested by at least one of these pests during their cultivation. Cannabis plants that have been infested for any length of time are considerably weakened and their flowers less potent. Outdoor-cultivated crops may also suffer attacks from slugs and snails, aphids, caterpillars, and whiteflies.*

A myth among cannabis cultivators in the 1970s was that spider mites when hatched were already carrying viable eggs. Today, these mites are better understood and infestations can be avoided by hygienic techniques.

A broad mite is an extremely small mite, only $^1/_3$mm in size. They infest over 60 species of plants, including cannabis. They are so small that cannabis growers sometimes miss them when inspecting their crops, and mistakenly believe the damage is more likely due to a virus.

Pests, such as fungus gnats, produce larvae that attack cannabis roots and can weaken the plant. Adult gnats can get trapped by trichome resin, sticking to the finished flower. Thrips are jumping insects that suck sap and weaken cannabis plants. There are as many as five different types of thrips that attack cannabis. A cultivation facility under attack by insect pests can drive cultivators to employ toxins that should never be used on medical cannabis. It's better to source your cannabis medicines from cultivators who understand that a rational pest management approach can institute preventive measures which eliminate pests before they become a serious issue.

Hair

The most common adulterant in medical cannabis is pet hair sticking to resinous bud, with human hair coming in second place in the adulterant derby. Because some cultivators occasionally keep pets around areas where harvested cannabis is trimmed and processed, hair remains an issue. Patients should refuse medications with pet hair, because accepting it sends the wrong message to those who sell it. Anybody trimming cannabis should wear a hairnet and long sleeves to avoid contaminating medicine with his or her own hair.

Odd Cannabis Adulterants

There are plenty of stories about strange things being found in bags of medical cannabis, from the occasional scary razor blade in a pound bag, which must have been left behind by a careless trimmer, to a small broccoli floret that somehow ended up in one patient's ounce. From live spiders to buckshot, it is clear that that the medical cannabis industry still lacks the regulatory oversight associated with other agricultural crops, and this means that unwelcome surprises will occasionally pop up.

Edible Cannabis Spoilage and Inaccurate Labeling

Edible cannabis products, such as cookies, and chocolate, can spoil, and most will, given enough time. Look for manufacturing and expiration dates on these perishable goods. And use common sense—for example, if a home-baked cookie only lasts for a week or so before it's too stale for consumption, why should a cannabis cookie be any different? The most common problem with edibles is deceptive labeling, which may lead to overdosing. If the label of a cannabis edible says "4x," it is assumed that "x" equals the dose. But what is a cannabis dose? The answer is: there is no standard. Some manufacturers of edibles claim that a dose is 50 milligrams, or 25 milligrams, or 10 milligrams of THC. The reality is that the dose varies by patient and there is no standardization. Fifty milligrams might be a single dose for one patient and 10 doses for another. Support those makers who label their edible products with accurate information about the amount of cannabinoids that the products contain. The safest approach for a patient is to calculate from the label the correct fraction of the edible that would contain five milligrams of THC and start with that as an initial dose. Five milligrams is a good starting point since it is commonly considered the threshold of psychoactivity for a dose of THC and is rarely too much for any patient. Once the patient knows what to expect from a five-milligram dose, the dose can be further adjusted for the level of symptomatic relief desired.

Fakes, Analogues, and Simulants

There isn't a huge amount of outright fake cannabis sold in dispensaries in California and Colorado. Mislabeled cannabis varieties are much more common, typically out of ignorance, but sometimes to deceive in the hope of passing off inferior cannabis varieties as better ones. However, synthetic cannabis products have become more common in the United States and Europe in the last decade, and a number were briefly legal in the United States, until their over-the-counter sales in convenience stores led to serious side effects in young people searching for a "legal high." Originally, synthetic cannabinoids were developed in the 1990s as part of legitimate research efforts at several universities to develop molecules different in their effects than the classical cannabinoids derived from the cannabis plant. Researchers quickly realized the problems that could arise if they remained unregulated, however, and warned of potentially dangerous side effects. By 2010, over 10,000 visits to emergency rooms in the U.S. were linked to the use of these synthetic cannabinoids. Unlike natural cannabinoids, very few of these synthetic cannabinoids have been widely used by humans and testing for their safety has not been conducted. The likelihood of clinical trials on humans remains remote, given the number of adverse effects already associated with them.

Medical Cannabis Quality Assurance—Analytical Testing

The most common form of analytical testing that cannabis undergoes is for cannabinoid potency, which is analyzed using a process called chromatography. It involves separating a mixture by passing a prepared sample of material in the form of a liquid or gas through a medium where the component chemicals in the mixture will move at different rates, allowing them to be identified by this rate of movement. The molecules within the sample have different interactions with the medium through which they are passing, which

Cannabinoids are identified (qualified) by a chromatography instrument and measured (quantified) by a mass spectrometer.

separates the different molecules and groups them based on their interactions with the medium. The molecules that display stronger interactions with the medium tend to move more slowly through it than those with weaker interactions. In this way, different types of molecules within the mixture can be separated from each other. Chromatographic separations can be carried out using a variety of media including silica on glass plates, volatile gases, paper, and liquids. Currently the most popular forms of chromatography among cannabis laboratories are gas and liquid chromatography.

Chromatography can help identify which cannabinoids and terpenoids are present in a cannabis sample, for example THC or CBD. Another instrument such as a mass spectrometer can tell how much of a particular substance is present in the sample.

The most important testing that medical cannabis can undergo is safety screening for pathogenic fungi, bacteria, and pesticide residues. For fungi and bacteria, these tests often consist of culture plates inoculated with samples of the cannabis, while pesticides are typically detected by chromatography.

The most common form of analytical testing that cannabis undergoes is for cannabinoid potency. Potency testing is useful for helping doctors and patients calculate dose. Nearly all of the analytical laboratory testing of cannabis is performed on chromatography instruments. Chromatography studies the separation of molecules based on differences in their structure and composition. Make certain that your testing laboratory is using independently validated testing methods.

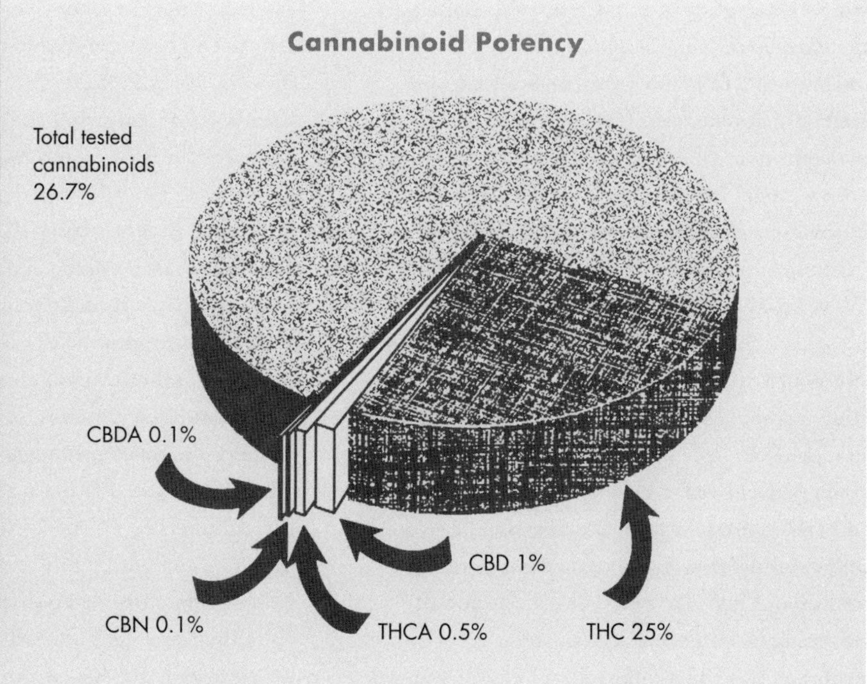

FORMS OF CANNABIS

In arid climates, such as Afghanistan or the Beqaa Valley of Lebanon, harvested cannabis has for centuries been dried and sieved to collect its cannabinoid-rich gland heads. This collected resin powder is pressed into hashish. In India, fields of unpollinated female cannabis flowers are cultivated to produce ganja, a potent marijuana preparation of these dried flowers. In the 1960s, hippies returning to California from India brought with them this Indian technique for producing seedless cannabis, dubbing it *sinsemilla* (see pages 22–23).

In Afghanistan in the early 1970s, the Brotherhood of Eternal Love, a group of smugglers composed of surfers originally from Huntington Beach, California, employed the extraction technologies developed back in California to make ultra-concentrated oil from Afghan hashish. Hash oil, being more concentrated, was easier to smuggle than conventional hashish. Forty years later, this innovation would spark the "dabbing" craze—inhaling vaporized cannabis oil—among West Coast medical cannabis patients.

Flowers

Many cannabis varieties are harvested outdoors in California in September and October, and some tropical varieties do not finish flowering until the winter solstice. Flowers are harvested and carefully dried and manicured to remove extraneous leaf. However, the definition of "extraneous" is controversial, since some patients prefer all leaf to be removed, while others insist that keeping the leaves intact helps to protect delicate trichomes. The "correct" approach typically depends on whether the cost of keeping those leaves is an issue. The money-is-no-object approach keeps the smaller leaves to protect the flowers. Keeping these leaves intact reduces the likelihood of rupturing the trichomes on the dried cannabis flowers, which hastens spoilage.

Outdoor Cultivation Cannabis loves sunshine. The cannabis plant flourishes outdoors from Alaska to Brazil, from Vietnam to Chinese Turkestan, to Humboldt County in California. A large number of indigenous cannabis varieties, called landrace varieties, have acclimated outdoors to different locales around the globe. These landraces exhibit a much wider range of characteristics than the common medicinal varieties currently cultivated in the United States. Some tropical outdoor landraces of cannabis, such as Thai or Colombian varieties, are not ready for harvest until weeks after the

Ganja to *Sinsemilla*—From India to Humboldt

All medical cannabis plants in the United States, Europe, and Israel are seedless females. Unfertilized, seedless flowers of the female cannabis plant produce far more medicinal resin than fertilized females. Female flowers produced with this technique are called *sinsemilla*, or ganja in South Asia where the approach was developed. The technique of preventing female pollination, which was developed in India in the early nineteenth century, consists of culling any male plants before they release pollen. This approach was brought to the United States in the late 1960s and became more widespread in Western countries by the late 1970s. Today, this technique of producing seedless cannabis is widely used, from the Manali slopes of northern India to GW Pharmaceuticals' secure, high-tech greenhouse located in a military research facility in the United Kingdom.

Trichome-laden female flower

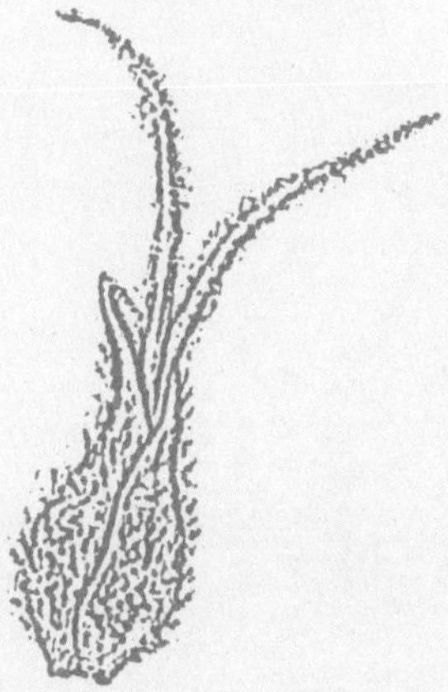

The relative heights of the two cannabis species following the three different methods of cultivation. Height depends on many factors, so heights are based on averages.

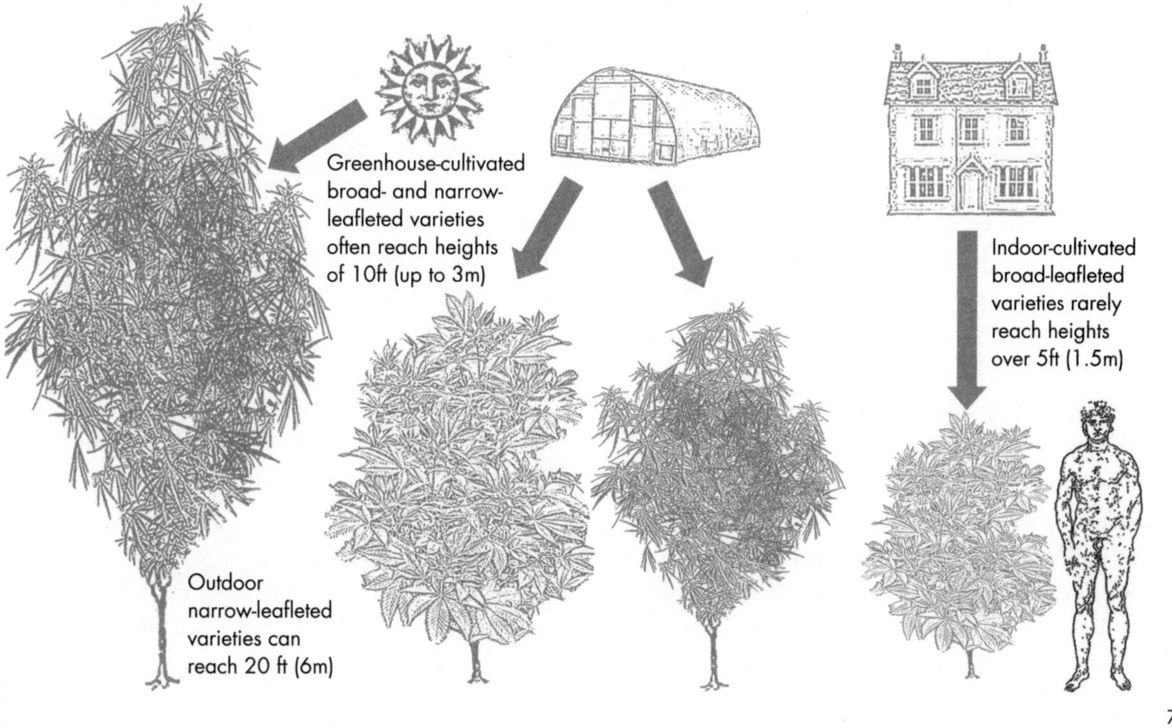
Greenhouse-cultivated broad- and narrow-leafleted varieties often reach heights of 10ft (up to 3m)
Indoor-cultivated broad-leafleted varieties rarely reach heights over 5ft (1.5m)
Outdoor narrow-leafleted varieties can reach 20 ft (6m)

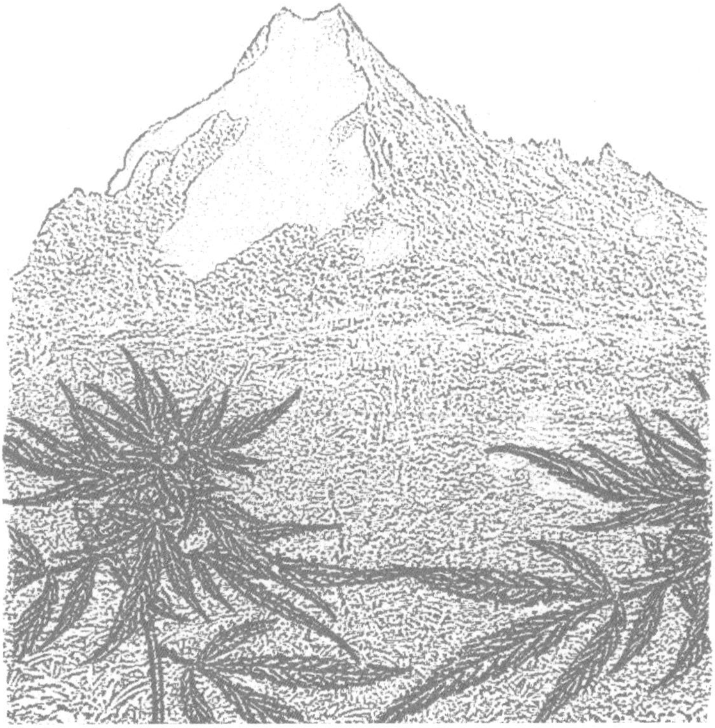

Historically, some countries have, at times, fostered immense outdoor crops. For example, plots in remote valleys of Nepal in the early 1970s covered hundreds of acres, with cannabis plants stretching as far as the eye could see.

winter solstice. These tropical varieties are often extremely tall by harvest time, which makes indoor cultivation challenging at best, and at worst impossible. Prohibition of cannabis ensured that smaller cannabis varieties, with shorter flowering times, would become more popular simply because they were safer to cultivate than their tropical relations. Furthermore, these fast-flowering cannabis varieties can be cultivated at much higher latitudes since they are ready for harvest before early frosts.

Outdoor cannabis plants can grow to over 20 feet (6 meters) high and yield over 5 pounds (2.3 kilograms) per plant of flowers from one single annual crop. There have been claims that one advantage of outdoor cannabis cultivation over indoor growing is that the cannabis plant may actually require the full spectrum of sunlight in order to produce particular terpenes, and perhaps even certain rare cannabinoids. Outdoor cannabis plants consistently host higher levels of bacteria and mold than their indoor counterparts, but outdoor plants are typically healthier and more robust. Currently, larger-scale outdoor cultivation in the United States tends to be sequestered away in remote mountains or valleys, where the need for discretion limits the size of such harvests.

While outdoor and lower-grade commercial cannabis are often lumped together, the reality is that the highest-quality outdoor cannabis will equal the quality of most indoor cultivation. It's worth noting that since sun-reared outdoor cannabis will by its very nature have higher microbial and fungi levels than other forms of cultivation, patients with immune disorders may wish to monitor these biological counts by only using lab-tested medicines.

Greenhouse Cultivation Within a secure greenhouse in the Porton Down military research facility in Wiltshire, U.K., GW Pharmaceuticals cultivates over 10,000 medical cannabis plants. These are harvested and extracted to make Sativex, a sublingual prescription cannabis spray sold in Europe and Canada. Controlled environment cultivation in a greenhouse provides the happy medium between indoor and outdoor approaches to medical cannabis cultivation. Supplemental electric lighting within the greenhouse can ensure that even the longest-flowering tropical variety can be cultivated in the short days of England's temperate winters. Up to three crops per year can be produced in a greenhouse: one conventional outdoor crop and two indoor crops of smaller plants produced with a combination of winter sun and supplemental lighting. This approach has been applied successfully in both the Netherlands and Canada.

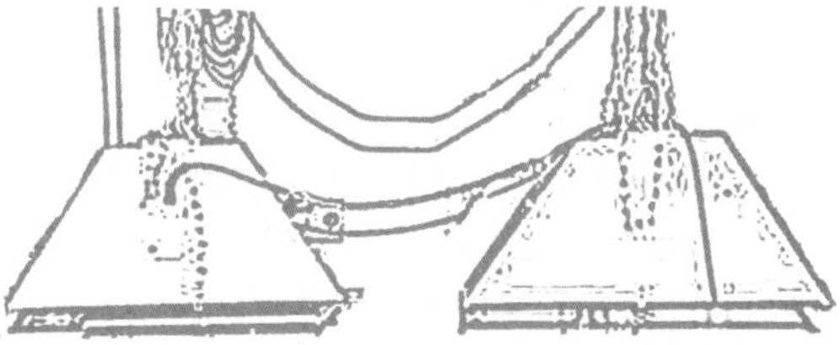

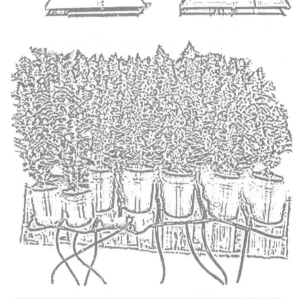

Indoor Cultivation Indoor cultivation is driven principally by prohibition, since it is considerably more challenging to detect indoor agriculture, and far easier to spot outdoor or greenhouse grows. Growing cannabis indoors has become an

Indoor cultivation (above): It is difficult to estimate how much high-quality cannabis is produced indoors in the United States each year, but the number could exceed 1,500 tons. Greenhouse cultivation (below): It is believed that this cultivation method may be the future of cannabis flower cultivation, as it is for many types of flowers.

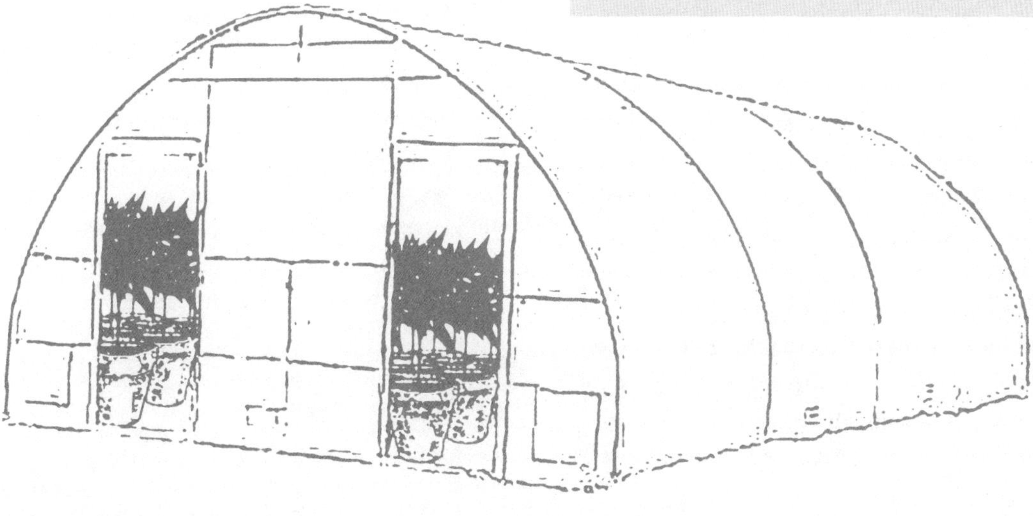

enormous clandestine industry. Hydroponics stores are found in every city in North America and Europe. Hundreds of cannabis-specific nutrient formulas are for sale in these shops. The primary advantage of indoor cultivation is that cannabis flowers and their resin-filled trichomes can be protected. Indoor cannabis cultivation is capable of producing the most pristine cannabis flowers, though not necessarily the finest. Conventional indoor horticultural lighting produces a limited spectrum of light that does not duplicate the wide spectrum produced by the sun. This spectral deficiency is believed to limit the number of chemical constituents that the plant can produce under artificial conditions. Recently, light-emitting diodes (LEDs) and plasma lamps have been introduced that may broaden the spectrum of indoor horticultural lighting for cannabis cultivation to better mimic sunlight. Additionally, these LED systems are more energy efficient.

Grading Cannabis Flowers Grading cannabis flowers is straightforward. First comes the aroma. High-quality cannabis will have a pungent aroma: it will rarely smell grassy or green, and at its best it will be a mix of fruit, spice, and unique to high-quality cannabis—a note of "skunk." While beer that smells like skunk has spoiled, cannabis with a similar aroma has not and is actually prized. The skunk aroma is associated with wide-leafleted *indica* cannabis and hybrids of these varieties. Even fiber cannabis varieties, of medicinal interest for their CBD content, will have an interesting pungent and grassy smell. Cannabis that smells like a freshly cut lawn is not properly cured; cannabis with a faint aroma is old or has been exposed to heat that has evaporated its terpenes; cannabis with no aroma can be quite potent, since cannabinoids have no smell—but once the terpenes are gone, so is their synergistic

Blending Cannabis Strains—Improving on Nature

Combining two or more cannabis varieties can create interesting blends, and this can broaden the available range of medicinal and psychoactive effects over that of a single cannabis variety. Prohibition has resulted in a reduction of cannabis diversity since it favors cannabis varieties suitable for indoor cultivation, which flower quickly and stay squat. Some of these small indoor plants retain chemical compositions from their larger, tropical cannabis ancestors. Narrow-leafleted varieties can produce significant amounts of terpinolene, a citrusy terpene, while wide-leafleted varieties can produce ocimene. By combining high terpinolene and ocimene varieties, the resulting blend has medicinal characteristics from both varieties, but can deliver synergistic terpene/cannabinoid effects that neither strain would produce on its own. This blending approach can effectively produce a chemotype of cannabis that is not found in nature.

To prepare a blend requires two or three oily, well-cured varieties of dried flowers. For precision formulation, laboratory analysis can provide guidelines for blending. Prior to combining, blends can be coarsely ground using a hand or spice grinder, but care should be taken to avoid overprocessing them. Although grinding cannabis can accelerate spoilage, ground blends of clean cannabis can be pressed into a small, airtight container and stored for up to a week in a cool, dark place.

A few cannabis varieties produce phenotypes that don't exude oil from the tips of their trichomes. These phenotypes carry a genetic defect that prevents them from producing functional secretory cells to exude cannabinoids and terpenes.

interplay with the cannabinoids. Cannabis with little aroma tends to have a generic, "one note" effect and is rarely of medical interest.

The second key to grading cannabis is visual inspection, for which you will need a 10–20× magnifying lens or loupe. Sunlight is the best light, since it exposes any discoloration. The plant material will range in color from deep to light green, with tinges of gold, yellow, and, more rarely, red. Some varieties of cannabis produce anthocyanin, a pigment that adds a purple or blue cast. Odd discoloration or browning can be a sign that the cannabis has spoiled.

Indicators of high-quality cannabis are trichome gland head size and density. They should be topped with tiny heads of cannabinoid and terpenoid oil secreted from specialized cells at the tip of the trichome. Look for large, intact trichome heads—the more of them, the better. These heads should be primarily clear, but a few of them should also be milky. Amber heads mean that the cannabis was likely harvested after maturity. Bright white tendrils on the sugar leaves, the tiny trichome-encrusted leaves surrounding the flowers, are typically a sign of powdery mildew, while gray fuzz is a symptom of gray bud mold. If possible, break a bud to inspect its interior for visible mold. Tapping a bud on a white sheet of paper can dislodge some other types of mold spores onto the paper, so that they can be more easily detected. With a loupe, it should also be possible to detect a number of pest infestations,

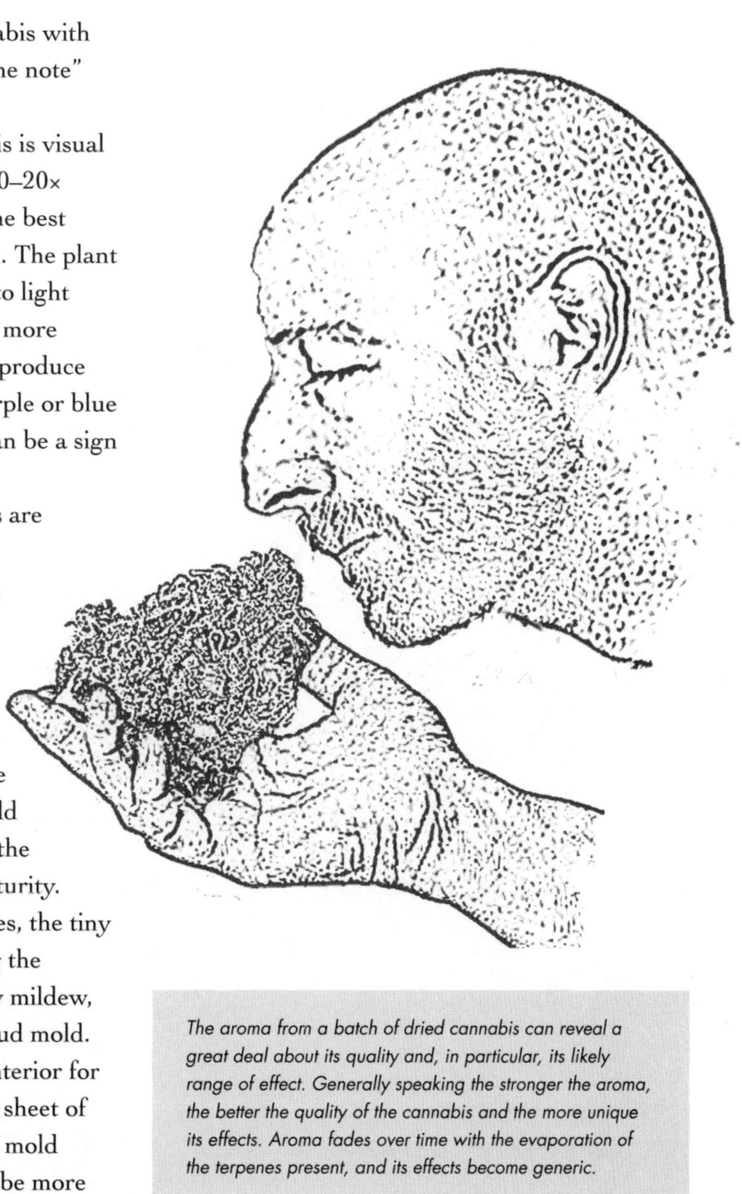

The aroma from a batch of dried cannabis can reveal a great deal about its quality and, in particular, its likely range of effect. Generally speaking the stronger the aroma, the better the quality of the cannabis and the more unique its effects. Aroma fades over time with the evaporation of the terpenes present, and its effects become generic.

since aphids, mites, and gnats are easily trapped by sticky trichome resin.

The third characteristic is the *feel* of the cannabis, which introduces the crucial concept of curing. Curing is the process of properly drying harvested cannabis so that chlorophyll, carotenoids, and other plant chemical constituents break down. This technique was developed with other plants, such as tobacco. The process of curing greatly improves the taste of cannabis when smoked. The key to successful curing is the concept of "low and slow." When cannabis is first harvested, the plant still contains a lot of residual water. The initial drying process should be relatively rapid with the goal to reduce the drying plant's water content below 15 percent. Once below 15 percent water weight, the cure begins, with the goal to reduce the water content to between 8 and 9 percent and maintaining as much essential oil content as possible. Certain varieties of cannabis, such as OG Kush, will benefit greatly from a month of slow cure. High-quality, well-cured cannabis is oily, but has a nice snap when crushed. The aroma of high-quality cannabis when crushed should be intense and rich.

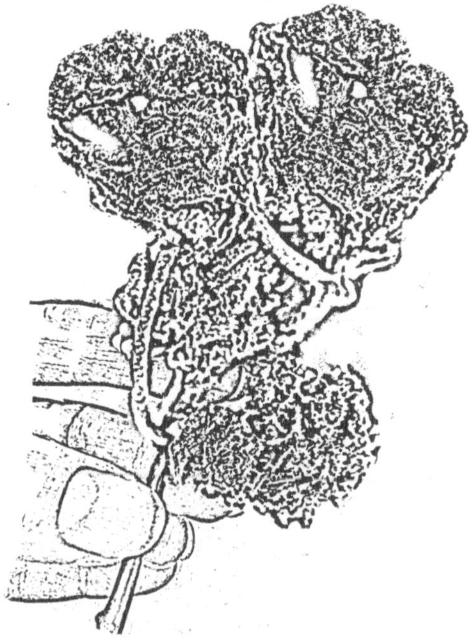

In correctly dried and cured cannabis, the smaller stems of the plant growing off the main stem—sometimes referred to as the "fishbone" stems—should break cleanly when snapped in two.

Visual inspection does not replace laboratory safety screening, but it can identify basic cultivation issues.

The fourth characteristic to detect is the taste of the smoke. The first inhalation should be floral and spicy, with no bitter or chemical aftertaste. A funny aftertaste is usually a sign of residual nutrients. High-quality cannabis flowers are flushed of those nutrients before harvest. An expert trick for judging the flavor of cannabis smoke is to pack enough cannabis into a clean glass pipe for two inhalations. Take one inhalation, exhale, and see how long the floral taste lingers. Fine-quality cannabis smoke remains on the palate for over 15 minutes. But the key to outstanding quality cannabis flowers is whether the second inhalation approximates the first in its floral character. Most mid-grade cannabis tastes burned on the second inhalation.

Vaporization can also be used to gauge herbal cannabis quality. The vapor of dried cannabis flowers should be expansive and extremely floral, with no trace of harshness or "chemmy" aftertaste.

Laboratory analysis for terpenoid and cannabinoid content is the final step in gauging cannabis quality. It's very useful to compare lab results of the variety being graded with direct observation and experience.

Wisdom and Nonsense from the Cannabis Underground

The marijuana underground is full of opinions on what constitutes high- or low-quality cannabis. In the 1970s, before laboratory testing was available to cannabis cultivators, one common rule of thumb was that a peppery aroma was an indicator of high-potency cannabis. Legendary varieties such as the Punta Roja from Colombia and Panama Red both smelled strongly of pepper. Today, we know that the smell of pepper is actually associated with the presence of beta-caryophyllene, the primary constituent of black pepper oil.

During the Vietnam War, it was commonly believed that Thai Stick, cannabis flowers from Southeast Asia that were tied to a short bamboo stick with lengths of fiber, were commonly dipped in opium, which explained the potency of Thai Stick effects. While some Thai marijuana could have been sprayed with byproducts of local opium or heroin production within the Golden Triangle of Thailand, Burma, and Laos, it is much more likely that those exposed to high-potency Thai cannabis thought it had to be adulterated, when the reality was that Thai cannabis was just stronger than anything that these users had ever previously experienced. Tropical narrow-leafleted cannabis is extremely psychoactive, and often five to 10 times more potent than commercial Mexican cannabis, which was the most widely available cannabis in the U.S. during the Vietnam War. A variant of the same myth extended to black hash, which sometimes had a white layer inside that was claimed to be opium. The reality was that this white substance was mold that grows in poor-quality, hand-rubbed hashish. Opium does not burn like hashish and is rarely combined with it.

Where the underground got it right was in its descriptions of high-quality cannabis. High trichome density was described as "a lot of crystals," which is an excellent indication of high-quality cannabis. Other descriptors that became associated with high-quality cannabis such as "piney," "citrus," and "mango" turned out to be descriptive of pinene, limonene or terpinolene, and myrcene, respectively (see pages 47–49). And these descriptions predate by decades the use of headspace analysis to confirm the presence of these terpenes.

Hashish and *Kif*—Dry and Water Extractions

The highest-quality hashish can reach 55 percent THC by dry weight. Many countries that have traditionally cultivated cannabis varieties on a large scale, as in Lebanon and Morocco, produce extractions from their cannabis harvests, rather than using the plant's dried flowers. These extractions are used to concentrate cannabinoids and terpenes from field crops of lower-potency cannabis varieties—producing very strong hashish. The future of herbal cannabis in Western countries will likely shift from dried flowers toward these extractions. The advantage of well-produced cannabis extractions is in their pure, rich taste when smoked or vaporized. But according to Robert Connell Clarke in his book *Hashish*,[1] few people have ever sampled world-class cannabis extractions since they are very difficult to produce. In many traditional hashish-producing regions, fields of different cannabis varieties are bulked together and extracted into hashish. With the advent of indoor cultivation, small-scale hashish production has focused on hashish that is extracted from an individual cannabis variety. These varietal extractions concentrate the individual attributes of the cannabis chemotype used. The varieties can also be blended to produce a wider range of effects, similar to blends made from dried and ground cannabis flowers. All hashish must be produced under sanitary conditions and carefully stored to reduce the risk of mold and spoilage.

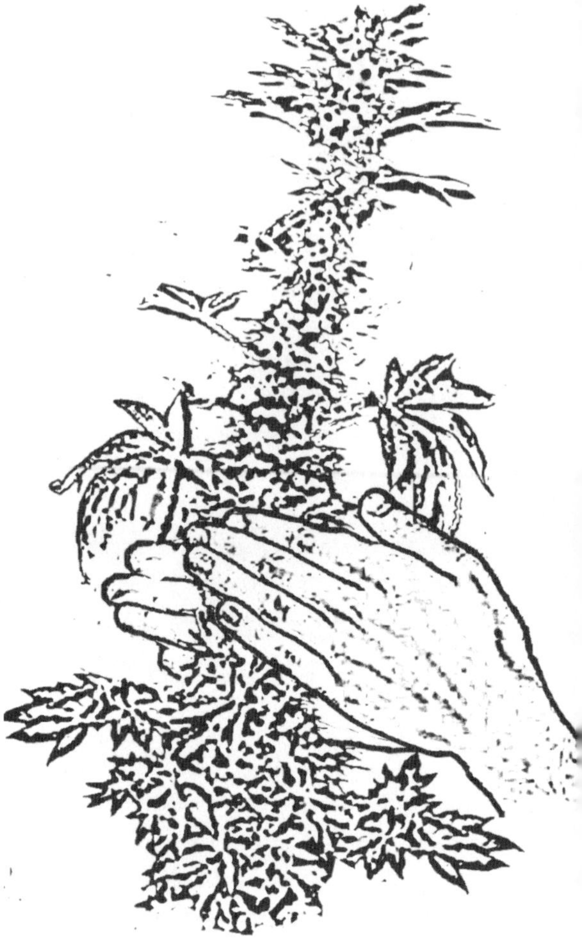

In Nepal and India, the flowering tops of cannabis plants are rubbed between the palms of the hands in order to collect their resin. The process creates friction and even a little heat, making the resin stick to the palms. The resin is then rolled and scraped from the palms into balls of fragrant hashish.

Rubbed Hashish Typically, cannabis grown in humid climes will never get dry enough to make sieved hash. Humid regions, such as India and Nepal, produce small-scale cannabis extractions by rubbing cannabis plants by hand, so that its resin sticks to the palms. While dry-sifted hashish is made in the West, hand-rubbed hashish is not, chiefly because fewer people are willing to toughen their hands so that resin can be scraped from their palms after rubbing.

Rubbing the ripe, flowering tops of live cannabis plants quickly coats one's palms in resin. In India, this rubbing technique produced the first concentrated cannabis, called *charas*. In the Himalayan foothills of India and Nepal, rubbed *charas* is formed into Manali and Nepalese Temple Ball hashish. In the West, trimmers manicuring cannabis flowers collect resin as it accumulates on trimming tools and fingers to make a form of rubbed hashish called scissor hash.

According to Clarke, the finest-sieved hashish was said to be the "bat-pressed" Primo hashish produced in Afghanistan in the early 1970s.[2] *This hashish was made from the finest resin powder compressed by pounding the resin with cricket bats.*

Sieved Hashish Very dry cannabis flowers can be sieved through a fine mesh to collect cannabis resin powder, which in Kashmir is called *garda* or *gurda*. The mesh size is selected to let cannabis trichome gland heads pass through the mesh, while leaving the stalks and plant material behind. These gland heads make up the bulk of high-quality cannabis resin powder. Sieving is best accomplished in cold, dry climates, therefore sieved hashish is produced in the high valleys of Pakistan, Afghanistan, Lebanon, and Morocco. Sieving is a superior method for making hashish because it keeps cannabis gland heads intact and prevents their cannabinoid and terpenoid contents from oxidizing or evaporating. Once the resin powder (*kif*) is collected, it is typically warmed very gently and immediately pressed into blocks of hashish. Most hashish connoisseurs consider the finest-sieved hashish to be the ultimate form of cannabis.

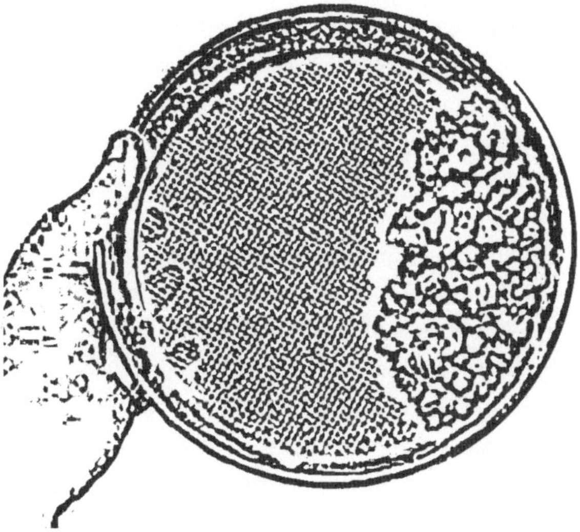

For the best results, the cannabis plants must be very dry before sieving. They are crushed first, and the main stems and thicker stalks removed. Each batch can be sieved and re-sieved dozens of times to produce the finest-quality resin powder. The ideal resin powder contains only trichome resin heads.

Water and Ice Hashish In the 1970s, a technique emerged that used cold water and/or ice to help extract gland heads and resin from cannabis. Dried cannabis was submerged in very cold water, which made the trichome stalks and resin heads become brittle. When the water/cannabis mixture was agitated, the trichomes and gland heads separated and could be sieved from the liquid through nylon mesh bags. The resulting extraction is called water hash. Typically, the mesh bags used to make water hash have pores at a fixed size, between 60 and 150 microns. Depending on the variety of cannabis, the optimal mesh size will vary. After extraction, water hash must be dried gently but thoroughly to avoid mold growth. Water hash can be pressed for storage, but must never be pressed while residual water remains, or else the extraction will quickly spoil. The drawback to water hash extraction is that brittle gland heads can rupture during the agitation process, releasing the lighter monoterpenes into the water. These terpenes form a slick on the water and can rarely be recovered. Only the coldest extractions with minimal agitation can protect these terpenes from being lost.

Bubbles and Melts Arguably, the highest grade of hashish is pure gland heads without any trichome stalks or plant material. This grade of hashish is typically achieved by obsessively sieving and re-sieving dry resin powder, but in such miniscule quantities as to be extraordinarily difficult to obtain. G. W. Guy, founder of GW Pharmaceuticals, refers to this level of extraction as "100-meter hash," since it is such a remarkable product that it was always consumed within 100 meters (330 feet) of where it was produced.[3] Since pure gland heads are so rare, the highest grades of hashish available are categorized as bubble hash or full melt. Well-made, full-melt extractions consist of cannabis oil, plant wax, and trichome stalks, typically extracted using ice water and filtered through carefully selected meshes. While it is possible to extract water hash that consists solely of trichome heads and no stalks, from a practical standpoint this is extremely difficult.

When heated, full melts bubble. Some of the bubbling is likely due to decarboxylation, whereby the raw acidic cannabinoids release carbon dioxide bubbles as they are converted into their bioavailable neutral form. Full melt water hashish is perishable and should be kept away from light. Ideally it should be stored frozen, at 25°F (-4°C) until used.

Kif In the United States, *kif* typically refers to unpressed resin powder collected by sieving dried cannabis. In the Netherlands, this resin powder is called *polm*. *Kif* is often collected using a mechanical silk screen tumbling device. This technique was pioneered in the Netherlands and the first marketed device was called "the Pollinator." The dried cannabis is placed inside a 120- or 150-micron drum made of silk screen, then gently tumbled. The resin powder falls through the fine mesh and lands on a glass or metal sheet where it can be scraped up and collected. Like all dry-sieved products, *kif* can be rich in aromatic terpenes, but if left unpressed these terpenes will rapidly evaporate or oxidize.

Will the Use of Cannabis Flowers Become Quaint? Flower vs. Hashish Cultures

The scale of most indoor cannabis cultivation in the United States is too small to support any large-scale production of hashish. But as the legalization and thus regulation of cannabis spreads throughout the United States, the size of the areas of open cultivation will increase. With this increase, the manufacture of cannabis extractions such as hashish will likewise expand. High-tech methods will inevitably emerge for improving the harvesting of cannabis trichome gland heads, the purest form of hashish. And well-made extractions have a longer shelf life than dried cannabis flowers. Such extractions also have richer organoleptic qualities—in layman's speak, they taste and smell better. Among cannabis connoisseurs, hashish has always been considered the pinnacle of cannabis forms. It is likely that the United States will slowly witness an increase in the popularity of high-quality hashish as the medicinal form of choice, eventually surpassing dried flowers in popularity, if electronic hash oil pens don't ultimately overtake both in popularity.

Grading Hashish Until very recently, the opportunity to choose from multiple varieties or grades of hashish was rare, except at Dutch cannabis coffee shops. In the Netherlands, most hashish is graded by its country of origin and production method. In California, hashish is graded by whether the cannabis was produced indoors, in a glasshouse, or outdoors. In West Coast dispensaries, the rule is: the lighter the color and the more aromatic the odor, the better the hashish. Water hashish technique has become very advanced in the medical cannabis community, with the result that high-quality hashish is readily available. Great hashish, whether it is made by dry sieving or water extraction, should smell like the variety from which is it was extracted, albeit less "grassy."

Solvent Extractions—Oils, Butters, Waxes

Since the first hash oils were made in Southern California in the early 1970s, they have been controversial. This controversy is primarily centered on the use of industrial solvents such as naphtha to accomplish the extraction. More recently, butane gas has become the most commonly used solvent to extract cannabis oil. The use of flammable solvents to make cannabis extractions will occasionally produce accidental explosions that have injured people. Thus, solvent extraction of cannabis is controversial in the United States. While solvent extraction may produce cannabis medicines of the greatest concentration and highest potency, the use of such solvents involves manufacturing methods whose processes can seriously injure or even kill. While many solvents, such as butane, are extremely flammable, other solvents, such as liquid carbon dioxide, pose asphyxiation risks, as well as the attendant dangers of working with compressed gas. A few solvents, including hexane, are toxic. Making these extractions is a risky proposition and the courts in California have declared that the solvent extraction of cannabis remains an illegal form of drug manufacture, even when the extraction is intended for medicinal use under California law.

Solvent extraction of cannabis was the method used in Afghanistan in the 1970s to make the first hashish oil. This crude hash oil was on occasion refined to make even more concentrated red oil. When California passed its medical cannabis laws in the mid-1990s, the first dispensaries began to stock hash oils. They remained a niche product until 2010, when the advent of tools designed to efficiently vaporize these oils and other solvent extractions launched the "dabbing" movement. On some levels, these ultra-concentrated cannabis extractions remain somewhat unrefined when compared with traditional extraction methods. Laboratory testing of solvent-extracted cannabis concentrates with highly sensitive "electronic nose" headspace analyzers typically detects solvent residues in these extractions.

Supercritical Carbon Dioxide (CO_2) Extraction Supercritical carbon dioxide extraction involves pumping highly pressurized liquid CO_2 though cannabis. The extract is separated from the CO_2, and the CO_2 is recovered and passed back though the cannabis several times until the extraction process is complete. The pressure and temperature of the gas can be manipulated to change its behavior as a solvent. The drawback to high-pressure CO_2 extraction is that the pressures and temperatures involved can break delicate molecular bonds that influence medical cannabis efficacy. The biggest advantage of CO_2 extraction is that it leaves no harmful residues in the resulting product. If performed by experts, CO_2 extraction can produce extremely high-quality cannabis extractions.

Butane and Hydrocarbon Extractions
Butane honey oil (BHO) has become highly controversial in recent years, because of explosions resulting from its illicit, unregulated manufacture, some of which have caused injury to workers. When made in professional, closed-loop solvent extraction systems, butane extraction is a safe and perfectly clean method for extracting medicine from botanicals, including cannabis. Butane is a relatively nontoxic gas, although it is difficult to completely remove it from cannabis extractions. Along with cannabinoids and terpenes, butane also extracts plant fats, which can rapidly oxidize and turn the extraction rancid.

Other hydrocarbons can be used for cannabis extractions. Hexane is very effective at extracting cannabinoids, but hexane residues are neurotoxic. Because of its toxicity, hexane is rarely used for cannabis extractions, except at professional labs possessing the equipment required to remove its residues. Propane and pentane are occasionally used for extracting cannabis oil because they are inexpensive solvents, but are extremely flammable and pose significant risk of injury if mishandled.

Rick Simpson Oil or Phoenix Tears Rick Simpson, a Canadian medical cannabis patient, promotes a solvent extraction method that produces an oil he calls "Phoenix Tears." Simpson reports that his Phoenix Tears cannabis extraction has cured the cancers of many people. His claims are anecdotal evidence and generalizing them to all forms of cancer is unwise. Although cannabinoids are being investigated for their antitumor activity in many cancers, there is little clinical evidence to support Simpson's broad claims. There are anecdotal reports that Phoenix Tears may help for some cancers, but the mechanism needs to be better understood. Simpson's approach primarily uses light naphtha as a solvent, which is often used as paint thinner. Light naphtha is excellent for extracting cannabis, but difficult to purge from the finished extraction. Simpson claims that the healing power of his oil can overcome the risk of solvent residue exposure. Anyone considering Simpson's approach would be advised to purge all solvent and seek confirmation of the resulting oil's purity from a reputable lab.

"Solventless" Extracts In 2012, a new class of extractions became available in California, which are produced without solvents in a high-pressure chamber. They look like butane honey oil or wax, but laboratory testing has shown them to be free of any trace of solvent residue. The extracts remain highly perishable and should be refrigerated or frozen until required for use.

Solvent extraction of cannabis does not have to be dangerous, but to be safe requires professional equipment and training.

Grading Solvent-Type Extracts Grading any of these extracts without recourse to laboratory analysis is not advised. Any ultra-concentrate should be tested to ensure that it contains no solvent residues. Since these types of extractions can also extract and concentrate pesticides and mold toxins, it is recommended to put them through a complete laboratory safety screening. Most importantly, with regard to solvent extractions: don't attempt to make your own. This is not extraction chemistry that should be done at home or in the backyard.

Synthetics & Pharmaceuticals

Marinol Marinol is the brand name for dronabinol, a synthetic THC prescription medicine which was the first FDA-approved cannabinoid available in the United States. Marinol is chemically identical to the THC produced by cannabis, although it is synthesized in a laboratory rather than extracted from the plant. The THC in Marinol is dissolved in sesame oil within a gelatin capsule. Marinol is typically prescribed for intractable nausea from chemotherapy and also to treat weight loss (cachexia) in HIV/AIDS patients. Because Marinol contains only THC, at higher doses it can produce a range of adverse effects, including rapid heartbeat, memory problems, anxiety, and panic attacks. Many patients who have used both herbal cannabis and Marinol claim that herbal cannabis produces fewer and milder adverse effects. Marinol is now available in the U.S. in generic form, in 2.5-, 5-, and 10-milligram dosages.

Sativex Unlike Marinol, Sativex is a pharmaceutical cannabinoid medicine that is extracted from whole cannabis plants. The medicine is formulated as an oromucosal spray; that is, it is designed to be squirted beneath the tongue or on the inside of the cheek. It is prepared with almost equal amounts of THC and CBD, and patients report that it produces fewer adverse effects than Marinol.

Sativex is approved in many European countries, Canada, and New Zealand, and it is currently undergoing trials for approval in the United States. It is used to treat spasticity due to multiple sclerosis, as well as neuropathic and cancer pain. Sativex is produced by GW Pharmaceuticals, a company founded in 1998 that

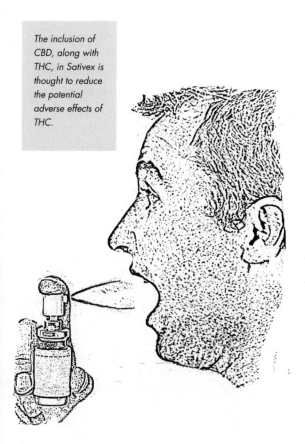

The inclusion of CBD, along with THC, in Sativex is thought to reduce the potential adverse effects of THC.

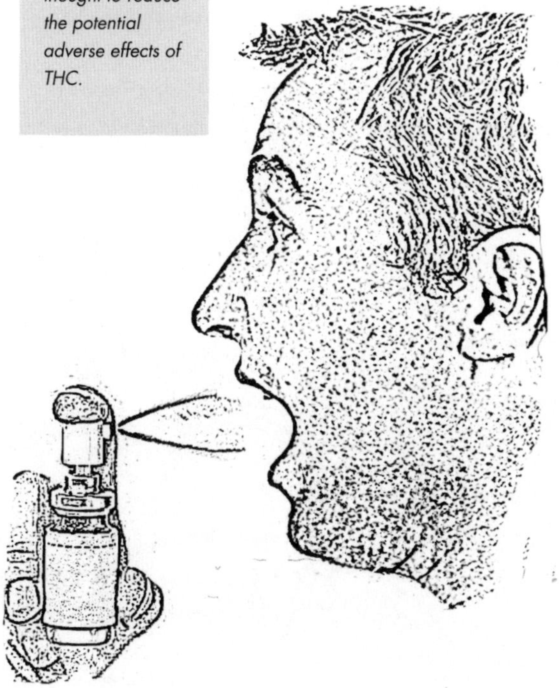

Why Marinol Is Not Cannabis

Marinol is the synthetic form of THC, a single constituent in herbal cannabis. Marinol represents the "single drug/single target" approach to drug design that is optimized for the FDA drug approval process. Drug designers moved away from combination multidrug therapies in the 1980s toward this approach. The single drug/single target tactic sidesteps the problem of figuring out the complex mixtures and interactions of whole plant medicines such as cannabis. Herbal cannabis has multiple active ingredients, which interact with numerous targets throughout the body. Recently though, more researchers have called for studies of multi-target drugs in cancer and metabolic disease therapies because of the network of processes that underlie these diseases.

Terpenes found in herbal cannabis can reduce some of THC's side effects (see pages 34–38). Some parts of the world that use cannabis medicinally—for example, India—produce cannabis that contains significant amounts of both THC and CBD. In addition to reducing the side effects of THC, CBD minimizes the buildup of THC tolerance. Studies by clinicians working with both herbal cannabis and Marinol report that herbal cannabis produces fewer side effects in patients. And when vaporized, the herbal cannabis dose can be easier to achieve than when using orally administered Marinol.

has spent 16 years researching cannabinoid medicines. GW Pharma produces Sativex by extracting proprietary cannabis varieties—a high-THC variety and a high-CBD variety—with liquid CO_2, then formulates these two extracts into Sativex. One spray of Sativex delivers 2.7 milligrams of THC and 2.5 milligrams of CBD.

Nabilone Sold in the U.S. under the brand name Cesamet, nabilone is a synthetic cannabinoid used to prevent vomiting and provide pain relief. As a Schedule II drug (per the U.S. Controlled Substances Act), its use is severely restricted in the United States.

Rimonabant Rimonabant was a synthetic cannabinoid pharmaceutical that was developed as a treatment for obesity. It was the first drug to be released that blocked the activity of a cannabinoid receptor. At one point, rimonabant was available as a diet drug in over 50 countries. Studies started to link the drug with instances of acute depression and suicidal thoughts, and it was withdrawn from the market in 2009.

Future Forms of Cannabis Medicine

Most varieties of cannabis currently available are high in THC, with a few terpenes and not much else. Cannabis can produce dozens of different cannabinoids, and the medical use of cannabis is inspiring the search for alternatives to THC. Cannabis varieties containing cannabinoids such as CBD are now becoming available, with THCV, CBDV, CBC, and CBG varieties expected to become increasingly accessible over time.

Sieved cannabis concentrates have been around since the nineteenth century, but more recently high-tech innovations—such as ultrasonic transducers and stacked graduated sieves—have emerged to increase the efficacy of the process. Soon hashish of the legendary "100-meter" quality should become more accessible.

Currently, ultra-concentrated cannabis is both dangerous to make and difficult to dose. As cannabis prohibition relaxes, higher-quality extractions, without any solvent residue, will be developed to match the complex chemistry found in the best cannabis varieties.

Topical and transdermal delivery methods may deliver the true future of cannabis medicines. Innovative techniques that enable cannabinoids and terpenoids to be absorbed through the skin more rapidly could revolutionize the ways in which cannabis is used to treat a wide range of conditions, from headaches to cancers.

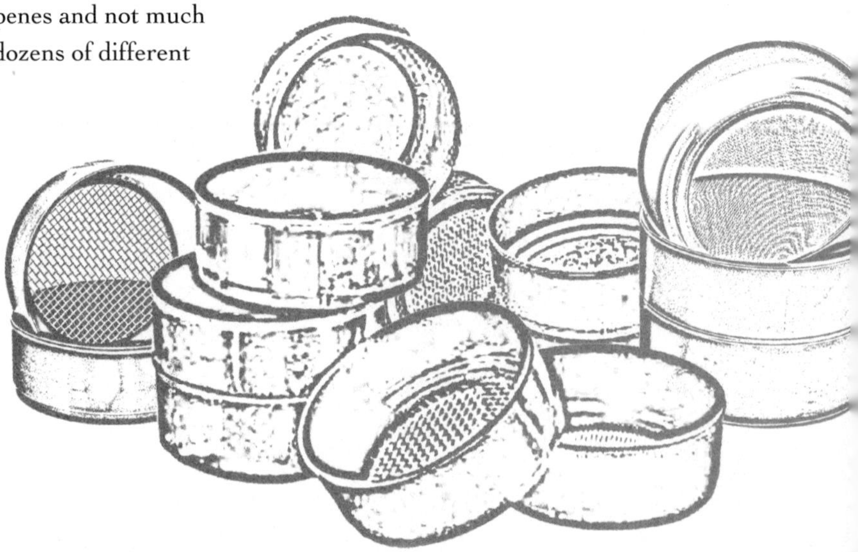

Palm-sized stacked sieves, where each has a smaller mesh than the one above it. These sieve sets enable the collection of fine-grade hashish powders consisting primarily of resin glands.

DELIVERY AND DOSING

From the clay chillum pipes of Goa, India, to miniature electronic vaporizers, there are hundreds of choices for delivering cannabis into the body. The most appropriate medical approach is the one that provides the most precise dose, for the desired duration, in the appropriate form, with the fewest side effects. That is quite a range of challenges, which cannot be addressed easily. Each delivery method has its own advantages and drawbacks. For example, smoking delivers a very wide range of cannabis constituents to the bloodstream within seconds. Delivering a precise dose is easy for most patients to learn, but the principal drawback is that combustion produces toxins, and those toxins can injure delicate lung tissue.

Vaporizing and e-pens are recent approaches to delivering cannabis medicines, and avoid some of the issues of smoking by keeping the temperature of cannabis below the level at which it combusts. Vaporization converts the medicine into an inhalable vapor. Most patients who use vaporizers, however, don't understand that the different active ingredients in cannabis boil at different times during the process. The method is only truly effective if the patient can learn how the process works. Eating cannabis medicines predates smoking and vaporizing by thousands of years. Oral cannabis medicines deliver their effects for twice as long as their smoked or vaporized counterparts. Because ingested cannabis is transformed in the liver, oral cannabis medicines take longer to take effect, and the duration of those effects varies widely between individuals.

Smoking

Smoking is the most common method of delivering a dose of herbal cannabis. Smoking cannabis causes rapid elevation of THC levels in the bloodstream, which are measurable within five seconds of inhalation. Peak blood levels of cannabinoids are achieved within five to 10 minutes. Because of the rapid rate of delivery, patients can easily and quickly learn to control dose by smoking cannabis. Patients can learn to control their smoked dose by simply titrating the dose one inhalation at a time, then waiting a few minutes between each inhalation.

Smoking cannabis is the process of heating cannabis to combustion temperatures, then inhaling the solid and liquid particulates and gases that are created in the combustion process. While unheated cannabis contains over 700 different

Smoking cannabis will begin to decline in popularity as vaporization technology becomes more portable and efficient and its cost declines.

compounds, when cannabis is smoked those raw compounds are converted into the thousands of combustion compounds contained in cannabis smoke. While it may seem that the practice of cannabis smoking is ancient, it is likely a relatively recent practice, going back to the fifteenth-century European discovery and exploration of the New World (viz the Americas). Robert Clarke and Mark Merlin believe that smoking was introduced to Europe after Columbus's transatlantic voyage in 1492. The local Taino people of Cuba introduced Columbus's sailors to tobacco smoking. Cigars in Central America had been smoked since at least the ninth century CE. Some of Columbus's crew became addicted to tobacco and brought their habit back to the Old World. Tobacco smoking became a craze during the half century following Columbus's return. At first, smoking was such an unusual sight it was described as "fog drinking." Cannabis smoking is believed to have become popular only after the introduction of tobacco smoking.

While some researchers claim that there is archaeological evidence in Ethiopia for cannabis smoking in the thirteenth century (in the form of pipes containing cannabis residue), this claim remains disputed. By the mid-fifteenth century, cannabis resin (in the form of hashish) was being smoked in the Middle East, often mixed with tobacco, though occasionally not.

A Controversial Form of Delivery

The practice of smoking medicinal cannabis remains controversial because smoke contains noxious substances, some of which are linked to pulmonary disease and cancer in tobacco users. According to University of Mississippi research, cannabis smoke contains 1,500 different chemicals, including some known carcinogens. However research at UCLA, led by Donald Tashkin, found that long-term chronic smokers of cannabis did not have increased incidence of head, neck, or lung cancers. In this study, with no concomitant tobacco use, cannabis smokers had a lower incidence of these cancers than nonsmokers. A more recent population study among chronic cannabis smokers appears to show a higher incidence of one type of lung cancer among those that deeply inhale and hold cannabis smoke into their lungs. And while smoking cannabis appears to be linked to the tissue changes associated with emphysema, it does not appear to lead to the development of the disease.

Preparing Cannabis for Smoking

Cannabis should be chopped carefully for smoking. Breaking the cannabis up using the fingers removes too much resin from high-quality flowers, so scissors are recommended. The most extraordinary (and breathtakingly expensive) scissors for chopping cannabis are the small, solid-

A wide range of tools is used to deliver cannabis as a medicine. The key to using cannabis properly as a medicine is leveraging these tools to deliver a precise cannabis dose.

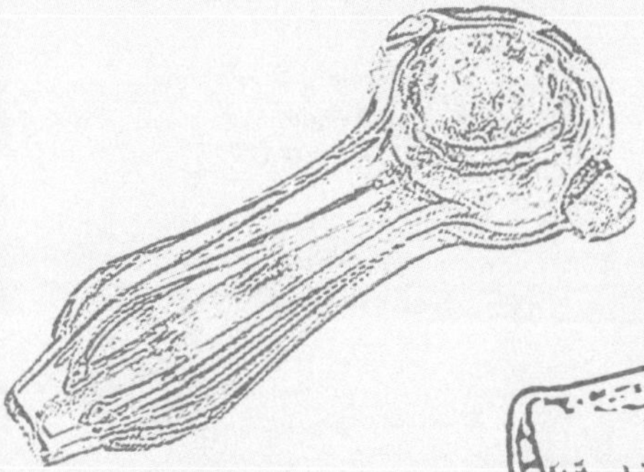

Spoon Pipe

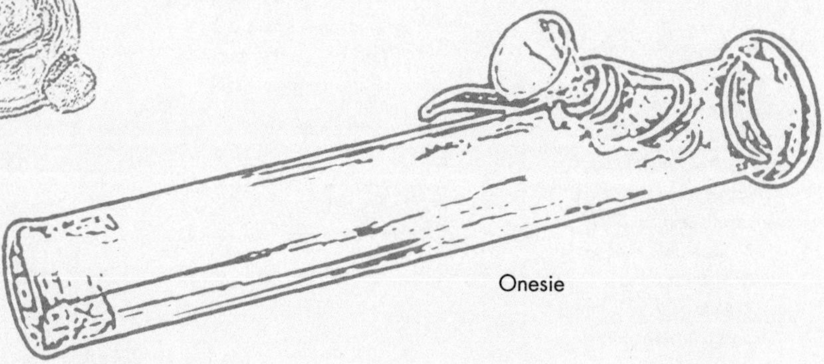

Onesie

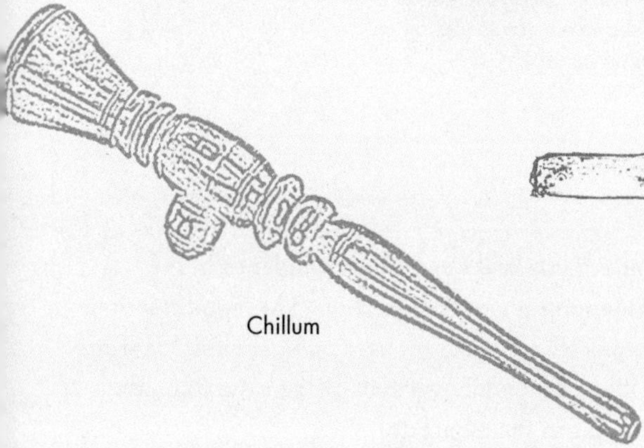

Chillum

Joint

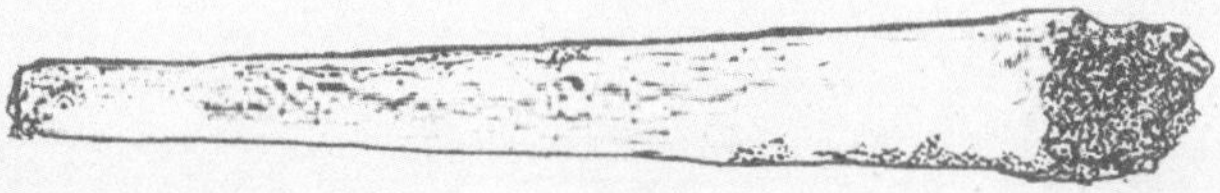

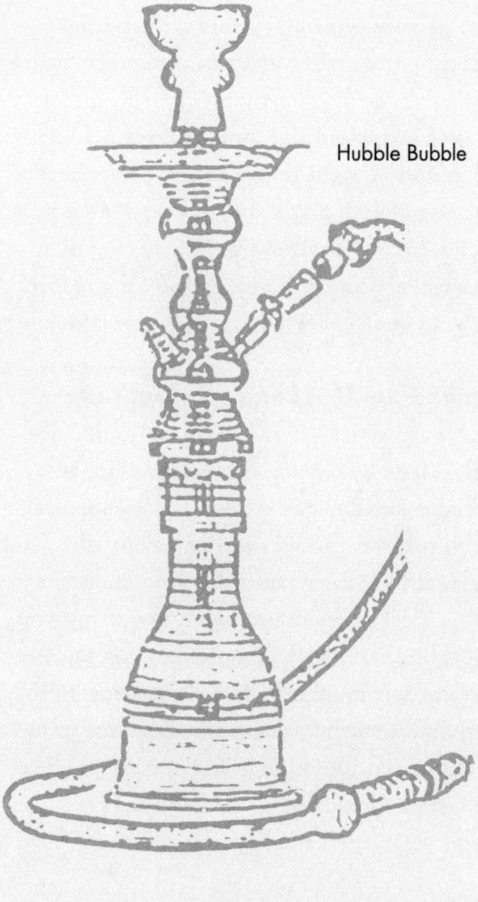

Hubble Bubble

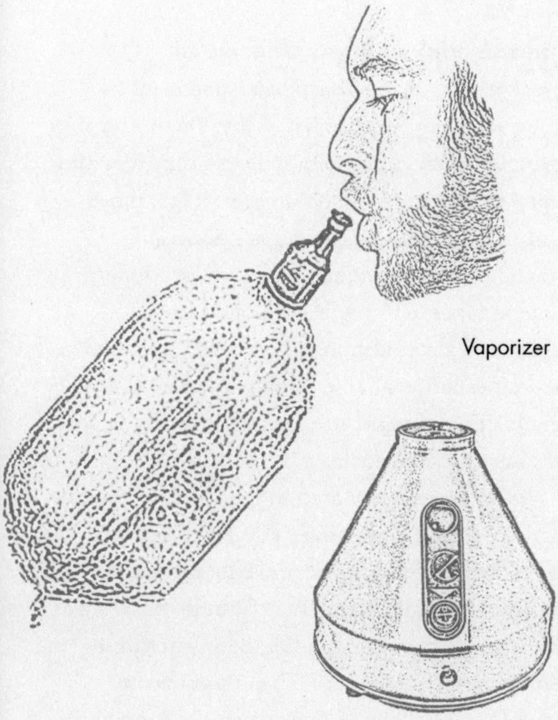

Vaporizer

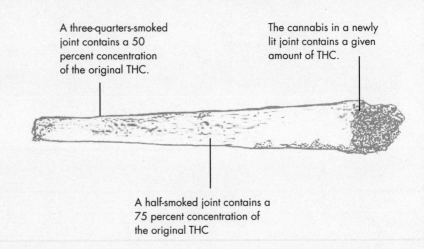

The potency of the cannabis in a joint increases as it is smoked, and as the cannabinoid-rich tars condense in the remaining portion of the joint. This makes dosage tricky when smoking a joint, since each inhalation is more potent than the last one.

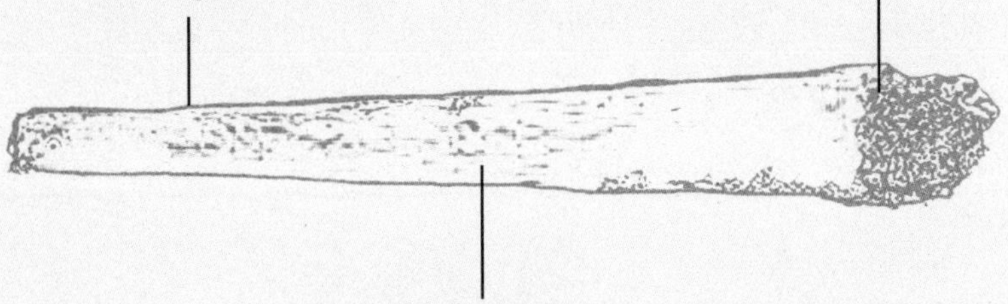

A three-quarters-smoked joint contains a 50 percent concentration of the original THC.
The cannabis in a newly lit joint contains a given amount of THC.
A half-smoked joint contains a 75 percent concentration of the original THC

steel Masakuni Type C bonsai trimming shears from Japan. Scissors should be cleaned regularly with 91 percent isopropyl alcohol, then dried.

If using scissors is too time-consuming, Space Case titanium grinders are a quick, high-quality alternative for preparing cannabis for smoking. Avoid grinder designs that separate and collect *kif* since it's always preferable to keep the *kif* in the grind. In any case, *kif* that is collected by a grinder will almost certainly dry out long before enough has been collected to make it worthwhile.

Joints and Spliffs—Cannabis Cigarettes Cannabis cigarettes—also known as "joints" and "spliffs"—have somewhat declined in popularity as cannabis potency has increased. Few medical cannabis patients can, or need to, smoke the entire length of a cigarette of high-potency cannabis. Because cannabis cigarettes require no additional tools beyond a flame, they can be very convenient as a multidose delivery system. In the United States, medical cannabis cigarettes rarely contain tobacco, although in Europe the practice remains widespread and is unhealthy. As a cannabis cigarette is smoked, the active ingredients will continually condense in the remaining unsmoked portion. This condensation means that the last quarter of a cannabis cigarette will contain well over half of the cannabinoids present in the cigarette.

Cannabis Pipes—From Onesies to Megabongs Cannabis pipes come in all shapes, sizes, and forms, from tiny "one-hitters" to enormous water pipes with multiple filtration and cooling stages. Depending on the design, pipes are often much more efficient for delivering cannabinoids than cannabis cigarettes. Modern cannabis pipes are chiefly fashioned from borosilicate glass, although metal, ceramic, and wood pipes are available. Some of the most exotic cannabis pipe designs use a water system to cool and filter the smoke.

Water pipes originated in the Gansu Province of northwestern China over 400 years ago, just after tobacco smoking was introduced to East Asia from the Silk Road. This Chinese design was subsequently simplified in bamboo water pipes used by country folk across Southeast Asia. Alfred Dunhill claimed that water pipes were

How to Roll a Cannabis Cigarette

Make your own medical cannabis cigarettes in four easy steps

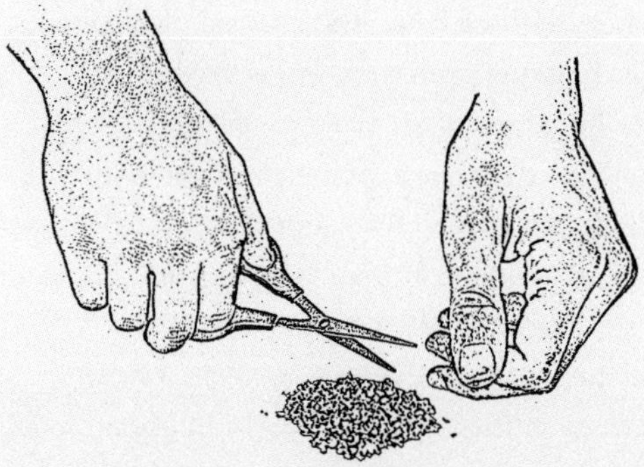

1 Finely chop half a gram of cannabis flowers for the cigarette. Take a gummed, regular rolling paper and cup it with the pad of your thumb, lengthwise along your index finger. Sprinkle the chopped cannabis evenly.

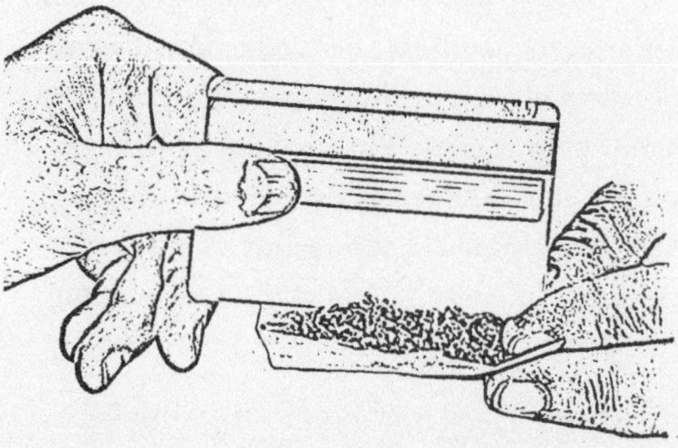

2 Slide a credit card between the cannabis and the rolling paper on the finger side. Press the cannabis against the card along the length of the cigarette through the paper with your thumb. This is to evenly distribute the cannabis in the cigarette.

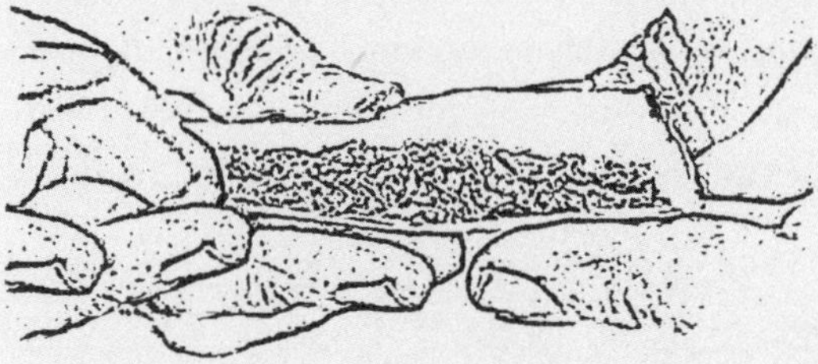

3 Remove the credit card, lick the gum on the paper, and roll the cigarette until it is sealed along its length. Pinch each end of the joint. Light one end, and then gently inhale from the other.

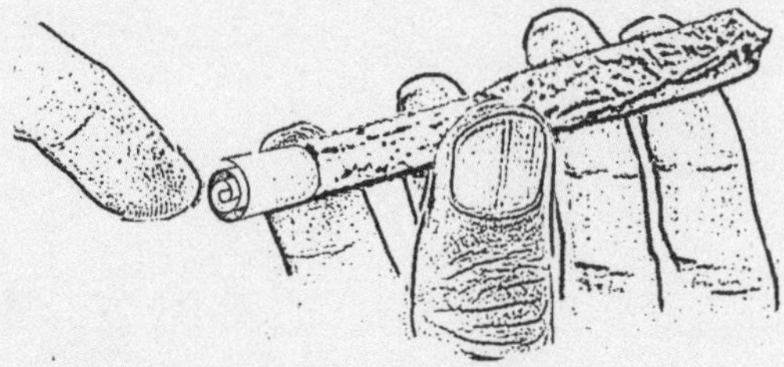

4 It is common to insert a bit of rolled card stock into one end of the cannabis cigarette, to serve as a mouthpiece. Expert rollers will often switch to ungummed Club brand papers.

actually invented in Africa by the San people, the earliest inhabitants of South Africa, before tobacco reached China.

Modern cannabis pipe design is epitomized by color-changing glass pipes. This movement is documented in the film *Degenerate Art: The Art and Culture of Glass Pipes*, which recounts how a hippie glassblower named Bob Snodgrass fumed silver metal onto a glass pipe, thus inventing glass that changed color as cannabis was smoked through the pipe. Snodgrass began selling color-changing pipes at Grateful Dead shows and an entire subculture of modern artistic glass-pipe-making was launched.

A small "spoon" pipe. Current trends have seen the emergence of all manner of glass designs that include sculptural, sometimes amorphous forms in a swirl of different colors and patterns. Many are real works of art.

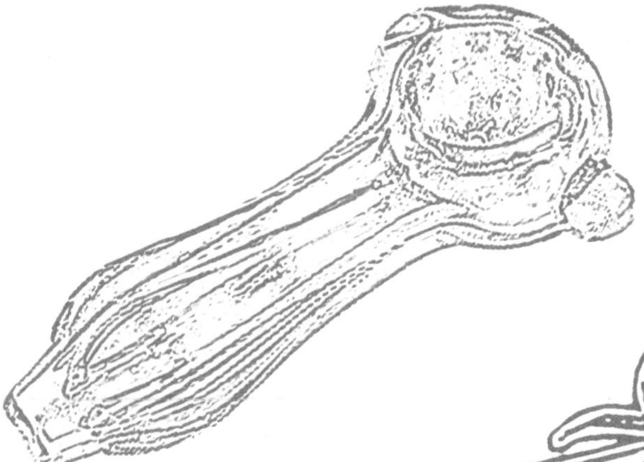

Today, glass pipes are categorized as art glass or scientific glass. Art glass pipes emphasize glassblowing techniques, colors and finishes, and sculptural form. Scientific glass pipes feature sophisticated functionality and form with their ash-catchers and intricate percolation designs. Many cannabis patients enjoy the aesthetic pleasure derived from using an art glass pipe. Other patients prefer the innovations that scientific glass pieces bring to smoked cannabinoid delivery. Some glass companies, such as Illadelph, combine art and scientific glass pipe design to produce extraordinarily complex water pipes featuring chilled condenser coils, sophisticated percolators (percs) that create hundreds of thousands of tiny bubbles and cool the smoke as it streams through the pipe's water reservoir, and exotic sculptural ornaments. Other companies such as RooR, Mobius, Salt, and Dave Goldstein continue to push the envelope of glass design.

The simplest glass pipe designs are one-hitters and spoons. One-hitters are intended to deliver a single inhalation of cannabis. These "onesies" are excellent for controlling dose, and highly recommended for novice patients who wish to smoke cannabis to treat their condition. Because onesies are available for as little as a few dollars,

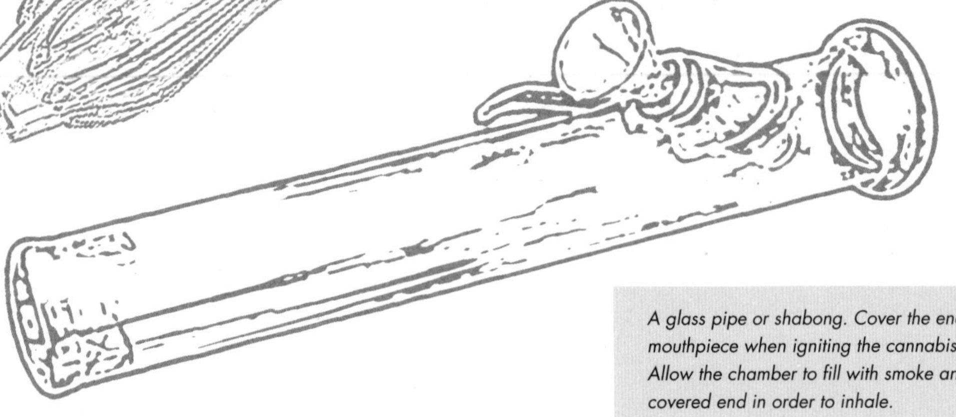

A glass pipe or shabong. Cover the end opposite the mouthpiece when igniting the cannabis in the bowl. Allow the chamber to fill with smoke and release the covered end in order to inhale.

they are also very cost-effective. Spoon pipes are the most common cannabis pipes. They are larger than onesies and because of the increased size do a better job of cooling cannabis smoke.

How to Light a Pipe Bowl Initially, use the flame to gradually heat the cannabis in the pipe, preferably from the edge of the bowl, until the lighter terpene molecules in the cannabis begin to vaporize. This technique results in the best-tasting, least-irritating inhalation. Take care to avoid igniting the cannabis, since if cannabis burns with a visible flame its terpenes are being burned off along with some of the cannabinoids. Oily cannabis flowers ignite quickly and it's important to tamp down any flame the instant it appears. Go slow. Quickly incinerating the bowl of cannabis with the flame destroys too many active ingredients. Cheap butane lighters tend to make smoked cannabis taste terrible. A more palatable alternative is a torch lighter designed for cigars, but torches burn so hot that incinerating the cannabis becomes more likely. Developing a light touch with a torch takes some practice. An alternative to using a flame can be provided with a ceramic soldering iron, like those used for working on electronics. The Hakko 15-watt N452 heats the cannabis to just under 700°F (371°C), which is low enough for it to vaporize, but not

Cleaning Pipes

Always keep glass pipes spotlessly clean. While there are many products available at smoke shops for cleaning glass pipes, a simple approach is kosher salt in 91 percent isopropyl alcohol. The salt will not dissolve in this alcohol, so it functions as a mild abrasive to remove accumulated tar. Alcohol is highly flammable, so exercise caution. With a small pipe or onesie, put enough alcohol and salt into a sealable plastic freezer bag to completely submerse the piece, add the pipe, then alternately soak and shake until the piece is clean. Use pipe cleaners to reach crevices beneath the pipe's bowl. Once the piece is sparkling clean, rinse the pipe thoroughly with warm water and leave to dry completely before using again.

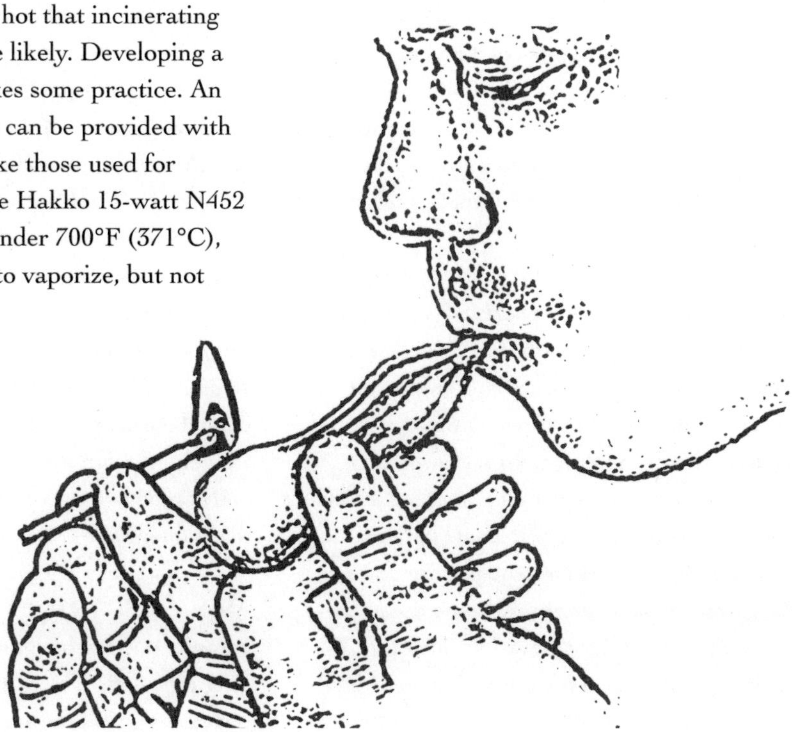

Lighting a spoon pipe. The trick is to heat the cannabis without actually igniting it.

burn, the cannabis. However, tools like the Hakko pose fire risks and caution must be strictly observed when using such a device.

Calculating a Smoked Dose of Cannabis
Different smoking techniques have varying efficiencies in delivering a dose of cannabis. One study conducted by Dale Gieringer, of nonprofit organization California NORML, indicated that a cannabis cigarette only delivered approximately 27 percent of its available THC. Glass pipes are more efficient. By carefully lighting a pipe and taking care not to incinerate the cannabis, efficiencies over 50 percent may be achieved. Begin with a match-head-sized dose, enough for a single inhalation. If a reliable laboratory has tested the potency of the cannabis, a smoked dose may be roughly calculated by the weight of the dose and the efficiency of the smoking method. One-thirtieth of a gram of cannabis containing 15 percent THC contains five milligrams of THC. In a glass pipe with 50 percent efficiency, this dose would deliver 2.5 milligrams of THC to the patient, which is the threshold at which most patients will feel the dose. Note that deeply inhaling and holding cannabis smoke in the lungs may prove harmful over time. Inhale, then quickly exhale cannabis smoke.

Smoking Cannabis Extractions Smoking concentrated cannabis extractions, such as hashish, can reduce exposure to combustion byproducts produced by burning plant material. The downside to smoking extractions is that dosage can be more challenging, making it easier to overmedicate, especially for new patients. It is especially useful to know the precise potency of an extraction in order to calculate dose. To prepare pressed, dry, or sieved hashish for smoking, gently warm the edge of the hashish with a lighter. This gentle heating will soften the resin and allow it to be fluffed back into its pre-pressed *kif*. Take a small amount of this fluffed resin powder and place it in a small glass bowl atop a steel or glass screen. Very gently light the edge of the powder, taking special care not to set it aflame. If the powder catches fire, immediately extinguish it. Ideally, the resin powder should smolder like incense, not burn like a log. Because hashish is considerably more potent than cannabis flowers, it is important to take a very small inhalation and thoroughly gauge its effect before smoking more.

Chillums, Hubble Bubbles, and Sebsis
Chillums are smoking devices designed for cannabis *charas*, the rubbed hashish popular in India and the Himalayas. Chillums and *charas* are associated with sadhus, holy men that follow the Hindu god Shiva. Chillums are usually made of fired clay, sometimes metal. Smoking a chillum is traditionally is a two-person job: one person holds and smokes the chillum, while the other person lights it. Chillums are never supposed to touch the mouth, so a wet piece of cloth is wrapped around the mouthpiece. This moist rag cools the smoke and prevents embers from being inhaled.

Hubble bubbles are the traditional Afghan water pipe used to smoke hashish. They deliver a prodigious amount of smoke and can pitch the unsuspecting person into paroxysms of coughing. Hubble bubbles and their Persian cousin the shisha (or hookah) are rarely used for medicinal cannabis since the dose is difficult to control. Porsche Design introduced a high-tech shisha water pipe at their outlet in Harrods, the London department store. Its price: £2,000 ($3,000)…

Sebsi pipes are the favored hashish pipe in Morocco. Sebsis feature a very small metal or ceramic bowl, which makes dosage easier, and a long pipestem. The metal bowl and long stem combine to cool the smoke.

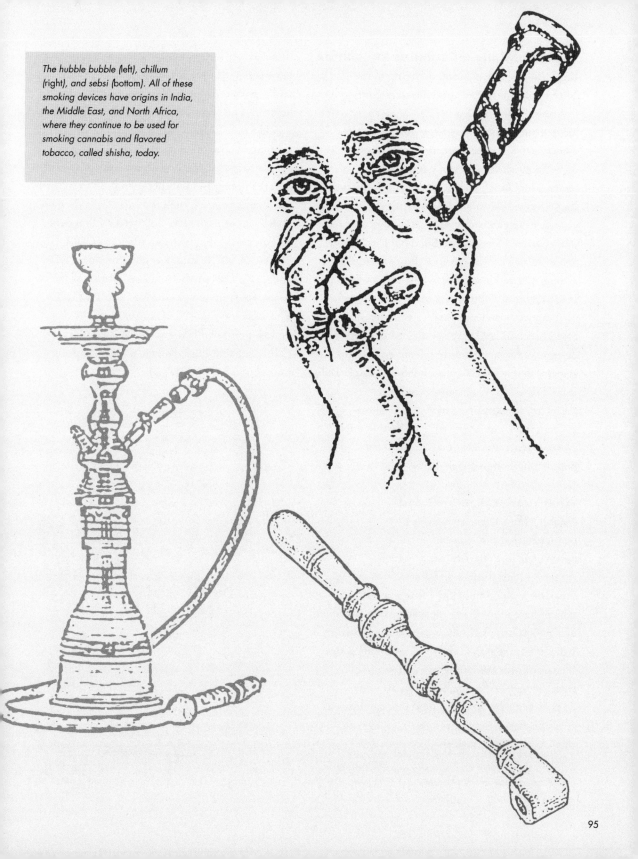

The hubble bubble (left), chillum (right), and sebsi (bottom). All of these smoking devices have origins in India, the Middle East, and North Africa, where they continue to be used for smoking cannabis and flavored tobacco, called shisha, today.

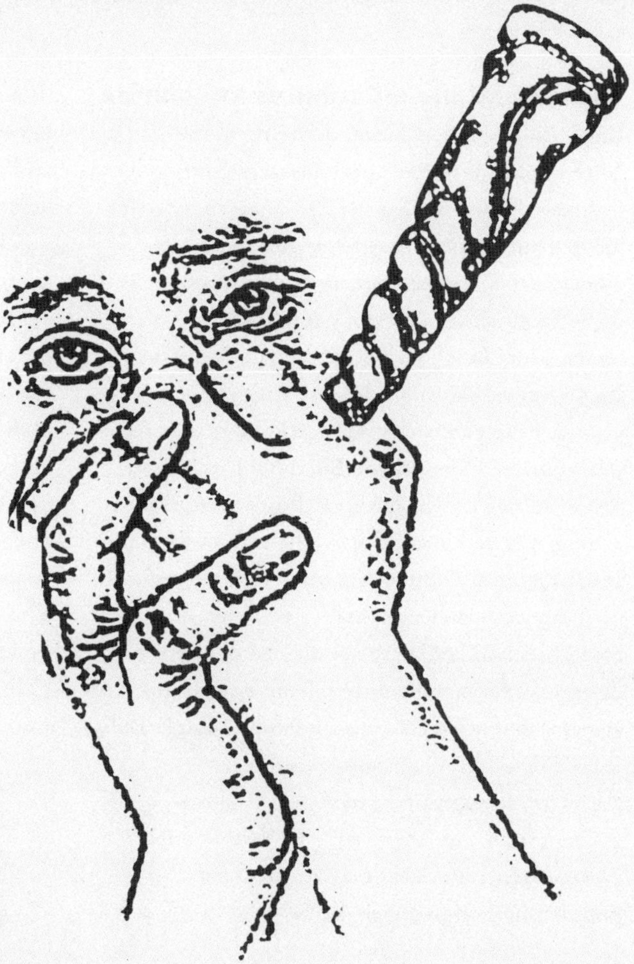

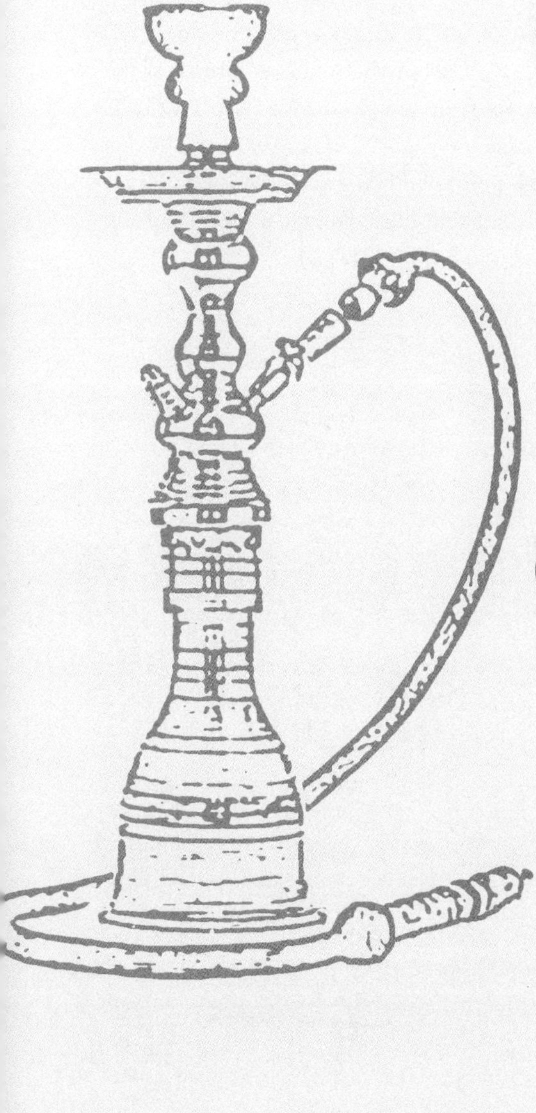

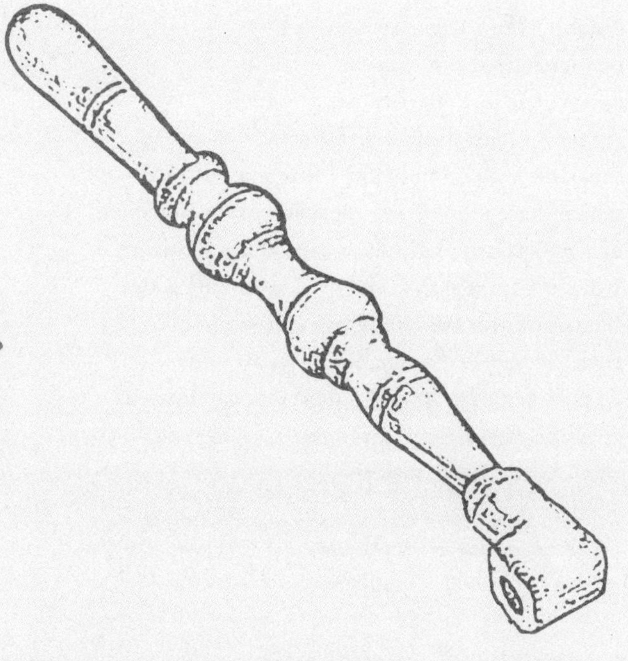

Vaping and the e-Cannabis Revolution

Eagle Bill, a Native American living in the Netherlands, invented cannabis vaporization in the early 1990s. A friend of Bill's had suggested using a hot-air paint-stripping gun to heat cannabis to a temperature at which the active ingredients would boil off, but below the temperature at which the cannabis combusts. Eagle Bill would catch the resulting vapor in a jar. His heat-gun magic was a trick that amazed everyone for whom Eagle Bill demonstrated it. The resulting cannabis vapor didn't taste like smoke; it tasted like flowers. The effects were like smoking cannabis, but they were also *different*.

Vaporization technology is evolving at a rapid pace. Today, there are dozens of vaporizer designs being manufactured, from hot-air gun systems that are direct descendants of Eagle Bill's first design, to tiny lithium-cell-powered e-cigarette designs used to vaporize ultra-concentrated cannabis hash oils. Within a few years, e-pen vaporizers may be the most popular method to ingest cannabis.

What Vaporization Does and Doesn't Do Vaporizers work by heating herbal cannabis or extractions to a temperature at which the active ingredients boil off and form an inhalable vapor, but below the temperature at which these ingredients approach precombustion or combustion. Typically, a cannabis vaporizer will not exceed 428°F (220°C), since this is the temperature at which the two cannabinoids with the highest boiling points, CBC and THCV, vaporize. When cannabis is combusted, thousands of compounds are formed including benzene, polycyclic aromatic hydrocarbons, and carbon monoxide. Vaporization delivers terpenes and cannabinoids to the bloodstream as quickly as smoking. With a minimum amount of training, a dose of medical cannabis vapor can be simple to gauge. Vaporization works in stages, in that the lighter monoterpenes boil off first, then the sesquiterpenes, then the cannabinoids such as alpha-pinene and THC, followed by limonene and myrcene, then the cannabinoids CBD and CBN, and finally the cannabinoids THCV and CBC. Carbon monoxide is formed at the precombustion temperature of 448°F (231°C). The issue for vaporizing (or "vaping") at the boiling point of THCV and CBC at 428°F (220°C) is that naphthalene, a toxin, boils off cannabis at 424°F (217°C).

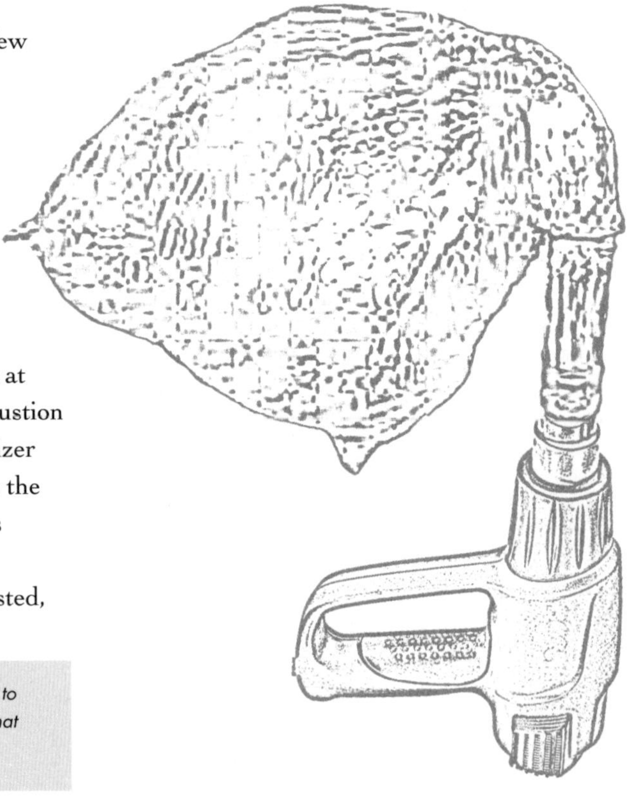

Eagle Bill's adaptation of a hot-air, paint-stripping gun to make the world's first cannabis vaporizer is a model that has been copied several times over.

The wide variation of boiling points in cannabis constituents means that precision temperature control is important. Arno Hazekamp of Leiden University in the Netherlands conducted a study for the manufacturers of the popular Volcano vaporizer. The purpose of the study was to learn the optimal temperature setting for vaporizing the cannabis variety Jack Herer. Hazekamp demonstrated that optimal extraction took place at 393°F (201°C), which is hot enough to boil off all of the terpenoids and cannabinoids except for CBC and THCV. Neither of these cannabinoids were available in common medical cannabis varieties when Hazekamp conducted his study.

Optimizing the Vaporization Process

The technique of using a vaporizer is straightforward: inhale, hold for three seconds, and then exhale. If the patient coughs, it is often a sign that the vaporizer's temperature setting is too high and the vapor is too rich. Because vaporization is incremental, it can take three or four inhalations to exhaust the cannabinoids and terpenoids from a single vaporizer load of ground cannabis. The cannabinoids have no taste when vaporized, but the floral terpenes which can be tasted are pharmacologically active.

Calculating Dose with a Vaporizer Studies conducted with the Volcano vaporizer indicate that the filling chamber should be loaded with one-quarter gram of cannabis. With 15 percent THC cannabis this is equal to 37.5 milligrams of THC. For the first four bags filled by the Volcano with this load, each contained just under six milligrams of THC in vapor, with the exception of balloon number 3, which peaked near seven milligrams. For a novice patient, this means that three-quarters of the first balloon would likely be a sufficient dose. If the patient were to inhale all four bags from a 250-milligram load of ground cannabis, the patient would receive a dose of nearly 22 milligrams of THC, which could result in unexpectedly strong psychoactivity.

Using a vaporizer: Hot air passes through dried cannabis flowers deposited in the filling chamber. As it does so, the bag attached to the filling chamber fills with vapor, ready to inhale.

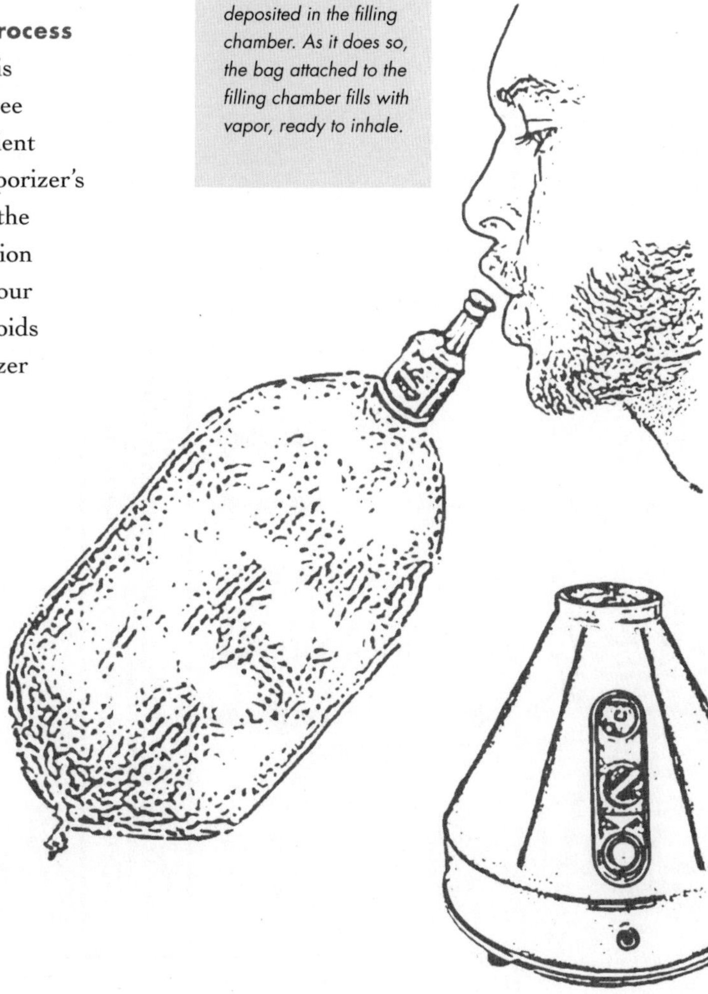

Types of Vaporizers The earliest vaporizers, such as Eagle Bill's, were based around industrial heat guns used for paint stripping, such as the Steinel Professional Heat Guns that feature LCD temperature displays with precise adjustment. The vaporizer setup included a glass bong fitted with a modified glass bowl wide enough for the air nozzle of the heat gun. The heat gun would be placed on the bowl, switched on, and the hot air would stream through the ground cannabis in the bowl until the boiling points were reached for the active ingredients. Although these heat gun vaporizer setups were precise, many of them required a lot of extraneous equipment and so were cumbersome.

Designers looked to develop vaporizers that were standalone with integrated heating elements. The next vaporizer style to become popular with patients was the "whip-style" vaporizer. A whip is a flexible tube with a glass bowl fitting to hold the ground cannabis. The fitting is loaded with cannabis and placed atop a heating element. The patient sucks hot air over the element, through the cannabis, and the resulting vapor is drawn into the tube and inhaled. Whip-type vaporizers start at around $100. Most whip vaporizers have analog temperature controls, so practice is required to use them efficiently. One advantage of whip vaporizers is that their mechanism is simple, so they tend to be reliable and long-lived devices.

Each of the cannabinoids and terpenoids present in cannabis has a different temperature at which it boils, with CBC and THCV needing 428°F (220°C).

The Boiling Points of Cannabinoids and Terpenoids

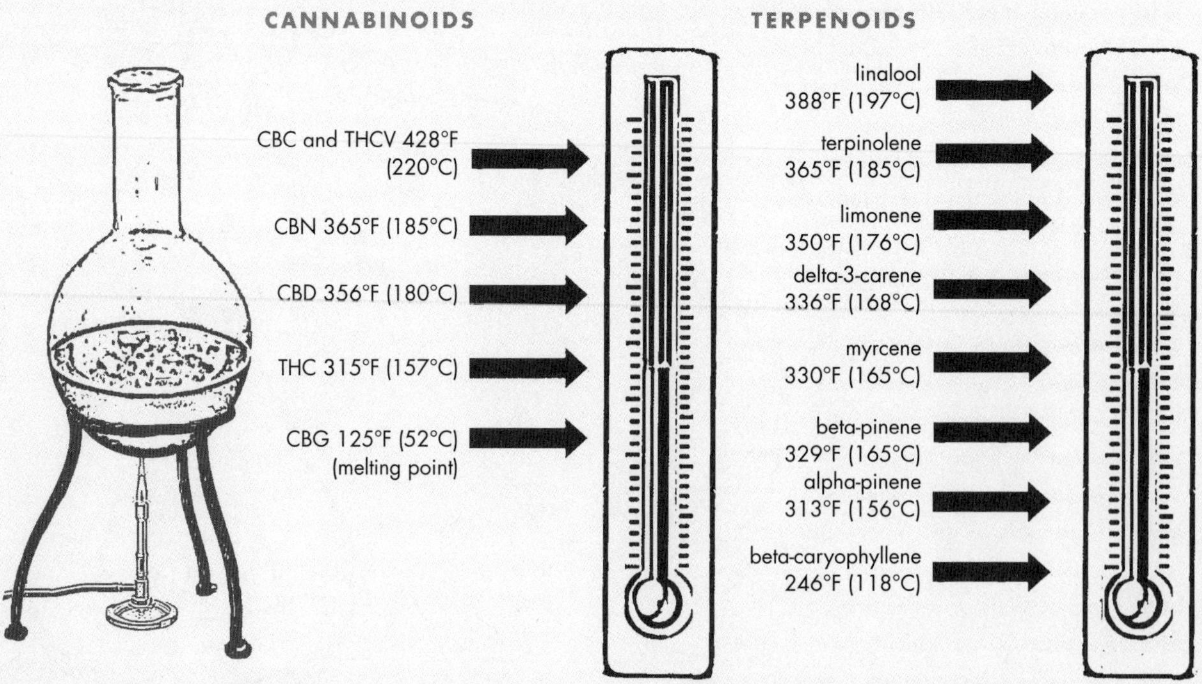

The Volcano Storz & Bickel, a medical equipment company in Tuttingen, Germany, was established in 2000 to develop the Volcano, a new vaporizer named after its conical shape. The Volcano was designed to fill a bag with cannabis vapor, which could then be detached from the unit and inhaled by the patient.

The Volcano is the best-studied vaporizer currently available. It has been used in clinical medical cannabis studies in Europe and the United States. The advantage to this research is that using the Volcano vaporizer with precision is quite well understood. The first Volcano model had an analog dial to adjust its heat output. The subsequent model, the Volcano Digit, featured an LED display that provided the selected temperature setting and the current heat output temperature. Recently, in Europe and Canada, Storz & Bickel have released a newer model, the Volcano Medic, which can vaporize herbal cannabis and also cannabinoid solutions. Such technology is not inexpensive, with the top-of-the-line Volcano Digit costing over $600.

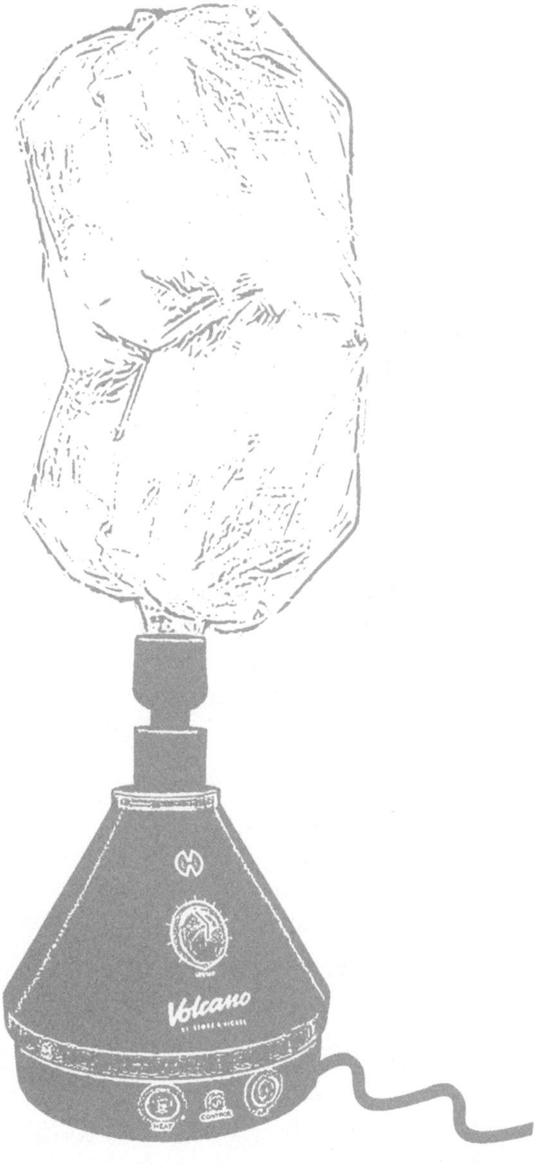

When using an analog Volcano vaporizer, the most robust vaporization of THC and CBD will occur when the device is set between 6 and 8.5 on the temperature dial.

Portable Vaporizers and e-Cannabis

Heating elements draw a considerable amount of electrical current, so first waves of vaporizer designs required AC power. In the past five years, lithium-ion batteries have enabled a range of portable vaporizer designs. Alternative portable vaporizers that use butane heating elements have been developed in Ireland by Iolite. The Iolite vaporizers were some of the first portable designs that could vaporize ground cannabis flowers. The latest trend in portable vaporizers for cannabis medicines has been adapted from the electronic cigarette market.

The idea for the electronic cigarette goes back to the mid-1960s, but the concept would not be commercialized for another 35 years. In 2003, a Chinese pharmacist patented a device that used ultrasound to create a mist of nicotine dissolved in a propellant that could be inhaled. The use of a propellant, usually propylene glycol, in e-cigarettes is controversial, since few studies have been conducted to examine whether inhaling this propellant is safe. The first cannabis e-cigarettes or e-pens delivered hashish oil suspended in a propylene glycol/glycerin carrier. More recent models of e-pens claim to be able to vaporize just hash oil. One advanced portable vaporizer, currently on the market in 2013, is the Pax vaporizer from Ploom. The Pax is designed to vaporize ground herbs. It has four different temperature settings, which makes it versatile across a range of cannabinoids and terpenes, and costs $250. The latest e-pen designs are rapidly gaining market share, because they are discreet and very easy to use. There is concern that some of the "carriers" used to dissolve the cannabinoids for use in e-pens may not be safe for inhalation, though more study is required to confirm this concern. FDA guidance on e-cigarette safety expected shortly may significantly impact on this class of product.

An inexpensive vaporizer for cannabis flowers, rather than cannabis oils, is the Magic Flight Launch Box. It looks like a tiny box-shaped wooden pipe and is powered by a single AA battery, which is inserted into a slot on the side of the device. The vaporizer market is rapidly evolving and new models continue to emerge.

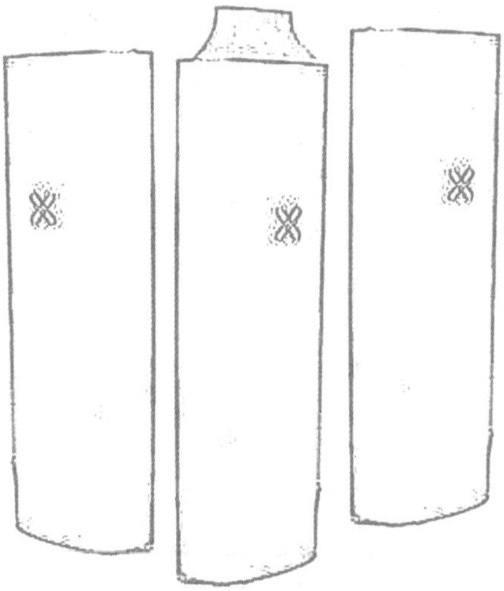

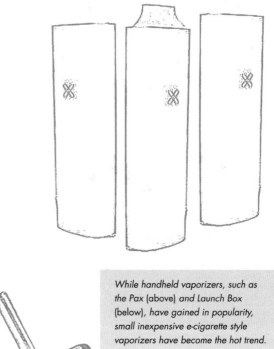

While handheld vaporizers, such as the Pax (above) and Launch Box (below), have gained in popularity, small inexpensive e-cigarette style vaporizers have become the hot trend.

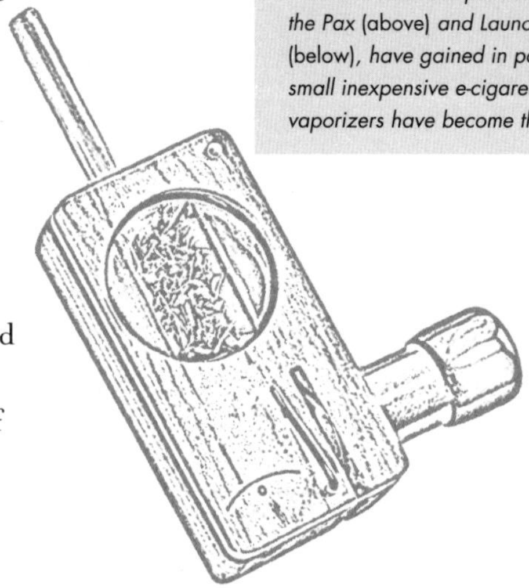

The Downside to Vapor—Dosing

The primary risk of vaporizing medical cannabis is overmedication. Cannabis vapor is floral and more easily tolerated by many patients than cannabis smoke. Because vapor is not as acrid as smoke, patients tend to inhale more of it and hold it in their lungs for longer, which can deliver a higher dose of cannabinoids than anticipated. One small study in Britain showed that "street cannabis" could produce significant levels of ammonia (200 parts per million) when vaporized. This could be due to high levels of residual nitrogen from poor horticultural technique. Interestingly, when herbal cannabis—provided by the U.S. government's cannabis cultivation program at the University of Mississippi—was vaporized in the same study, the ammonia level was far below dangerous levels (10 parts per million).

Dabbing Ultra-concentrated cannabis medicines such as hashish oils and waxes are easy to ignite, wasting the medicine as it goes up in flames before it can be inhaled. Since 2008, techniques have been developed to vaporize these concentrates with a modified water pipe or bong. The key to the pipe modification is a metal plate called a nail, which can be heated with a torch lighter. The nail sits where the pipe bowl typically would on a regular glass water pipe or bong. Once the nail is hot, a dab of the oil or wax is scooped up on a needle and spread across the hot nail. When the oil contacts the hot nail, the oil instantly vaporizes and is inhaled though the water pipe. This vaporized oil is absorbed incredibly quickly through the lungs. The onset of a dab is intense and felt within seconds. This rapid effect is extremely disorienting to some patients and can also be overwhelming. It is easy to overmedicate when dabbing, which can result in the development of tolerance to the effects of cannabis. Also, any adverse effects of THC tend to be amplified for some patient when dabbing, so dose control becomes crucial.

Sublingual Tinctures—Using Cannabis in the Mouth

Long ago, the word tincture meant a substance used to dye or tint something. Today, it refers to an alcoholic, medicinal plant extract. Tinctures use solvents such as ethanol to dissolve active ingredients from medicinal herbs such as cannabis. Soaking cannabis in very high-proof ethanol, such as Everclear neutral grain spirits, forms the basis of most cannabis tinctures. The cannabis is often soaked in this alcohol for over a month, and then the soaked plant material, called the menstruum, is pressed and the resulting tincture collected. Well-made cannabis tinctures can reach nearly 80 milligrams of cannabinoids per milliliter. This makes them extremely potent and great care must be exercised to avoid overmedication.

There is some evidence from conventional herbal medicine that terpenes such as those found in cannabis may be more efficiently delivered by mouth than by smoking or vaporization. This is because the heat associated with smoking and vaping breaks down the terpenes, rendering them less effective. Many terpenoids can be very effectively delivered in tincture form.

Dosing Tinctures Dosing cannabis tinctures beneath the tongue or applying them to the buccal tissues that line the mouth gets cannabinoids into the bloodstream much more quickly than swallowing them. Sublingual absorption delivers more of the experience of smoking or vaping, rather than eating, cannabis medicine. When a cannabis tincture is placed beneath the tongue, the cannabinoids and terpenoids pass through the epithelium tissue. Because the tissues beneath the tongue contain a huge number of tiny blood vessels, cannabinoids quickly diffuse into these capillaries and the bloodstream. Sublingual administration of cannabinoids has advantages over oral administration because the active ingredients get into the bloodstream more quickly, thus avoiding the digestive tract where the cannabis medicine will be broken down by stomach acid, bile, and digestive enzymes. Sublingual absorption also avoids the liver transformation of orally administered THC into the metabolite 11-hydroxy-THC.

If the tincture is lab tested for potency, a dose of 2.5 milligrams of THC should be calculated from the test results as an initial dose. GW Pharmaceuticals recommends that new patients starting Sativex, their proprietary cannabinoid mouth spray, begin with one spray in the evening for the first two days, then two sprays in the evening for the next two days, then on the fifth day adding one spray in the morning. After this, one spray may be added per day to the dosing schedule. This approach gives the patient the opportunity to adjust to the medicine and minimizes adverse effects.

Some tinctures are made with glycerin, though cannabinoids will not stay in a glycerin solution unless a laboratory homogenizer is used to blend them.Using a small lab homogenizer will produce a more shelf-stable product.

Making an Ethanolic Tincture

Start with 1 ounce (28 grams) of high-quality cannabis flowers of tested potency.

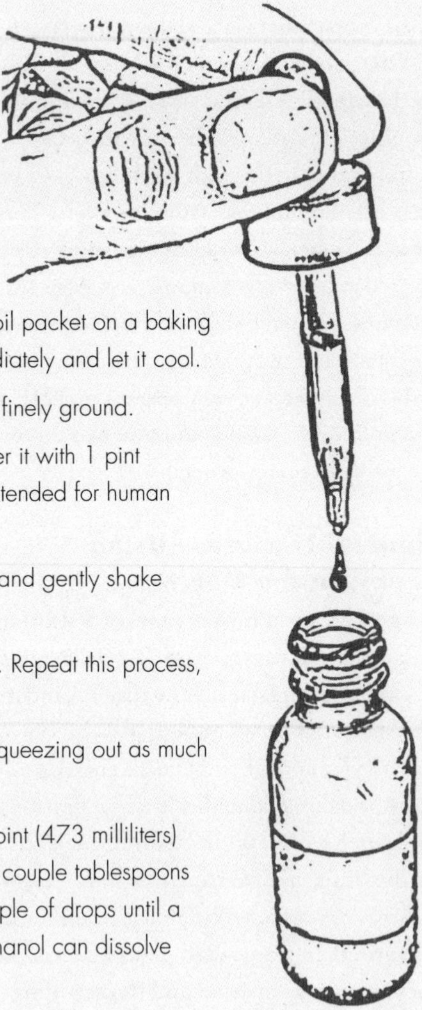

1 Place the cannabis in a bowl, and put in a frost-free freezer for 24 hours, in order to thoroughly dry the cannabis.

2 The next day, remove the cannabis. It should be so dry as to crumble to the touch. Tightly seal the cannabis in aluminum foil so that it forms a packet of ¾ of an inch (1.9 centimeters) thick.

3 Preheat an oven to 315°F (157°C). Place the aluminum foil packet on a baking sheet and heat in the oven for seven minutes. Remove immediately and let it cool.

4 Put the cannabis into a spice grinder and pulse it until it is finely ground.

5 Pour the ground cannabis into a small mason jar and cover it with 1 pint (473 milliliters) of ethanol, Everclear, or high-proof alcohol intended for human consumption.

6 Put the jar in the freezer. Let it sit for an hour, then remove and gently shake the jar for five minutes.

7 Put it back in the freezer for three hours, then shake again. Repeat this process, during waking hours, for a few days.

8 When complete drain the mixture through a coffee filter, squeezing out as much ethanol as possible from the cannabis.

Starting with 15 percent THC cannabis, this should yield a pint (473 milliliters) of very potent tincture. If the ethanol burns the mouth, add a couple tablespoons (30 grams) of raw honey to the tincture. Start with just a couple of drops until a reasonable dose is established. Store in a glass bottle as ethanol can dissolve some chemicals in plastic.

Ethanol in tinctures can aggravate the delicate tissues of the mouth, so care should be observed to avoid irritation or mouth ulcers. One technique to minimize this irritation is to place the tincture on the tongue, let the alcohol evaporate a bit, then let the remaining liquid flow beneath the tongue where it can be absorbed.

Cannabis tinctures should be stored and tightly sealed in a lightproof bottle, preferably in the refrigerator.

Topical Application of Cannabis and Cannabinoids

Cannabinoids can be absorbed through the skin and have been shown to provide an anti-inflammatory response in animal studies.[4] Additionally, there are a large number of cannabinoid receptors in the skin and topical application may help treat some skin conditions such as eczema and psoriasis. Hemp oil creams infused with cannabinoids and terpenes may provide significant therapeutic relief. Care must be observed when using cannabis-based treatments on the skin because a small number of patients are allergic to topical preparations. It's recommended to first apply a tiny amount of the cannabis cream or preparation, then wait a day or so to see if any sensitivity or rash develop. The majority of patients tolerate topical cannabis preparations very well. It is rarely psychoactive, if at all, but extremely high topical cannabinoid doses may result in psychoactive effects.

The anti-inflammatory nature of many of the cannabinoids makes topical cannabis very soothing to the skin. Donald Abrams, the noted oncologist, has stated that he personally uses concentrated cannabis oil to treat an occasional precancerous lesion on his own skin.[5] Many people who use cannabis oil find that it is effective in healing a variety of local skin blemishes and lesions.

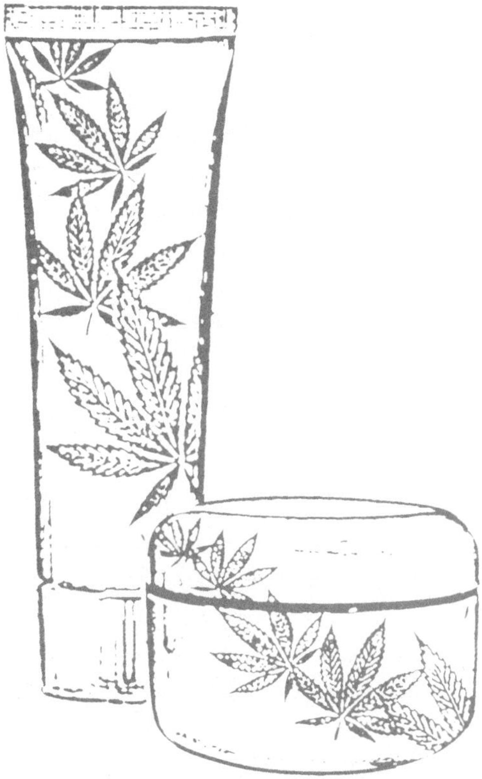

A wide variety of products are available that include hemp oil—hand creams, body lotions, bathing oils, and more. Always test a small area of skin before using frequently.

Endocannabinoids are linked to the regulation of oil production in the skin. Ethan Russo suggested that the cannabinoid CBD, in combination with cannabis terpenes limonene, linalool, and pinene, might form the basis of a novel topical treatment for acne.[6] CBD is absorbed through the skin and reduces the overproduction of sebum—a fatty lubricant matter secreted by the skin's sebaceous glands—which is linked to the complaint. The three terpenes cited by Russo are also potent antibiotics against the primary bacteria associated with acne.

Eating—Oral Administration of Cannabis

Oral cannabis has several advantages over smoked or vaporized cannabis, primarily in increasing the duration of medicinal effect produced. There is a very wide range of responses to oral cannabis, and patients given 20 milligrams of oral cannabis will each absorb it at different rates and metabolize it with varying efficiencies.[7]

Risks of Oral Cannabis A rule of thumb is that orally administered cannabis delivers an effect that lasts twice as long as smoked cannabis. Absorption of oral cannabis is slow and erratic. Onset of effects can be highly variable among patients, ranging from extremes of 15 to 180 minutes. In the majority of patients, onset takes 30 to 90 minutes. Peak plasma ranges vary from 75 minutes to seven hours. Compared to inhalation, oral cannabis effects last longer and fade more slowly over a period of five to eight hours. The biggest risk is using oral herbal cannabis products is overmedication, which can result in frightening levels of psychoactivity and anxiety. And while these symptoms pass in a few hours, it can be a difficult experience to endure.

The First Form of Medicinal Cannabis Eating cannabis as a medicine goes back 2,500 years to ancient China and likely much earlier. *Ma-Fên*, or "ground hemp" from female cannabis flowers, was recommended in the earliest known Chinese herbal to treat malaria, rheumatism, and menstrual pain. The same herbal warns that hemp seeds can cause those that eat them to see demons.

Cannabis is a cornerstone in traditional Indian medicine. Sharma calls it the "penicillin of Ayurvedic medicine."[8] *Bhang*, the traditional Indian cannabis drink, is taken as a general tonic across India (see opposite).

Variations on Oral Cannabis With the increasing availability of cannabis varieties that contain cannabinoids other than THC (such as CBD), oral cannabis preparations can be made with modified, reduced, or no psychoactivity—depending on the ratio of CBD to THC in the preparation. An eight to one ratio of CBD to THC typically eliminates THC psychoactivity altogether. A three to two CBD to THC ratio will have some psychoactivity, but of a distinctly clearheaded variety.

These ranges are noteworthy because patients consistently note that these ratios are excellent for reducing anxiety. Alternative cannabinoids, such as CBD and THCV, may also be of interest to patients for whom conventional THC psychoactivity may be a problem. Many experts consider these alternative cannabinoids to be the future of herbal cannabis medicine.

Suppositories and Exotic Methods of Administration

As odd as it might sound, a cannabis suppository has several medicinal advantages. The dose in a suppository form can be efficiently absorbed without any loss of cannabinoids to digestive acids or enzymes. The suppository form also bypasses liver metabolism of the cannabinoids, so the experience feels identical to smoked or vaporized cannabis. The suppository can also be formulated to be time-released so that the effects last longer than smoking. The patents for cannabinoid suppositories are held by a small company affiliated with the U.S. government–contracted cannabis cultivation project at the University of Mississippi. There is no cannabis suppository currently available on the market.

Patchtek—The Cannabinoid Transdermal Patch Lawrence Brook, the founder of General Hydroponics, has developed

Making Bhang

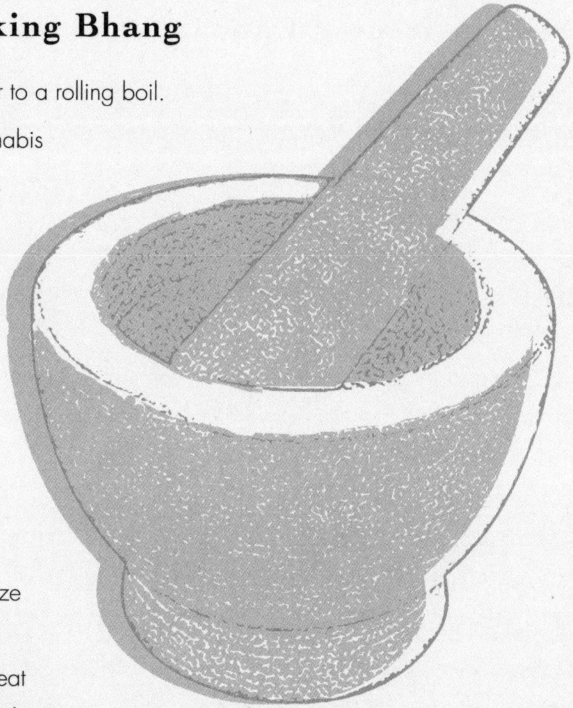

Start by bringing 2 cups (237 milliliters) of water to a rolling boil.

1 Put 1 ounce (28 grams) of fresh, undried cannabis flowers in a teapot and cover with the boiling water.

2 Wrap the teapot in a towel and let the cannabis tea steep for eight minutes.

3 Strain the tea through a fine mesh strainer. Press the cannabis to remove all tea. Reserve the cannabis and set the tea aside.

4 Put the cannabis in a mortar and add 3 tablespoons (45 grams) of warm milk (whole or soy) and mash the cannabis with the milk.

5 Put the mash into a piece of muslin and squeeze out the milk.

6 Put the cannabis back into the mortar and repeat this process several times with more warm milk (using a total of 4 cups or 946 milliliters) until you've got ½ cup (118 milliliters) of cannabis milk. Remove and place in a separate container.

7 Discard the cannabis.

8 Add 2 tablespoons (30 grams) of chopped, blanched almonds to the mortar and cover with milk.

9 Grind with the pestle, then squeeze the almond milk through some fresh muslin; repeat with more milk a few times.

10 Combine all the liquids: the tea, the cannabis milk, the almond milk, and the rest of the milk.

11 Add ⅛ teaspoon (0.6 grams) garam masala, ¼ teaspoon (1.25 grams) powdered ginger, and ½ teaspoon (2.5 grams) rosewater. Add sugar or honey to taste.

These instructions yield 12 doses. Keep the *bhang* refrigerated and shake well before serving. The cannabinoids in *bhang* are only slightly decarboxylated, so typically this recipe is not very psychoactive. Heating the cannabis to 315°F (157°C) for seven minutes will decarboxylate it and make the *bhang* extremely potent when taken orally.

Making Infused Cannabis Oil for Cooking

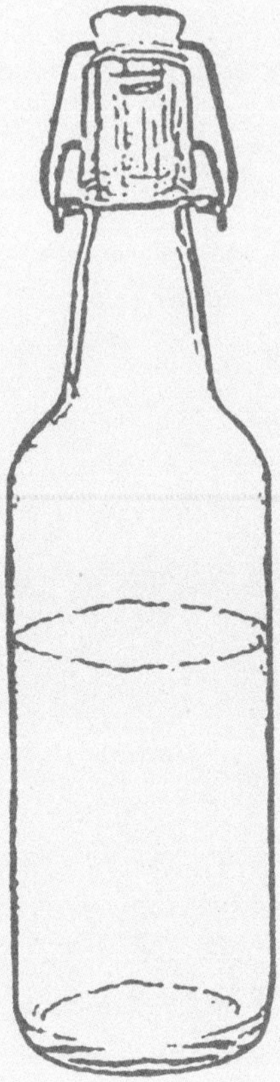

Cannabis-infused cooking oil is very versatile and can be incorporated into a range of recipes. While cannabis flowers can be used to make infused oil, cannabis extractions are a better choice.

1 To prepare, put 2 ounces (57 grams) of lab-tested cannabis dried flowers or 1 ounce (28 grams) of hashish; 4 cups (946 milliliters) of water; and 1 cup (237 milliliters) of canola, sesame, or olive oil into a slow cooker. Heat for 8 hours.

2 Use a coffee filter and press to squeeze the oil and water from the cooked cannabis. Pour the liquid into a bowl and freeze overnight. The infused oil will float to the top.

3 Wear gloves to scrape the oil from the bowl. Discard any brown, frozen water.

4 Keep the oil in the freezer, as it will go rancid quickly if not frozen.

The oil will be quite potent and great care should be observed to avoid accidental ingestion. If made with 15 percent THC dried cannabis, the oil can contain (adjusted for loss in the extraction process) approximately 6 grams of THC. Just 1 teaspoon (5 grams) of this infused oil should provide approximately 10 to 12-milligram doses of THC.

and patented a transdermal patch called Patchtek, which delivers cannabinoids through the skin. Patchtek is undergoing preclinical studies for use in the treatment of neuropathic pain, nausea, vomiting, anorexia, and multiple sclerosis spasticity. As a drug delivery approach for cannabinoid medicines, this technology is much more likely to gain acceptance from the conventional pharmaceutical community.

Namisol and Solving Cannabinoid Solubility Issues One of the biggest issues with delivering cannabinoids orally is that cannabinoids love fat and hate water. This makes them difficult and erratic to absorb (see page 56). Echo Pharmaceuticals in the Netherlands has developed a technology for increasing the absorbability of cannabinoids, called Alitra. Alitra is used by Echo to produce a THC pill called Namisol, which is much easier for the body to absorb. Some Finnish researchers have taken cyclodextrin, a ring made of sugar molecules, and inserted a cannabinoid molecule into the ring, which increases its solubility dramatically. A cyclodextrin-cannabinoid formulation might some day make it possible to take a spoonful of cannabis medicine and simply stir it into a glass of lemonade.

Time of Day and Medical Cannabis Use

While cannabis is noted for interfering with the perception of time, does time of day have an effect on how cannabis works? Perhaps. Especially when it comes to nighttime. THC is known to interfere with dreaming and sleeping cycles. In order to avoid this effect, it's recommended not to take cannabis medicines within at least four hours of bedtime. Conversely, to encourage this effect—in the case of persistent night terrors or post-traumatic stress disorder nightmare syndromes—taking cannabinoids close to bedtime can break this cycle. Chronic anxiety can be extremely fatiguing and the use of CBD in the morning may help reduce anxiety that would normally result in mid-afternoon exhaustion. The timing of taking cannabis medicines is still under investigation, but because cannabinoids mimic the body's own homeostatic regulators, it makes sense that timing a cannabinoid dose could go far in helping to stabilize an imbalanced system.

Nanotech and Cannabinoid Medicine

Researchers at Complutense University in Madrid, Spain, have embedded THC and CBD into microparticles for deployment within brain tumor cells. This innovative technique allows for the sustained release of the cannabinoids, at a high level of concentration, directly at the tumor site. Cannabinoids appear to be a promising treatment for glioblastoma multiforme, one of the most common and deadly forms of brain cancer. The essential issue in using cannabinoids in this way lies in getting them directly to the tumor and successfully releasing them at the site. The initial animal studies with this technology, however, appear very promising.[9]

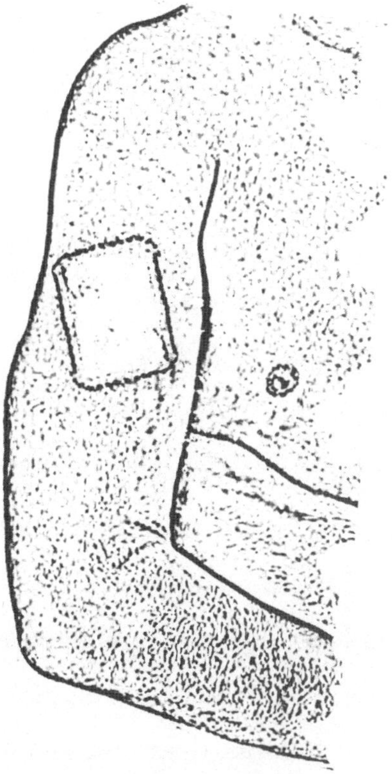

The use of a transdermal patch to deliver cannabis medicine is still in its infancy.

USING MEDICAL CANNABIS IN THE WORKPLACE

Even though a patient using medical cannabis may not use it at work or come to work under its influence, many corporate zero-tolerance drug policies make no accommodation whatsoever for these patients. Zero-tolerance workplace rules prohibit any detectable amount of illegal drugs in an applicant or employee's blood system, and this prohibition is typically extended to medical cannabis. Many state medical cannabis statutes fail to provide accommodation for this issue, and because THC metabolites can be detected long after a user is impaired or influenced by the use of cannabis, users may still lose their employment if cannabis use is detected through mandatory drug testing.

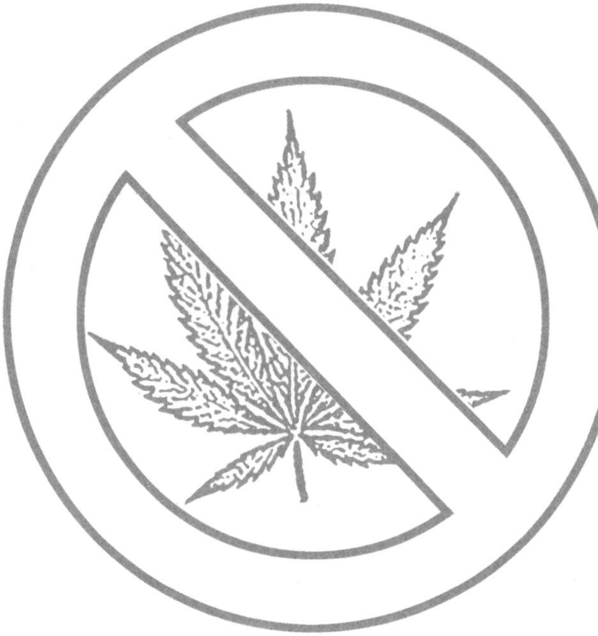

Using cannabis in the workplace can be very difficult if the employer decides not to permit it. Employers are allowed to ban cannabis use in the workplace and to date the courts consistently have ruled with employers on this issue. In September 2012, the Sixth Circuit U.S. Court of Appeals sided with Walmart in the company's termination of a Michigan brain cancer patient using medical cannabis, in violation of the company's substance abuse policies.[10] The court said that Michigan's medical cannabis law did not change the state's at-will employment law, nor did it create any basis of a claim for wrongful discharge. Medical cannabis laws in Arizona, Connecticut, Delaware, Maine, and Rhode Island specifically protect medical cannabis patients from hiring discrimination. Arizona and Delaware prohibit businesses from refusing to hire applicants or disciplining employees on the basis of drug tests that uncover cannabis components or metabolites. However, there is no protection in these states if the patient is "impaired" from their use of medical cannabis. There are no reliable guidelines for defining impairment based on blood levels of THC or other cannabis constituents or metabolites. There are exceptions to these rules in which, for example, the employees are "impaired" by cannabis while on an employer's property or during work hours. But it is difficult to prove impairment beyond anecdotal reports of "drugged" behavior.

United States government agencies such as the Department of Health and Human Services and the Department of Transportation demand that businesses with federal contracts have a written policy prohibiting the use of medical cannabis by its employees.

Obviously, employees need to be honest about any impact that the use of medical cannabis could have on the quality of their work and whether workplace safety is an issue. Additionally, employment laws need to be revised to reflect the changing status of cannabis within society and its use as a medicine.

Driving and Medical Cannabis: Is It Safe?

Twenty-five percent of motor vehicle deaths involve drunk drivers, with many automobile accidents involving drivers that test positive for cannabis. It has been shown that combining alcohol and cannabis more severely impairs driving abilities. Impairment of driving ability by cannabis seems dependent on dose. In cognitive tests related to driving performance, cannabis has been shown to impair performance, with the level of impairment dependent on the dose of cannabis employed in the study. But a few tests on actual cannabis intoxication have been shown to only slightly impair actual driving performance. A 2009 review of cannabis driving research cited a number of studies where cannabis impaired one or more driving skills: "120 studies have found that in general, the higher the estimated concentration of THC in blood, the greater the driving impairment, but that more frequent users of cannabis show less impairment than infrequent users at the same dose, either because of physiological tolerance or learned compensatory behavior. Maximal impairment is found 20 to 40 minutes after smoking, but the impairment has vanished 2.5 hours later, at least in those who smoke 18 mg THC or less...."[11]

The effects of cannabis on driving vary individually due to differences in THC absorption, tolerance, and smoking method. Interestingly, cannabis appears to most negatively influence highly automatic driving tasks, such as staying within a lane, rather than more complex driving tasks, such as merging into traffic.

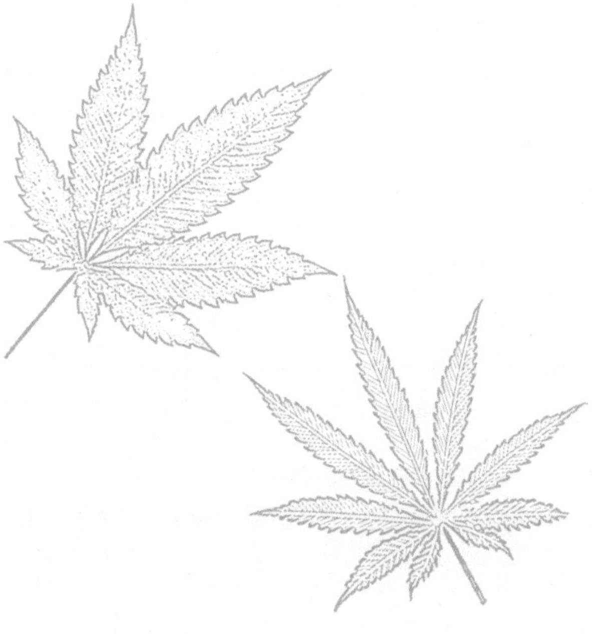

Varieties of Medical Cannabis

Acapulco Gold, Skunk, Thai Stick, and OG Kush are names associated with well-known cannabis varieties that have emerged from the marijuana underground since the 1960s. Some of these varieties were landraces originally native to specific regions—Durban Poison from South Africa or Guerrero Green from Mexico, for example. Others, including Haze and Blueberry, were bred on the West Coast. Each variety produces medicinal effects, which vary from one strain to the next. It follows that an understanding of the primary varieties of cannabis can be helpful in selecting the right cannabis medicine for a specific condition.

3

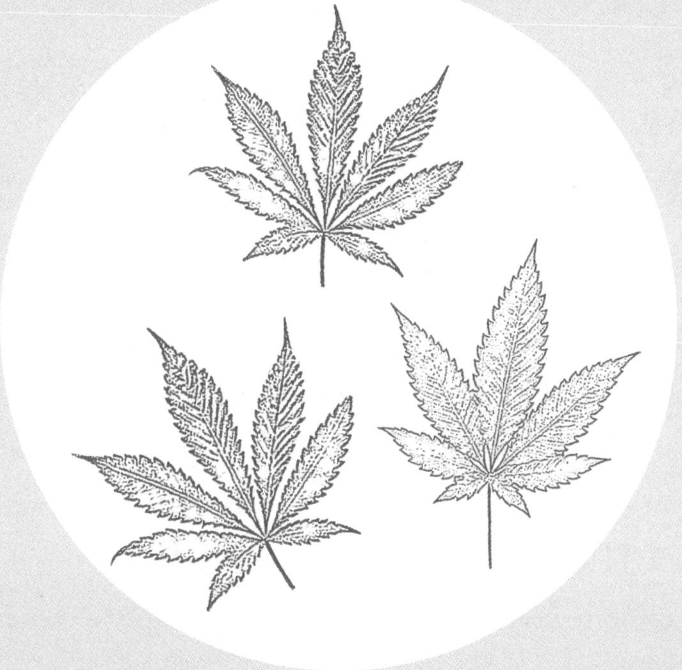

WHAT MAKES A CANNABIS VARIETY AND WHY IT'S IMPORTANT

Different cannabis varieties produce different medicinal effects, owing to unique variations in the chemistry produced by each individual variety. The medicinal effects can vary so dramatically among cannabis varieties that each one can effectively become a different medicine. Some cannabis varieties produce THC, while others produce CBD; some produce nearly equal amounts of both cannabinoids. Variation in terpene content also significantly modifies the medicinal effects of cannabis varieties.

Narrow-leafleted THC cannabis varieties were likely introduced to the Western Hemisphere by indentured laborers from India, when the British transported these Indian workers to Jamaica in the 1830s. The major expansion of cannabis varieties in the West did not begin until marijuana breeding became more widespread in the 1960s, however. In 2009, CBD-rich varieties were identified in the United States and the use of these CBD cannabis varieties could eventually spark another medical cannabis breeding revolution.

Name Games and Strain Identification

Pick up any alternative newspaper in San Francisco, Denver, or Los Angeles, and you'll see advertisements for G13 Kush, Blue Lightning, Charlie Sheen Kush, Obama Cookies, and so on. There are hundreds of medical marijuana varieties being marketed by storefront dispensaries and delivery services. The average person looks at this and thinks, "Where do they get these ridiculous names?" The answer is that they're made up. Then again, someone made up the name "Google," too.

The more important question about these medical marijuana varieties is: If the names are just made up, what are the chemically distinct varieties of cannabis that these companies claim to be selling? The fact of the matter is that nobody really knows, including the folks selling them. This ignorance is usually not malicious, and cultivators do try to make informed guesses as to the identities of the cannabis varieties they provide. But there aren't many standards or certification procedures in California or Colorado—although that is changing.

In 2013, legislation was introduced in Connecticut to regulate medical cannabis, and it requires products to have brand names. As a result of this, each batch of the cannabis product

The Pioneers at Hortapharm

In the late 1980s, Hortapharm, a Dutch company founded by David Watson and Robert Connell Clarke, began to study the chemistry of cannabis, looking specifically for varieties of medicinal interest. The founders of Hortapharm had collected landrace varieties in their travels around the globe, including cultivars that produced rare cannabinoids such as THCV. GW Pharmaceuticals subsequently acquired Hortapharm's cannabis genetics library, and under the guidance of Etienne De Meijer developed a new generation of medical cannabis cultivars.

must fall within a tight chemical tolerance based on its initial product specification registered with the state, or it loses the right to the product name.

Cannabis varieties can be chemically and genetically fingerprinted to identify them with precision. Chemical fingerprinting determines the normal range of terpenoids and cannabinoids produced by a specific phenotype of a single cannabis variety. For example, one phenotype of OG Kush (see pages 152–155) when cultivated under consistent conditions will produce 24 percent THCA, 0.8 percent CBD, 1.6 percent myrcene, 0.9 percent alpha-pinene, 0.7 percent limonene, and 0.8 percent beta-caryophyllene. These numbers comprise the pharmacologically active chemical fingerprint of this OG Kush. The genetic fingerprint of the same OG Kush phenotype could be the genes that control the plant's manufacture of these pharmacologically active substances. Each variety of cannabis contains genes that determine its specific chemical composition. The production of each essential oil and each cannabinoid by the plant is controlled by the expression of genes.

Optimization of a cannabis variety's ability to produce pharmacologically interesting substances requires this kind of fingerprinting to understand what each cannabis variety is capable of producing. This kind of understanding and precision is used for all kinds of herbs, spices, and produce on the market. Soon, it will be used for medical cannabis as well. With uniform product names will also come consistent composition and manufacture of herbal cannabis medicines. So the next Charlie Sheen Kush will be exactly the same as the last Charlie Sheen Kush… and they may have to pay a royalty to the actual Charlie Sheen, if he'll grant that right. One part of the great guessing game of medical cannabis will end. Others will remain.

The biggest mystery of modern cannabis is why varieties of cannabis produce different medicinal or psychoactive effects. While it is clear that these effects are profoundly influenced by the ratios of cannabinoids and terpenoids that are unique to each variety, the results of the interactions of these terpenoids and cannabinoids is extremely complex and still not completely understood. Through emerging approaches, such as principal component analysis of cannabis, an exploratory data analysis technique that helps scientists understand the complex interactions of multiple plant constituents, it will become possible to predict the effects of a cannabis variety more accurately, by mapping its chemistry precisely and understanding the interactions that arise because of that chemistry.

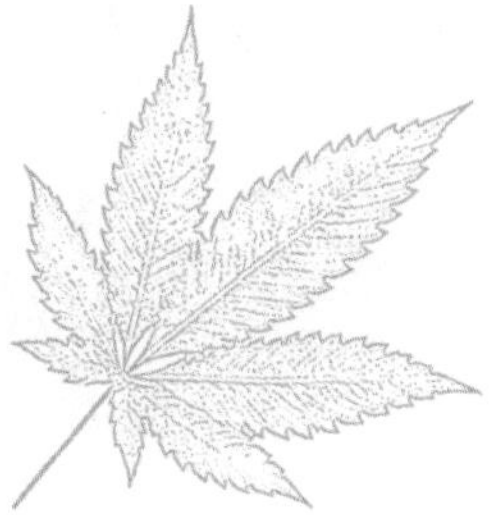

From Landrace Varieties and Adaptation to Modern Breeding

There are thousands of cannabis varieties from Korea to Mexico, from Uruguay to Malawi. All across Russia, Kazakhstan, Nepal… Cannabis is everywhere and everywhere each strain is different, slightly adapted to each specific locale. Individual varieties are called landraces—a term used to define the local variations of the cannabis plant. And it is from these landraces that modern medical cannabis varieties have been bred. In a few cases, such as Malawi Gold, the landrace has not been bred with another variety. For this unique strain, the plant remains exactly as found near villages along the banks of Lake Malawi in Africa.

In the 1960s, as illicit cannabis use increased in Western countries, hippie backpackers visited regions of the world where native varieties of cannabis could be found. Mexico, Jamaica, Colombia, Morocco, southern Africa, Lebanon, Turkey, Afghanistan, Pakistan, Nepal, India, and Thailand all produced landrace varieties that were brought back to form the genetic pool from which modern cannabis was bred. This illicit "bio-prospecting"—searching for local plant species of medicinal value, is actually prohibited in many of these countries today, because the landrace plants are now considered strategic national assets.

Most medical cannabis varieties in use today have been crossed to yield new varieties. They are descended from landraces, certainly, but the majority of them likely bear little resemblance to their ancestors. These new varieties have been chosen and bred for one thing: their ability to produce THC. And while this has made for some extraordinarily psychoactive varieties, it has also resulted in highly inbred cannabis. Marijuana from around the world exhibits some fascinating natural diversity, while modern, medical cannabis contains very little that is unique and quite a bit that is identical. In a word, these varieties are invariably cut from the same cloth.

Prohibition of cannabis has ensured that we know very little of the composition or ancestry of many pre-1965 varieties. And what we do know is often impossible to confirm. There are a lot of egos and faulty memories involved, as well as more than a little arrogance. Consider the legendary Santa Cruz variety called Haze (see pages 138–139)—a foundation strain in modern cannabis breeding that has been used to breed dozens, if not hundreds, of varieties of cannabis. David Paul Watson, a.k.a. Sam the Skunkman, a.k.a. Jingles, claims to have introduced Haze to the Netherlands in the 1980s and his claim is well supported. The Australian cannabis breeder, Neville Schoenmaker, a.k.a. Nevil, claims to have visited Santa Cruz himself, where he met the legendary Haze Brothers, who then gave him the variety. The actual story of Haze, the foundation of modern cannabis breeding, remains obscure. Those who know believe that Haze was more luck than skill. The only remaining evidence of the Haze project is a poster printed in 1976 in Santa Cruz signed "R.L.," discussing grow tips observed in its production. Sifting the truth from the legends is impossible.

There may be an occasion on which a breed of cannabis is designed to smell good or look attractive—but at the end of the day, it all comes down to cannabinoid and terpene content, and the cleanliness of the cultivation.

When it comes to the genetics of a particular variety, we often don't know what landraces were used to breed it, or whether said variety is anything more than an inbred mess with a big THC spike. Modern scientific testing has started to unravel the mysteries of how cannabis makes its constituents and, increasingly, which genes control the process. Soon we should be able to breed cannabis to suit our tastes and medicinal needs perfectly. Today's present mess will fade away. And from the remaining landraces and high-quality varieties we will create the next generation of medical cannabis. Breeders have been toiling away for decades, trying to improve the cannabis plant's ability to produce medicine. Some of the most successful efforts follow.

Selecting a Medical Cannabis Variety

The common descriptors used at dispensaries, *indica* and *sativa*, rarely determine anything beyond the most basic medicinal effects. Typically, *indica* is used to describe broad-leafleted varieties that produce terpenes such as myrcene and linalool. More sedating, they produce more lethargic "stone." *Sativa* characterizes narrow-leafleted varieties that produce terpenes such as caryophyllenes and pinenes, which are stimulating and tend to produce more of a cerebral "high." Selecting precisely the appropriate variety of medical cannabis requires an understanding of the variety's basic genetics and chemistry beyond simplistic *indica* and *sativa* designations.

The basics of cannabis chemistry manifest themselves in a variety's appearance and aroma. Certain aromas produced by cannabis provide a surprisingly reliable indication of the variety's effects. A piney scent is indicative of stimulating results. A lavender or grape aroma typically is associated with sedative varieties. Learn how to associate cannabis aroma with cannabis effects and you'll become informed very quickly.

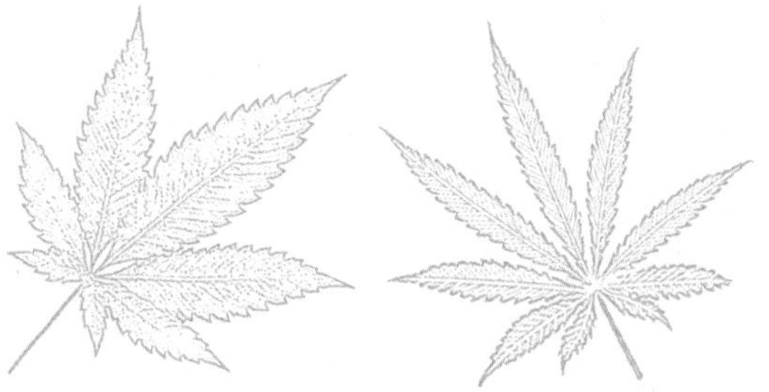

But judging cannabis simply by its variety name remains a gamble. There is a great deal of fraud, and even more innocent ignorance. For example, nobody really knows what varieties bred OG Kush. So what is real OG Kush? More importantly, what are the genetics and chemistry that make OG Kush an effective medicine? There are stories of the origin of OG—they may or may not be true. But they always run out of rope. Some say that OG Kush's parent first showed up as a seed in a bag of Chemdawg cannabis at a Grateful Dead concert. OK, but then what varieties bred the cannabis seed in that bag? No answer. Is this Chem '91 a version of some amazing Colorado variety? Or a Nepalese Thai cross? Or a landrace from Afghanistan? Nobody knows. What is known for certain is that OG Kush is a tall, broad-leafleted hybrid that typically produces upward of 20 percent THC and has an intense aroma of pine, citrus, and fuel.

Once you establish consistency in the varieties available to you, it's easier to decide among them. Simple, right? You just need to find someone who pays attention to their cannabis and looks for repeatable patterns in its structure and chemistry. Those patterns are definitely there, and with the help of laboratory instruments—which take precise measurements of your cannabis product's constituent elements—the uniqueness of your preferred medical variety may be revealed.

The following patterns and observations can help you determine the most suitable medical cannabis variety for the course of treatment recommended by your physician.

Modern Cannabis Varieties

The following pages consider 27 modern cannabis varieties and their medicinal properties. The locations in which they are grown are indicated on this map, as well as each variety's species type, whether *indica*, *sativa*, or hybrid.

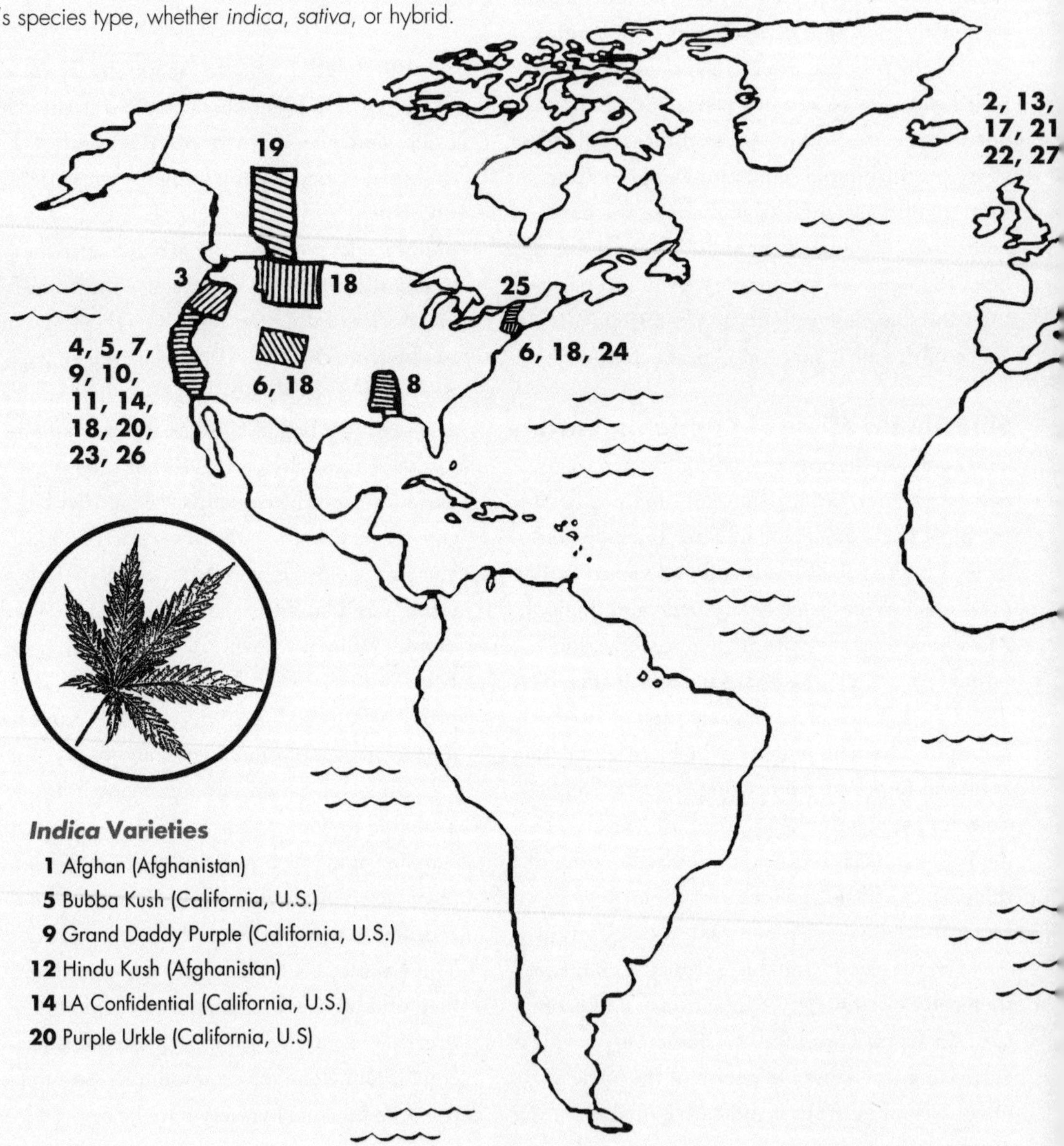

Indica Varieties

1 Afghan (Afghanistan)
5 Bubba Kush (California, U.S.)
9 Grand Daddy Purple (California, U.S.)
12 Hindu Kush (Afghanistan)
14 LA Confidential (California, U.S.)
20 Purple Urkle (California, U.S)

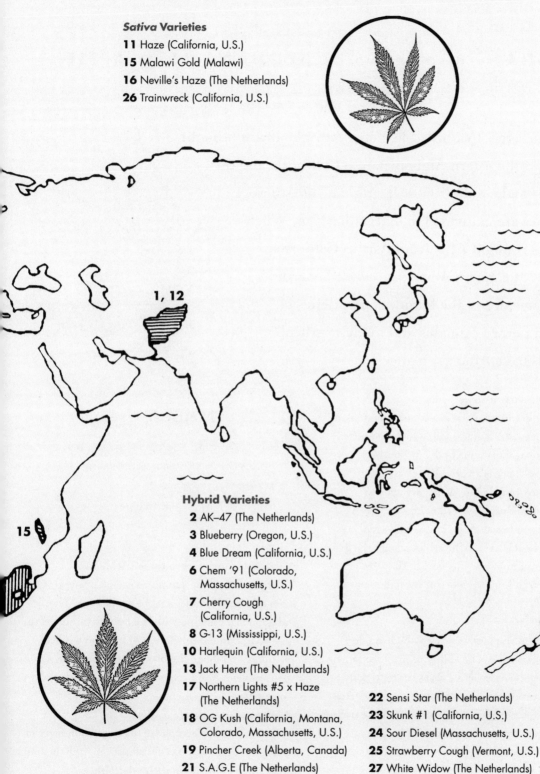

***Sativa* Varieties**

11 Haze (California, U.S.)
15 Malawi Gold (Malawi)
16 Neville's Haze (The Netherlands)
26 Trainwreck (California, U.S.)

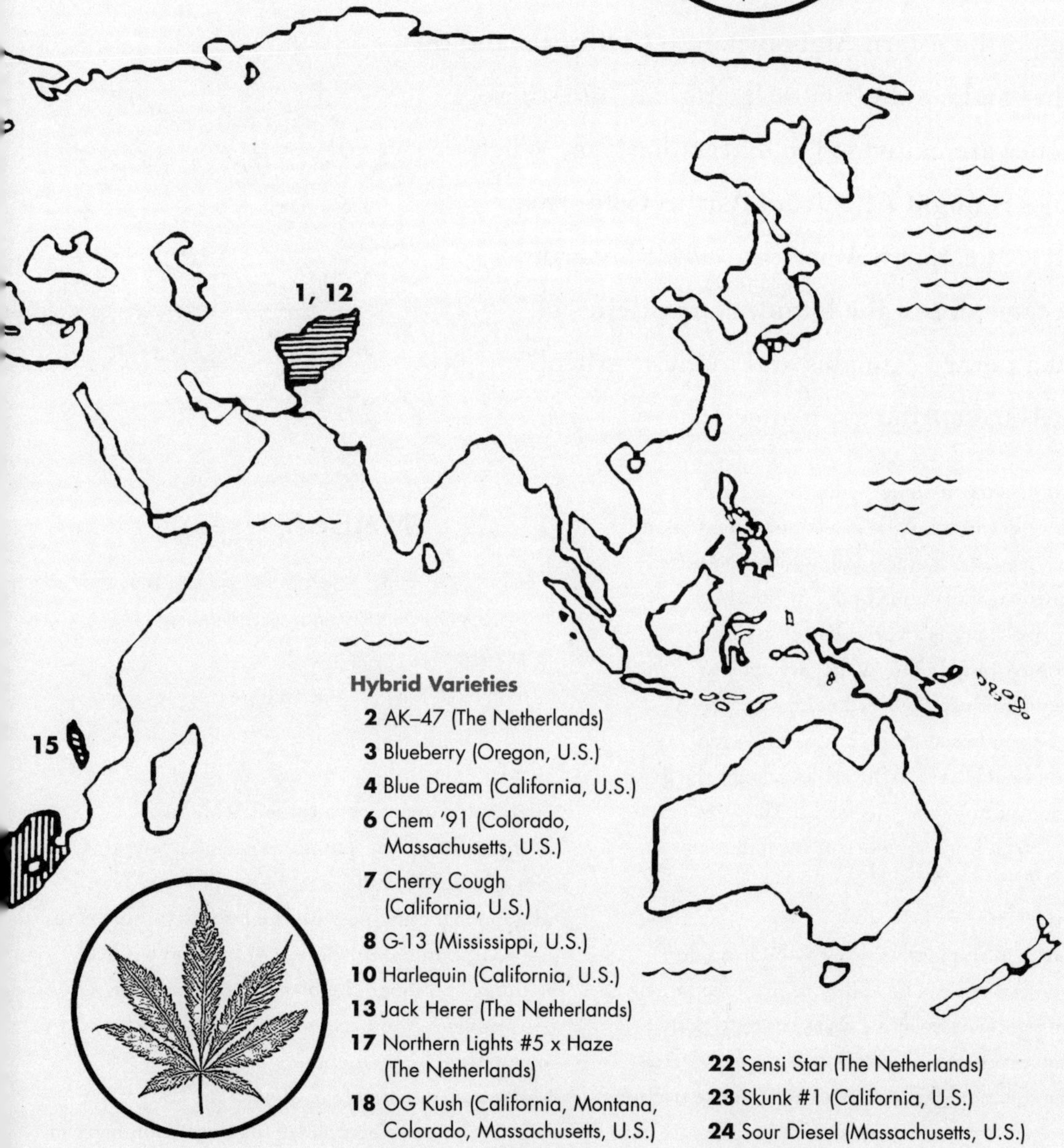

Hybrid Varieties

2 AK–47 (The Netherlands)
3 Blueberry (Oregon, U.S.)
4 Blue Dream (California, U.S.)
6 Chem '91 (Colorado, Massachusetts, U.S.)
7 Cherry Cough (California, U.S.)
8 G-13 (Mississippi, U.S.)
10 Harlequin (California, U.S.)
13 Jack Herer (The Netherlands)
17 Northern Lights #5 x Haze (The Netherlands)
18 OG Kush (California, Montana, Colorado, Massachusetts, U.S.)
19 Pincher Creek (Alberta, Canada)
21 S.A.G.E (The Netherlands)
22 Sensi Star (The Netherlands)
23 Skunk #1 (California, U.S.)
24 Sour Diesel (Massachusetts, U.S.)
25 Strawberry Cough (Vermont, U.S.)
27 White Widow (The Netherlands)

AFGHAN, also known as **AFGHANI #1** or **AFFIE**

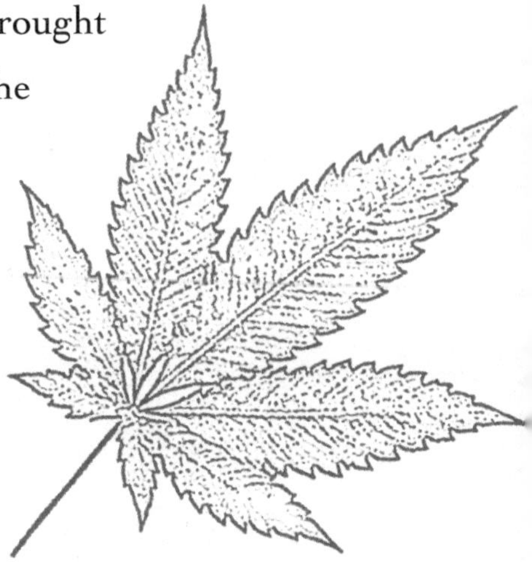

Afghan refers to a broad-leafleted *indica* landrace brought from northwestern Afghanistan to California and the Netherlands in the 1970s. In Afghanistan, these varieties are cultivated to extract hashish. When hippies brought Affie from Asia to California, it led to the North American "*indica* invasion." It became one of the foundation varieties of contemporary cannabis and today nearly all indicas have Affie as an ancestor.

Prized because it could be harvested in mid-October outdoors, Affie is a squat, bushy plant up to 8 feet (2.5 meters) tall, which produces a profusion of resinous buds. In Southern California there is a very rare, clone-only phenotype called "The Affie," which was subsequently used by seed company, DNA Genetics, to breed their "LA Confidential" (see pages 144–45). The Affie ranks among the great cannabis cultivars in the world. They are among the few true kush varieties of cannabis.

Medical Uses

Affies are great for pain and relaxation. They are also popular with patients with gastrointestinal, appetite, and nausea issues.

Notes

As a true hash plant, the key to high-quality Afghan cannabis is its ability to produce large amounts of psychoactive resin content. A true Afghan produces a heavy, stinky, greasy dried-flower cluster. Affie should exhibit dense trichome coverage even on its smaller leaves. Because of this trichome density, Affies are typically not as tightly manicured as other cannabis varieties—which helps to preserve these trichomes.

In Afghanistan, it's common to smoke cannabis from a hubble bubble, a large water pipe. The indigenous technique with the hubble bubble is to take a large initial inhalation of hashish to clear the lungs and dilate the bronchi, which often sends novices into paroxysms of coughing. This method likely increases the surface area of lung tissue available to absorb the drug. The second inhalation completes the dose. Commercial hash oil production was developed in Afghanistan using these cultivars in the mid-1970s.

TYPE: Pure broad-leafleted *indica*.

SPECIES: *Cannabis indica ssp. afghanica.*

BREEDING DATE: Landrace—Afghan hashish cultivars were likely developed in the nineteenth century. Afghanis #1, #2 (and a purple variant), and #3 first appeared in February 1981 in a *High Times* advertisement for the Sacred Seeds seed bank, one of the earliest commercial cannabis seed ventures.

GENETICS: Landrace, though considerably interbred since it was brought to the West in the late 1970s in Vacaville, California.

SIMILAR VARIETIES: LA Confidential, Bubba Kush (see pages 126–27), Hindu Kush (see pages 140–41), Purple Afghani, AfPak.

AVAILABILITY: Afghani #1 is available from cannabis seed bank Sensi Seeds, but Sensi has refined their version by breeding it with other Afghan cannabis genetics over the last several decades. "Affie," a very special Afghan phenotype still exists in Southern California, but is not widely distributed.

EASE OF CULTIVATION: Relatively easy. With little mold resistance among Afghan cultivars, climate control and low humidity are important to successfully cultivate Afghans, which are acclimated to semiarid Central Asia. Afghani #1 finishes outdoors in the third week of October. It has a 55-day flowering time indoors.

AROMA: Afghan cannabis flowers have a distinctive smell of skunk and spice, with some phenotypes delivering the rich scent of freshly roasted coffee. Affies are typically high in linalool and alpha-humulene, both relatively scarce terpenes in cannabis.

TASTE: Afghani #1 has an acrid, hashy smoke that is spicy, floral, and slightly tart when vaporized. It is never subtle!

POTENCY: Around 17 percent THC, with certain phenotypes over 20 percent. It has very low CBD content, and occasionally, Afghan phenotypes will produce THCV in addition to THC.

DURATION OF EFFECTS: It has long-lasting effects, except for THCV phenotypes.

PSYCHOACTIVITY: Narcotic with a strong "body effect," this type of broad-leafleted cannabis was responsible for the introduction of the "stony" effect. The irony is that Affie produces far less sedating myrcene than many of today's so-called *indicas*. Before these Afghan cultivars were brought to the West, cannabis was commonly thought to deliver more of a cerebral "high" associated with the Mexican, Thai, Jamaican, and Colombian cultivars.

ANALGESIA: Excellent, with a general numbing effect at moderate doses.

MUSCLE RELAXATION: Excellent.

DISSOCIATION: Strong.

STIMULANT: Little stimulation, except at micro-doses.

SEDATION: Strong.

AK–47

AK–47 takes its name not from the weapon, but from the rapid onset of this variety's psychoactivity. AK may also stand for "Afghan Kush." Ironically, AK–47 rifles flooded Afghanistan during the Soviet invasion in the 1970s, around the same time that the Afghan parent of this variety was brought from its home country to Amsterdam. It is likely that the Afghan wide-leafleted parent was bred into Dutch narrow-leafleted genetics, which explains why AK–47 can produce so many different phenotypes from its seed.

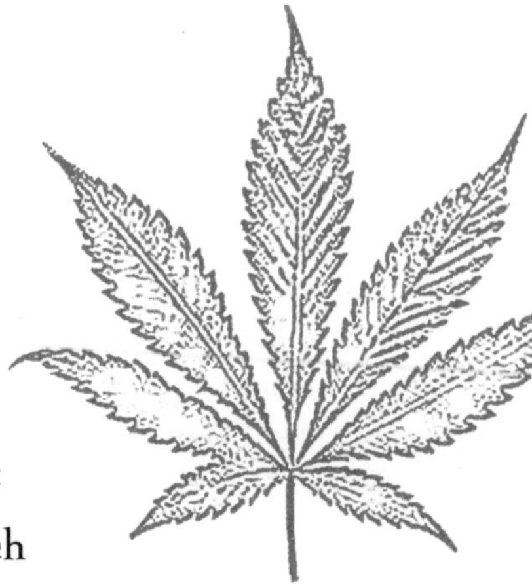

Medical Uses

AK–47 is a classic, ultra-potent THC variety and excellent medicine at low doses. At higher doses, it can overwhelm patients with its intense psychoactivity. Great for appetite stimulation and settling an upset stomach.

Notes

Simon, the chief breeder of AK–47 and founder of Amsterdam's Serious Seeds, was a biology teacher before he joined Alan Dronkers, operator of Amsterdam's Hash, Marihuana, and Hemp Museum and co-owner of Sensi Seeds. Simon did not smoke cannabis until he was 25, because he hated the customary Dutch approach of combining cannabis with tobacco. He wasn't offered pure cannabis until he was studying in Africa, where he fell in love with the plant.

Among cultivators of AK–47, there supposedly exists a rare and cherished phenotype, the Cherry AK. The Cherry AK is supposedly found once in every hundred germinated seeds. This phenotype is supposed to have an aroma reminiscent of ripe black cherries. Simon disputes this claim, stating that many AK phenotypes are fruity, but none that he has found smell distinctly of cherries. Simon's belief aside, Cherry AK remains one of the most sought-after varieties in California dispensaries. Cherry AK definitely smells fruity, but not particularly cherry-like. This may be an example of "priming," where a person's experience is primed by their expectation of the experience. In the case of Cherry AK, it could be that the cherry aroma is confirmed simply because of its objective, if indistinct, fruitiness. Or there may actually be a true Cherry AK out there, somewhere.

TYPE: AK–47 seeds produce both wide-leafleted and narrow-leafleted phenotypes. Because of this natural variation and its high potency, it is the only cannabis variety to have won separate Cannabis Cups for best *indica* and best *sativa*.

SPECIES: *Cannabis indica ssp. indica* × *cannabis indica ssp. afghanica.*

BREEDING DATE: circa 1994.

GENETICS: (Thai × Brazilian) × Afghan.

AVAILABILITY: Available from Serious Seeds Amsterdam and many other seed retailers in Europe and Canada.

SIMILAR VARIETIES: Ole–47, White Russian, AK–47 × White Widow (see pages 172–73).

EASE OF CULTIVATION: Easy, popular with novice cultivators. AK–47 can produce very large flowers and high yields.

AROMA: AK–47 is considered one of smelliest modern cannabis varieties. It reeks of skunk with a little rotting fruit.

TASTE: Not to everyone's taste, but AK–47 does have a distinct pungent flavor with a hint of fruit. Some complain that the variety tastes acrid, a trait associated with some Afghan varieties.

POTENCY: Very high, consistently around 20 percent THC when cultivated indoors. Somewhat notorious.

DURATION OF EFFECTS: Most patients claim that AK–47 has a longer than average high.

PSYCHOACTIVITY: Intensely psychoactive with an interesting combination of clear-headed high at some moments, interspersed with a profound disorienting "stone" as the terpenes—myrcene and beta-caryophyllene—duke it out.

ANALGESIA: Excellent, long-lasting distraction from pain.

MUSCLE RELAXATION: Good.

DISSOCIATION: AK–47 can cause absentmindedness and has contributed to many a visitor to the Cannabis Cup in Amsterdam losing their bearings.

STIMULANT: More disorienting than stimulating.

SEDATION: AK–47 is not particularly sedating, but is so strong that it can leave a patient glued to his chair for hours.

BLUEBERRY

Blueberry emerged in the late 1990s as one of the classic hybrid *indica* varieties. It launched the entire range of Blue genetics popularized by the Dutch Passion seed bank in Amsterdam—with varieties including the extraordinary Blue Moonshine, Flo, Blue Velvet, and many others. Blueberry won the 2000 *High Times* Cannabis Cup.

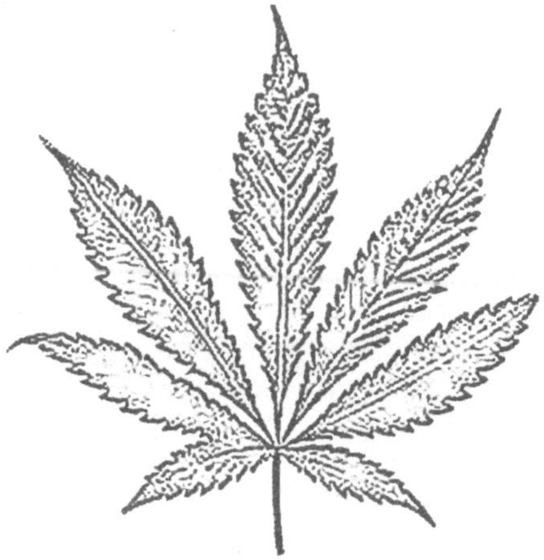

The Blue family of cannabis varieties was originally developed and refined by DJ Short, an Oregon cannabis breeder who began working with Mexican and Thai landrace genetics in the 1970s. With its distinctly sweet, fruit aroma and only a hint of skunk, Blueberry put to rest the criticism that Afghan-dominant varieties could only produce coarse- and acrid-smelling cannabis.

Notes

Today, great Blueberry is difficult to find, but it remains quite easy to recognize, since it smells very much like its namesake. One of the reasons that Blueberry is difficult to locate is a problem that plagues all contemporary cannabis breeding: maintaining stability of the genetic lines from seed. Creating a stable, true breeding variety is extremely time-consuming and labor-intensive. Growing out a few thousand plants in order to make selections is not a discreet endeavor, and it places the breeder at considerable risk. After Oregon passed its medical marijuana law, DJ Short teamed up with his son to revisit the breeding efforts that produced the original Blueberry. Their hope was to resurrect the magic of the early DJ Short crosses. The result was Whitaker Blues, a variety that many consider equal to his original Blueberry.

Medical Uses

Because Blueberry is potent without being overwhelming, it is often well tolerated by naive cannabis patients. Blueberry has often been cited for its ability to lift the spirits while ill. Patients note that Blueberry reduces anxiety, especially in social situations.

TYPE: 75 percent *indica.*

SPECIES: *Cannabis indica ssp. afghanica* × *cannabis indica ssp. indica.*

BREEDING DATE: 1980s.

GENETICS: "Juicy Fruit" Thai (landrace) × "Purple Thai" (Highland Oaxacan × Chocolate Thai) × Afghan. The genetics of Blueberry owe a lot to the great Thai Stick varieties of the Vietnam War period. The earlier Thai genetics from the mid-1960s often had a citrusy or fruity aroma, while the later Thai genetics smelled like cocoa. These varieties were pure tropical sativas cultivated within the Golden Triangle—an area in Southeast Asia known for its opium production. Burma, Cambodia, Laos, and Vietnam all produced cannabis of extraordinary quality through the 1970s. The Oaxacan region of Mexico produced Acapulco Gold and some narrow-leafleted cannabis that was among the first purple varieties brought to the United States.

SIMILAR VARIETIES: Blue Dream (sees page 124–25), Blueberry Sativa, Flo, Blue Velvet, Blue Moonshine, Whitaker Blues.

AVAILABILITY: Blueberry is available directly from DJ Short at his medical cannabis cultivation classes in the United States. Dutch Passion also still sells their version of Blueberry.

EASE OF CULTIVATION: Moderate—seven-to-eight-week flowering time.

AROMA: Blueberry and a little spice.

TASTE: Spicy fruit.

POTENCY: 14 to 16 percent THC.

DURATION OF EFFECTS: Long-lasting.

PSYCHOACTIVITY: All of DJ Short's genetics are noteworthy for the quality of their psychoactivity. Blueberry offers the epitome of a "functional high," and its effects are long-lasting. Even though the morphology of this plant is clearly Afghan-dominant, it retains the limonene effects associated with Blueberry's Thai and Oaxacan ancestors, with some relaxing *indica* myrcene in the mix.

ANALGESIA: Medium.

MUSCLE RELAXATION: Significant.

DISSOCIATION: None.

STIMULANT: Most patients find this variety to be creatively stimulating without being speedy. It is also great for appetite stimulation at low doses.

SEDATION: Gentle when used in the evening or before an afternoon nap.

BLUE DREAM, also known as **BLUEBERRY HAZE**

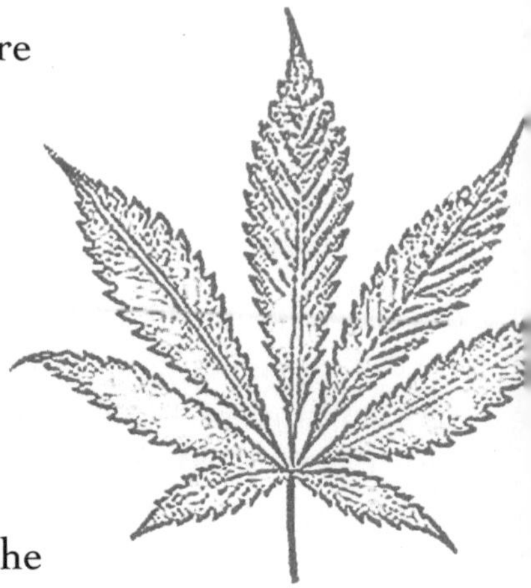

Two great cannabis varieties, Blueberry and Haze, were bred to produce this outstanding hybrid. Widely popular with medical cannabis patients for its potent and versatile broad-spectrum effects, and with cultivators for its big flowers and high yield, Blue Dream is found in nearly every dispensary on the U.S. West Coast. Blue Dream has exceptional trichome production and is very resinous. It is one of the few cannabis varieties that appeals to both the novice and the chronic care cannabis patient.

Medical Uses

A great choice for low and micro-doses. At higher doses though, it can "couchlock" nearly any patient. It's effective in elevating one's mood, and is an excellent choice for multi-target use—for example, pain and nausea or pain and insomnia. Blue Dream is an outstanding medicinal strain that rivals Jack Herer (see pages 142–43) in its wide range of medicinal applications. Patients with gastrointestinal issues consistently praise its effectiveness. It is rare to find an ultra-potent medication that is easy for patients to use at lower doses without becoming instantly overwhelmed. Its ability to help patients relax—but not become sedated—is very useful for daytime doses.

Notes

Among patients who prefer kush varieties, Blue Dream is the most popular non-kush choice. Why? It's likely because the Blue Dream variety expresses a lot of terpenes, producing an "entourage effect" similar to OG Kush (see pages 152–55). While it has yet to be confirmed, it may be that these terpene entourages reduce THC-tolerance buildup, and so regular users can use this variety effectively over long courses of treatment. Interestingly, Blue Dream has never fallen out of favor with patients, remaining consistently in demand over the last seven or eight years. Occasionally, a Blue Dream phenotype appears on a dispensary shelf with its customary high-THC content and an additional bonus up to 2 percent CBD—making it a real find.

TYPE: Broad- and narrow-leafleted cross—a true hybrid.

SPECIES: *Cannabis indica ssp. indica* × *ssp. afghanica.*

BREEDING DATE: Unconfirmed, but likely 2003 near Santa Cruz, California.

GENETICS: Between its two parents, Blueberry and Haze, this variety brings together Thai, Colombian, Indian, and Mexican genetics to impressive effect.

SIMILAR VARIETIES: Blueberry Sativa, Blue Dragon.

AVAILABILITY: Widely available as a cutting.

EASE OF CULTIVATION: As a big yielder and a hearty plant, it is reasonable project for talented novice patients.

AROMA: Often more "blueberry" than Blueberry, with a unique, spicy note of pepper and pine.

TASTE: Blue Dream is a classic combination of fruit and spice, with a haze aroma when smoked. It has a pure floral fruit flavor when vaporized. It is one of the best-tasting varieties of cannabis when the crop has been flushed of residual nutrients and properly cured.

POTENCY: Blue Dream approaches 25 percent THC on occasion, and is among the most potent varieties available.

DURATION OF EFFECTS: Long-lasting body and head effects for over two hours.

PSYCHOACTIVITY: At moderate doses, Blue Dream delivers a very potent combination of cerebral head high and relaxed body stone effects from lots of myrcene balanced by beta-caryophyllene and both pinenes.

ANALGESIA: It is excellent for distraction from pain and painful procedures. Its Haze parent helps to balance analgesia with alertness.

MUSCLE RELAXATION: Very relaxing; multiple sclerosis patients report that Blue Dream is effective for making spasticity and stiffness more tolerable.

DISSOCIATION: At high doses, Blue Dream's *indica* lineage takes over and the effect can become very stony.

STIMULANT: Because of its Haze lineage, it is a mild stimulant. It rarely causes anxiety, except at the highest doses.

SEDATION: As a very relaxing sedative, it is the choice of many insomnia patients. Blue Dream is appropriate for both evening and daytime use.

BUBBA KUSH

Bubba Kush is a classic broad-leafleted small *indica* that became one of the most popular medicinal cannabis varieties in California in the early 2000s. Bubba Kush is noteworthy for its moderate potency but narcotic effect. It shares many characteristics with Afghan varieties. In many ways, Bubba Kush may be as close to an exemplar kush as any variety widely available today. It is more refined than the early Afghans and produces a more interesting psychoactivity.

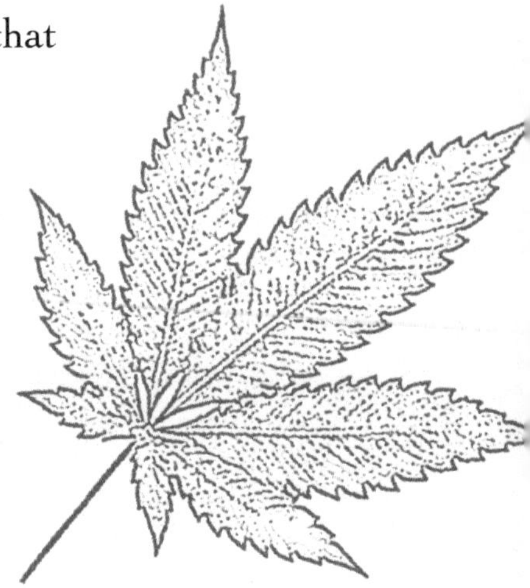

Medical Uses

Bubba Kush is an outstanding choice for pain and nausea. As such, Bubba has become the go-to variety for many chemotherapy patients. It can be challenging to titrate a proper daytime dose of Bubba Kush that avoids sedation, but is worth the effort. Its range of effects is well tolerated by most patients with cannabis experience, but novice cannabis patients may find it a bit too strong.

Notes

Bubba Kush is often overshadowed by OG Kush (see pages 152–55). The reality is that they are very different varieties. OG Kush is not a true kush while Bubba is more of a kush idealization, since it bears little resemblance to authentic kush landraces. Bubba is a perfect example of a cannabis variety with "bag appeal," the combination of look and aroma that catches the eye of the medical or recreational cannabis consumer. Fine-quality Bubba Kush is so covered with trichomes that it can actually be difficult to see the plant tissue beneath, as if the Bubba flower cluster is covered with pave-set resin diamonds. High-quality Bubba is very simple to identify: it looks and smells great. Beware of Bubba that has not been properly flushed of excess nutrients before harvest. This fault can be discerned by paying attention to the aftertaste, which should have no "chemmy" flavor—just clean floral spice.

TYPE: 100 percent *indica.*

SPECIES: *Cannabis indica ssp. afghanica*

BREEDING DATE: circa 1996.

GENETICS: Unknown, but likely of Afghan/Pakistani lineage.

SIMILAR VARIETIES: There are dozens of fine Bubba cuttings circulating within the medical cannabis community: Bomb Threat, Pre-98, Platinum, Presidential, etc.

AVAILABILITY: Cuttings only, readily available in western North America.

EASE OF CULTIVATION: Challenging! Bubba is often cultivated indoors with a "bonsai" approach, meaning the plants are flowered after a minimal vegetative growth phase, which keeps the plants very short. There is a 60-day flowering time.

AROMA: Sandalwood, pepper, balsam, citrus, coffee, spice, sour—never musty.

TASTE: Bubba has a very spicy, sour flavor when smoked. It has a strong floral hashish aftertaste with a note of B vitamins.

POTENCY: Despite extraordinary trichome coverage, its gland head size varies among cuttings. Its potency is widely variable under expert cultivation, from 14 to 20 percent THC.

DURATION OF EFFECTS: Bubba Kush is long-lasting with little ceiling, meaning that it will deliver increased effects with each sequential dose, instead of plateauing. A good variety for long-term medicinal use, and it may be that Bubba Kush's terpenoid profile slows the development of THC tolerance.

PSYCHOACTIVITY: Bubba Kush is considered to produce among the most stony psychoactive effects of any variety of cannabis. It tends to be mentally stimulating, while almost paralyzing the body. Time distortion is common: a hyperfocus effect alternating with drifting through clouds. Bubba Kush presents an extremely complex range of reactions and is a very "floaty" narcotic experience overall from its entourage of beta-caryophyllene, limonene, and myrcene. It has a reputation for being a "creeper," with the effects increasing in intensity over time. This was incorrectly thought to be due to the presence of CBD. As it turns out, Bubba Kush has virtually no CBD. Its creeper effects are likely due to its terpenoid or flavonoid (antioxidant) content, but more research is needed to confirm this hypothesis.

ANALGESIA: Very strong.

MUSCLE RELAXATION: Highly relaxing, nearly to the point of lethargy.

DISSOCIATION: Rare.

STIMULANT: It is mentally stimulating, but less so physically. It can cause anxiety at high doses.

SEDATION: High.

CHEM '91, also known as **CHEMDAWG**

Why the interest in the origin of Chem '91? Because it claims to be the closest ancestor of both OG Kush and Sour Diesel, two of the most popular cannabis varieties to appear in the last 20 years. The legend of the origin of Chem '91 is complex and begins in Montana, where the variety first appeared in the 1980s, supposedly under the name Chemdawg.

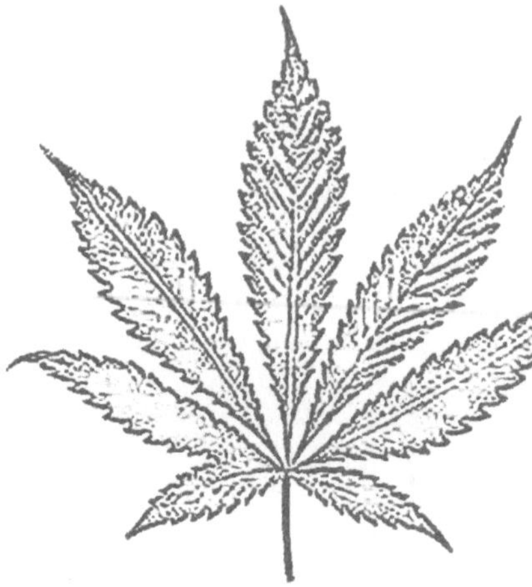

Chemdawg was popular in Montana because of its unique aroma and profusion of trichomes. A grower brought Chemdawg to Colorado where it became popular in the same circles as another legendary Colorado variety, the Paonia Purple Paralyzer, also known as P Bud. Chemdawg was supposedly seized in a raid in Montana and the variety is said to have survived within a small group of cultivators in Colorado. In 1988, two members of the Colorado Chemdawg circle went to a Grateful Dead concert in Noblesville, Indiana. There, they met a cannabis aficionado from Massachusetts who was extremely smitten with Chemdawg and secured an ounce from the Colorado boys for the lofty price of $500. The Massachusetts lad liked the Chemdawg so much that he later arranged to have more of it shipped home. In that shipment he discovered 13 seeds. Three years later, four of those seeds were germinated. Three females were found among those four seeds: Chemdawg '91, the Sister, and a third variety that was not kept. Chem '91 and the Sister were subsequently used as breeding stock for over a dozen varieties. OG Kush (see pages 152–55) was initially supposed to have been grown from some Chem '91 seeds found in a bag of Chemdawg buds in Lake Tahoe, California, in 1996. Sour Diesel (see pages 166–67) is supposed to have originated when a Northern Lights (see pages 150–51)/Hawaiian cross accidentally pollinated a cross of Chem '91 and Massachusetts Super Skunk. It is a surprisingly complex tale for a story involving an ultra-potent marijuana that tends to impair memory.

Medical Uses

Chem '91 is scarce and so few patients have been able to get hold of it that few medical uses have been found.

TYPE: Chem '91 is a relatively frail plant with moderately wide leaflets that underscore its hybrid lineage.

SPECIES: *Cannabis indica ssp. afghanica* × *cannabis indica ssp. indica.*

BREEDING DATE: Introduced sometime in the 1980s, likely in Montana.

GENETICS: Unknown. The landrace varieties used to breed the variety remain unknown, with Skunk (see pages 164–65, Afghan (see pages 118–19), Thai, and Northern Lights cited among its ancestors. Varieties with a fuel or diesel aroma, like Chemdawg, have been found in Nepal.

SIMILAR VARIETIES: OG Kush, Sour Diesel, Chem D, Double Dawg, Chem 4, Snowdawg.

AVAILABILITY: Available as cutting only. Not widely circulated.

EASE OF CULTIVATION: Difficult. Chem '91 is a tricky plant to grow, with little mold or insect resistance.

AROMA: Chem '91 has a unique aroma and not a particularly pleasant one. It has been described as a mix of diesel fuel and bad breath. There is definitely a note of something rotten in Chemdawg's aroma, likely from an uncommon sesquiterpene. Its fuel aroma comes from beta-caryophyllene and limonene atop a big myrcene content.

TASTE: Superb mix of floral hashish and sour citrus.

POTENCY: Potent, but not as potent as many of its progeny, such as OG Kush and Sour Diesel, but when its myrcene kicks in, you'll stay put.

DURATION OF EFFECTS: Fast onset and the subsequent effects last for several hours.

PSYCHOACTIVITY: The psychoactive effects of Chem '91 are very complex and much more than its THC content, since Chem '91 produces a wide range of synergistic terpenes.

ANALGESIA: Classically numbing, almost like an anesthetic.

MUSCLE RELAXATION: Only moderately relaxing.

DISSOCIATION: At higher doses, Chem '91 can send someone to Mars or a reasonable facsimile.

STIMULANT: Stimulating to a degree that can be anxiety-provoking for some patients.

SEDATION: The effects of Chem '91 tend to "crash," meaning that the high starts euphoricially, but can settle into a mildly narcotic stone after 90 minutes.

CHERRY COUGH

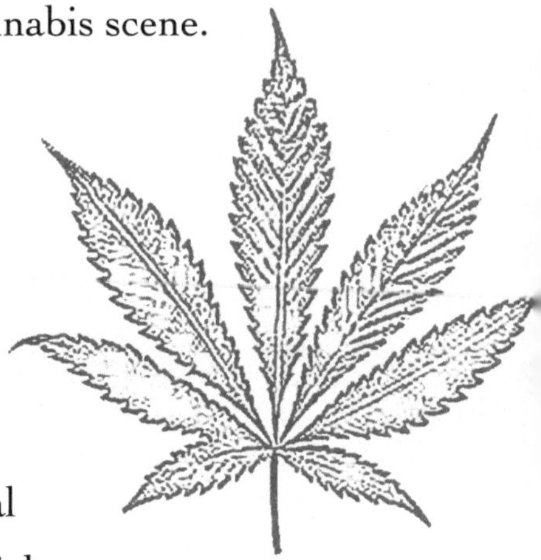

Cherry Cough is a recent arrival on the medical cannabis scene. It is a cross of a broad-leafleted Afghan with a narrow-leafleted Strawberry Cough. Such crosses tend to favor one parent. With Cherry Cough, its berry parent passed on its happy, mood-elevating effect but the Afghan contributed significant analgesia and relaxation. With clear intent, more and more varieties will be developed to fill medicinal niches. In the case of Cherry Cough, it's filled the niche for a mood-elevating med that also helps a patient sleep. This is a tall order however, since those characteristics rarely coexist in cannabis.

Medical Uses

From post-traumatic stress disorder to acute neuropathic pain, Cherry Cough is good for enforcing relaxation. It is also popular with older patients with chronic aches and pains, since it makes it very hard to focus on discomfort for any length of time. Cherry Cough is favored by insomnia patients and anyone recovering from surgery who is having a tough time falling asleep.

Notes

It is interesting to contrast this with Strawberry Cough (see pages 168–69). Strawberry has more THC, but Cherry Cough has significantly more sedative and "couchlock"-inducing abilities. Strawberry Cough won't interfere with memory, while Cherry Cough nearly guarantees that you'll temporarily misplace something. Cherry aromas on cannabis varieties only began to be discovered in 2010. They appear to be a combination of myrcene, terpinolene, and linalool. This terpene combination is often found on the much spicier and less fruity Bubba Kush (see pages 126–27), but here the proportions of each terpene are very different. Several patients have commented that Cherry Cough makes it nearly impossible to watch television because one quickly falls asleep.

TYPE: Broad-leafleted hybrid.

SPECIES: *Cannabis indica ssp. indica × ssp. afghanica.*

BREEDING DATE: 2010.

GENETICS: Broad-leafleted Afghan *indica* with a narrow-leafleted Strawberry Cough.

SIMILAR VARIETIES: Strawberry Cough, Cherry Pie, Grape Ape.

AVAILABILITY: Currently only available in a few California dispensaries.

EASE OF CULTIVATION: Not a beginner's crop, but Cherry Cough is a good long-term prospect for the more experienced enthusiast. It is an excellent yielder and easy feeder.

AROMA: Very pleasing fragrance of spiced cherry cough drops with a hint of castile soap.

TASTE: Cherry spice with a hashish exhale

POTENCY: Moderate. Cherry Cough is a good choice for a daytime, broad-leafleted variety that is not too strong. It typically hits around 16 percent THC.

DURATION OF EFFECTS: With very long-lasting effects, Cherry Cough seems to persist forever. This can be convenient for patients that are not given many opportunities to medicate. The length of effect might be due to the terpene linalool, which is a powerful and smooth muscle relaxant.

PSYCHOACTIVITY: Cherry Cough delivers a floating, dreamy psychoactivity accompanied by a smile. It does not induce a profound stone like a purple variety, and patients with mild depression have reported that it gently lifts the spirits.

ANALGESIA: Excellent distraction from pain and also good for painful outpatient medical procedures.

MUSCLE RELAXATION: Cherry Cough is a great variety for relaxing tight muscles or recovering from athletic strains or back pain.

DISSOCIATION: Cherry Cough is not conducive to concentration. Prepare to drift.

STIMULANT: Not much of a stimulant at all, it is much more of a chill pill experience.

SEDATION: Excellent for a quick nap or a long snooze.

G13

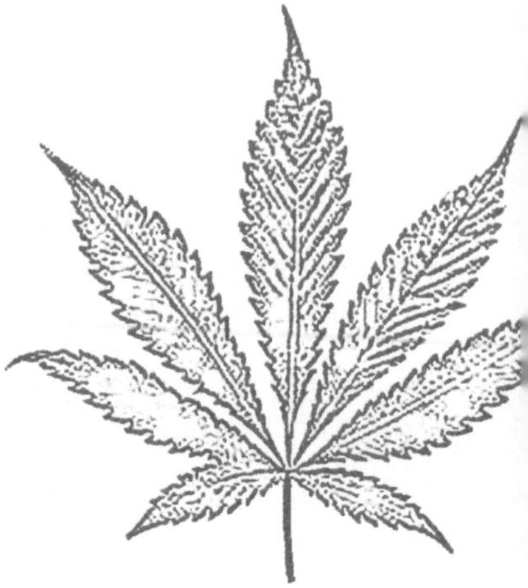

G13 is a cannabis variety with a movie star story. It is supposed to have originated in the 1970s within the confines of a top secret, secure U.S. government cannabis research facility. This special variety was alleged to have exceeded 29 percent THC. The reality is that the U.S. government does have an official secure marijuana plantation located at the National Center for Natural Products Research (NCNPR) at the University of Mississippi. Supposedly G13 was developed at NCNPR and liberated as a cutting through unknown means. Someone gave G13 to Neville, the Dutch breeder, and the legend grew. Today, G13 is typically used as a breeding plant, but it is also available in dispensaries.

Medical Uses

G13 is a good choice for a myrcene-dominant, sedative *indica* medicine. It is also popular with migraine patients both for prophylaxis and acute care, but overdosage can lead to "rebound" headaches.

Notes

In the 1999 film *American Beauty*, the actor Wes Bentley plays a young marijuana dealer who specializes in selling G13 for $2,000 per ounce, an insanely high sum. This supporting role in an Oscar-winning film has further cemented the variety's legend.

Since 1968, the U.S. government has exercised its monopoly on the production of all cannabis for domestic scientific and medical research through a contract with the University of Mississippi. The Drug Enforcement Administration (DEA) issues permits to a few researchers each year to receive some of this cannabis, most often for studies that emphasize some possible risk of marijuana use. Over the years, NCNPR has assembled quite a collection of seeds from U.S. Customs seizures and DEA drug raids. NCNPR grows these seeds and analyzes the results, while conducting fundamental research on the plant and its metabolism and chemistry. The NCNPR Marijuana Project also produces pre-rolled cannabis cigarettes for the Compassionate Investigational New Drug Program (IND), a project designed to study cannabis as a medicine. Even though the IND was shut down during the administration of President George H. W. Bush, four surviving medical cannabis patients still receive a tin of 300 marijuana cigarettes per month, and will do so in perpetuity under the terms of program.

So could G13 have originated with the U.S. government? The short answer is yes. It didn't have to be a 29 percent THC producer, though. In the mid-1970s, Afghan varieties were extremely rare and it is not preposterous to think that a graduate student might have been enticed to liberate a cutting. We'll never know, but the story is fantastic and the variety is good medicine.

TYPE: Broad-leafleted *indica.*

SPECIES: *Cannabis indica ssp. afghanica.*

BREEDING DATE: circa 1970s.

GENETICS: Unknown, presumed Afghan.

SIMILAR VARIETIES: G13 Haze, Amnesia G13.

AVAILABILITY: As a cutting, G13 is available in some dispensaries. As a seed, it can rarely be found on its own—though often in hybrids.

EASE OF CULTIVATION: Easy.

AROMA: Skunky and heavy with plenty of balsamic myrcene.

TASTE: Just average, according to many patients.

POTENCY: High, though not to the exalted level promised by the G13 legend. However, it often tops 21 percent THC.

DURATION OF EFFECTS: Long-lasting, up to three hours.

PSYCHOACTIVITY: Primarily body, with a narcotic and stony quality.

ANALGESIA: Very good, especially for nausea relief.

MUSCLE RELAXATION: Noted for its relaxing effects.

DISSOCIATION: Spacey and forgetful.

STIMULANT: Very little.

SEDATION: Good medicine for insomniacs.

GRAND DADDY PURPLE, also known as GDP

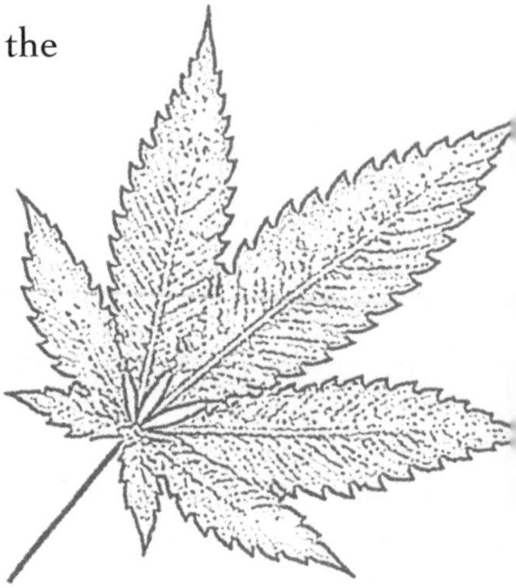

One of the best purple medical cannabis varieties on the U.S. West Coast, and especially popular around the San Francisco Bay Area, Grand Daddy Purple became available in the early 2000s. Many consider "Ken's GDP" to be the highest-quality cutting of this variety. Today, other purple medical cannabis varieties such as Purple Urkle and Girl Scout Cookies wrestle with GDP for the mantle of top purple. Many first trips to a medical cannabis dispensary have culminated with a Grand Daddy Purple purchase; the irresistible initial appeal of purple cannabis is its otherworldly appearance. GDP is dark purple with bright orange pistillate hairs, covered with glistening clear and milky trichomes.

Medical Uses

Purples are excellent for bed rest and recovery. They are too strong to produce anything but a healing inertia. Because most purples tend to make patients a bit forgetful, GDP is often recommended for post-traumatic stress disorder. Purples are also popular for chemotherapy-induced nausea and discomfort, including neuropathy. These varieties are also effective for any severe illness in which "just waiting it out" is part of the process.

Notes

Some strains of cannabis turn purple as a response to a stimulus. That stimulus could be cold, stress, or an infestation. Typically though, the stressor is cold temperature. The purple coloration is from the same pigment produced by blueberries, apples, and grapes—called anthocyanin. Purple varieties of cannabis, if left unstressed, won't turn purple, but can still reach and even exceed their potential potency.

The first purple cannabis was brought to California in the mid-1960s from mountains of Zacatecas, Mexico. The story goes that an American smuggler drove a load of purple cannabis up from Mexico to San Francisco. With 110 pounds (50 kilograms) of this purple sequestered in his trunk, his car broke down on Market Street downtown in the mid-afternoon. He pushed his car to a parking meter. Over the next five hours, using a nearby phone booth, he sold all 50 kilos, right from the trunk as he kept a close eye out for any police. Purple cannabis had never been seen before, and the Bay Area's love affair with this unique cannabis continues to this day.

TYPE: Broad-leafleted *indica* (80 percent).

SPECIES: *Cannabis indica ssp. indica var. afghanica* × *var. mexicana.*

BREEDING DATE: circa 2000.

GENETICS: Purple Urkle × Salmon Creek Big Bud.

SIMILAR VARIETIES: Purple Urkle, Girl Scout Cookies, Kryptonite.

AVAILABILITY: Cuttings only in dispensaries in California, Colorado, and Washington.

EASE OF CULTIVATION: Good single plant project for the novice.

AROMA: Grape, pepper, and skunk from a myrcene/beta-caryophyllene combo with hints of ocimene and linalool.

TASTE: Spicy and hashy with a hint of wine.

POTENCY: GDP consistently exceeds 20 percent THC.

DURATION OF EFFECTS: Long-lasting.

PSYCHOACTIVITY: Purple indicas deliver among the heaviest-hitting psychoactivity of any cannabis. Caution should be observed when trying it for the first time since its effects are rarely characterized as "functional." This is the wrong variety on which to drive, operate machinery, or attempt anything beyond the complexity of eating a banana and staring contently at the wall.

ANALGESIA: Excellent at moderate dose; numbing at lower doses.

MUSCLE RELAXATION: Excellent. Grand Daddy Purple is very synergistic with other pain medications.

DISSOCIATION: There are special terms for the effect of GDP, specifically "couchlock" and "stuck" for the tendency of these varieties to leave you precisely where they found you.

STIMULANT: During the initial onset only.

SEDATION: Great for sleep and relaxation.

HARLEQUIN, CANNATONIC, & HIGH-CBD CANNABIS

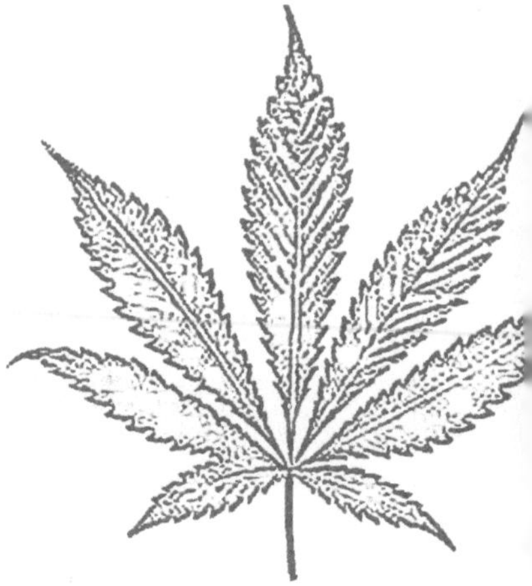

Cannabidiol (CBD) is the second most common cannabinoid produced by the cannabis plant. CBD is non-psychoactive, but produces a wide range of medicinal effects. Until recently, CBD was virtually impossible to find within medical cannabis varieties in the United States. In Europe, the Hortapharm team, and later GW Pharmaceuticals, were the first to recognize the incredible value of CBD. In the U.S., Martin Lee, Fred Gardner, and Sarah Russo helped to lead the search for high-CBD cultivars and promote their use through Project CBD. This non-profit was specifically established by Lee and Gardner to encourage the broader dissemination of CBD cultivars.

Medical Uses

Medical applications are potentially vast, but the effective doses for different medical conditions in humans are not well understood. Preliminary reports from patients treating anxiety indicate that CBD is effective at lower doses than THC, around 2.5 milligrams.[1] Extrapolating beyond that guidance is difficult. CBD is nontoxic, so in the absence of THC, higher doses are likely to be well tolerated. In the presence of THC, care must be observed with doses for naive patients.

Within a year, over a dozen varieties had been identified. Within two years, Harlequin, Sour Tsunami, Omrita Rx, Cannatonic, and others became available at a few dispensaries in California and Colorado. Cuttings were also being distributed of Harlequin and Cannatonic. By late 2012, the first nearly pure CBD cultivars began to emerge, including a Cannatonic C6 with a 35 to one CBD to THC ratio, also called ACDC.

Notes

With any claimed CBD genetics, always insist on seeing test results from a reputable laboratory.

TYPE: Narrow-leafleted hemp hybridized with narrow-leafleted and broad-leafleted drug varieties.

SPECIES: *Cannabis sativa × cannabis indica.*

BREEDING DATE: High-CBD varieties began to be identified by laboratories beginning in 2009.

GENETICS: All the high-CBD genetics are partially derived from hemp fiber varieties of cannabis, since these plants produce the enzyme that transforms CBGA into CBDA, the acidic precursor of CBD.

SIMILAR VARIETIES (COURTESY PROJECT CBD): Sour Tsunami, Harlequin, Omrita Rx3, Jamaican Lion, Cannatonic, Sugaree × Blue Diesel, Poison OG, Granny Durkel.

AVAILABILITY: Cuttings only, though Cannatonic is available in seed form from Resin Seeds in Spain.

EASE OF CULTIVATION: Easy to grow, but a little tricky to optimize for CBD production.

AROMA: These are typically not the most pleasingly aromatic varieties, since they were originally selected to produce rope, not dope. But that's changing… Harlequin, the most widely available of the CBD varieties, has a nice minty fragrance when well cultivated from its pinene and myrcene expression.

TASTE: There is wide variation in taste among CBD varieties. The general consensus is that most are not as flavorful as their high-THC counterparts.

POTENCY: The highest CBD percentage seen in 2013 was 22 percent in a Cannatonic. Harlequin can hit 15 percent CBD with 5 percent THC. Sour Tsunami has an identical three to one ratio of CBD to THC. Potency may not be nearly as important with CBD as the ratio of CBD to THC. One phenotype of Cannatonic was tested at 18.5 percent CBD to 0.6 percent THC, a ratio of over 30 to one.

DURATION OF EFFECTS: Most CBD varieties with only a tiny amount of THC will deliver a distinct CBD effect for several hours.

PSYCHOACTIVITY: In the near absence of THC, there is virtually no psychoactivity. The ratio of CBD to THC does appear to blunt the effects of THC. However CBD varieties produce something like psychoactivity, but different. It is possible that it's just the CBD drug effect being felt.

ANALGESIA: Effective, but too soon to tell if it is a better analgesic than THC.

MUSCLE RELAXATION: Very relaxing.

DISSOCIATION: The most accurate description of the CBD is that the patient feels protected by a layer of bunting. There is a slight dissociation.

STIMULANT: Never sleepy, but never truly stimulating either.

SEDATION: It is claimed in some research studies that CBD can produce "mental sedation" at high doses. This is characterized as a dulling of the mind. With reasonable doses (below 20 milligrams), CBD does not appear to interfere with cognition at all, though this needs to be more rigorously tested.

HAZE

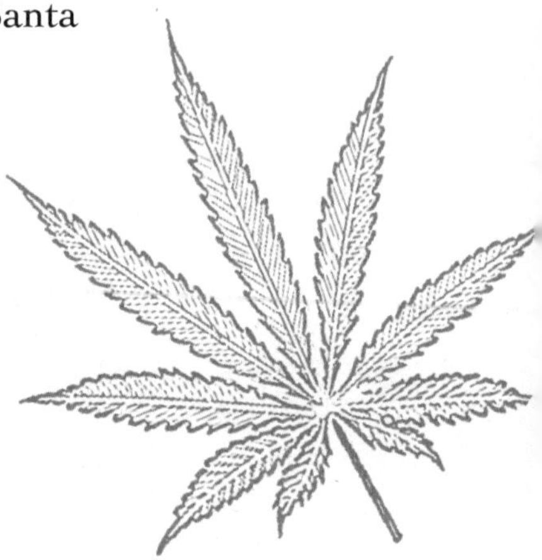

In the late 1960s and early 1970s, two friends from Santa Cruz began a short-lived outdoor cannabis breeding experiment that would profoundly influence all marijuana cultivation for the following 40 years. Their cannabis variety was called Haze and it combined the finest narrow-leafleted sativas gathered from Mexico, Thailand, India, and Colombia into the first superstar cannabis variety. Haze quickly gained a reputation as the world's finest cannabis. Each individual ounce of Haze was delivered in a redwood box emblazoned with a custom label. Each season a new version of Haze was introduced: Magenta, Gold, Silver, Purple, and Blue.

Medical Uses

Among medical cannabis varieties, Haze is a good choice for daytime use (at low doses) since it results in little cognitive impairment. It is an excellent choice for attention deficit/hyperactivity disorder, as it encourages hyperfocus at low doses. Its reputation as a "clean the house" med is well founded. Haze is a nearly perfect micro-dose cannabis medicine, since at this small dose range it seems to sharpen rather than dull the senses. At high doses, Hazes can induce profound, even uncomfortable, experiences.

As varieties hailing from tropical climes, the Hazes did not flower in greenhouses until mid-December. One variety flowered until mid-January. This long flowering time ensured phenomenal psychoactivity, but also risks to the cultivator. By the late 1970s, state and federal marijuana eradication programs made large-scale cultivation of long-flowering tropical varieties nearly impossible. A serious case might be made for Haze, along with Kona Gold, as consistently the greatest cannabis variety of all time.

Notes

Haze, a foundation of our cannabis past, is likely to form the basis of our future cannabis. As cannabis prohibition crumbles, tropical varieties that are impossible to produce stealthily will begin to reemerge into the marketplace. In the United States, commercial greenhouse production of Haze varieties is likely in the next five years.

TYPE: Pure narrow-leafleted tropical *sativa*.

SPECIES: *Cannabis indica ssp. indica*.

BREEDING DATE: 1971–76.

GENETICS: Colombian, Thai, Indian, and Mexican lineage.

SIMILAR VARIETIES: Hazes had a huge impact on the nascent Dutch cannabis scene of the 1980s. Celebrated cannabis breeder Neville used an original Haze to breed Neville's Haze (see pages 148–49). Super Silver Haze won three consecutive *High Times* Cannabis Cups. More recently, Lemon Haze has become popular on the U.S. West Coast.

AVAILABILITY: Several Dutch seed banks claim to maintain stocks of the original Haze germplasm brought to the Netherlands by David Watson, but this assertion is disputed. Watson has stated that the Haze that he delivered was better breeding stock than an actual candidate for cultivation. Recently some vintage Haze seeds have surfaced in both Santa Cruz and Oakland, California. Tissue culture techniques will be used in an attempt to rescue a few viable plant embryos from these very old seeds. But medicinal cannabis experts are extremely interested in this variety and want to incorporate it into the next generation of post-prohibition medical cannabis.

EASE OF CULTIVATION: Because of its tendency to grow very tall and its long flowering time, Haze is for expert cultivators. The closer to the equator it's grown, the better the result. The finest Haze in recent times was cultivated on one of the more remote Hawaiian Islands.

AROMA: When burned, Haze has a unique spicy character that makes it instantly recognizable. It does not smell like marijuana; *it smells like Haze*.

TASTE: Haze's taste is complex, with notes of licorice, pepper, soap, citrus, and cocoa. No sweetness, just sophistication.

POTENCY: For its time—unprecedented. Haze averages 20 percent THC, with claims of up to 2 percent CBD.

DURATION OF EFFECTS: Extremely long-lasting, although the effects of Haze diminish almost imperceptibly, avoiding the "crash" associated with some stimulating varieties of cannabis.

PSYCHOACTIVITY: Psychedelic at higher doses. This makes Haze of potential interest as an insight drug for use with end-of-life hospice patients.

ANALGESIA: Medium.

MUSCLE RELAXATION: Mild.

DISSOCIATION: Strong at moderate and higher dosages.

STIMULANT: Very stimulating and can cause anxiety in the susceptible.

SEDATION: Little.

HINDU KUSH

Hindu Kush is a true kush, which differs considerably from the top-shelf "Kush" that is currently the craze in U.S. dispensaries. In many ways, it is closer to an old-school landrace Afghan than even Afghani #1 (see pages 118–19). True kush varieties were not bred to be smoked as flowers; they are hash plants, intended to be dried and sifted for their trichome heads. So while Hindu Kush is an authentic representation of what is smoked in Central Asia, we don't smoke it as it smoked there.

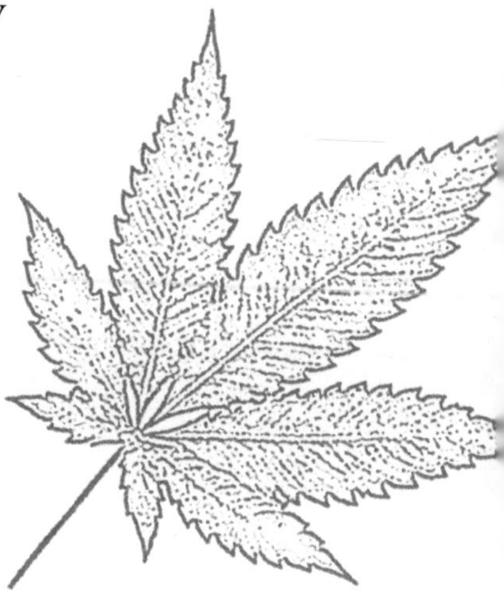

Medical Uses

Hindu Kush is used for the basics: back pain, sleep, and appetite. Some things haven't changed in centuries. Occasionally, Hindu Kush varieties will produce rare cannabinoids like CDBV and THCV. These strains are so rare in North America and Europe that virtually no laboratory can currently test for their presence. If eventually found in Hindu Kush varieties in the West, the medicinal significance to patients will increase dramatically.

To most Westerners, Hindu Kush seems a little coarse and rough. That is simply because, normally, Hindu Kush is refined through extraction. Smoking Hindu Kush flowers is a bit like eating raw garlic, then complaining that it's too pungent. Nearly all of Central Asia's cannabis varieties are grown solely for extraction.

Notes

Since this variety and its brethren were designed to make hashish, it can be a fun project if you have access to a small crop. In Central Asia, the hashish is dry-sifted through cloth screens. The cannabis is first carefully and thoroughly dried, to make it easier to separate the trichomes from the plant. Once this separation is complete, the resulting resin powder is resifted until as little plant matter remains as possible. The ideal: pure gland heads. If you attempt the extraction process, you'll definitely develop an appreciation for how much work sieving hashish requires.

There is not one Hindu Kush variety; it is likely that in the 1970s there were dozens of acclimatized kush landraces scattered from the Kashmiri border across Pakistan and into Afghanistan. Devout followers of fatwas condemning the use of cannabis resin may have destroyed many of these varieties, but some true kush varieties likely still survive.

TYPE: Broad-leafleted landrace.

SPECIES: *Cannabis indica ssp. afghanica.*

BREEDING DATE: Probably first cultivated in the thirteenth century.

GENETICS: Afghan or Pakistani hash plant.

SIMILAR VARIETIES: Afghan, AfPak, Hindu Skunk.

AVAILABILITY: Widely available as seeds and cuttings.

EASE OF CULTIVATION: Easy, but humidity must be controlled to avoid molds.

AROMA: A subtle scent of incense and spice, but primarily it smells like fresh hashish. Its terpenes include myrcene and beta-caryophyllene with a dollop of limonene. These varieties were never selected for their fancy fruit aromas, but there are some true kush landraces with a little Diesel tang.

TASTE: Hashy, earthy, and a little harsh.

POTENCY: While there are phenotypes of these kush plants that test over 20 percent THC, the most authentic specimens are between 12 to 16 percent THC.

DURATION OF EFFECTS: Very long.

PSYCHOACTIVITY: Not subtle—just a strong *indica* stone. Hindu Kush is not intended to do much beyond plaster the patient to the nearest surface. In Asia, this is the daily smoke in a harsh environment, so it takes the edge off without a lot of psychedelic insight.

ANALGESIA: Great for soothing those muscles as you trek up the Khyber Pass. This may sound arch, but making tough physical labor more tolerable is precisely what this plant was selected for.

MUSCLE RELAXATION: Good.

DISSOCIATION: Not much, except for a general thickening of thought.

STIMULANT: Negligible.

SEDATION: Works very well at night.

JACK HERER

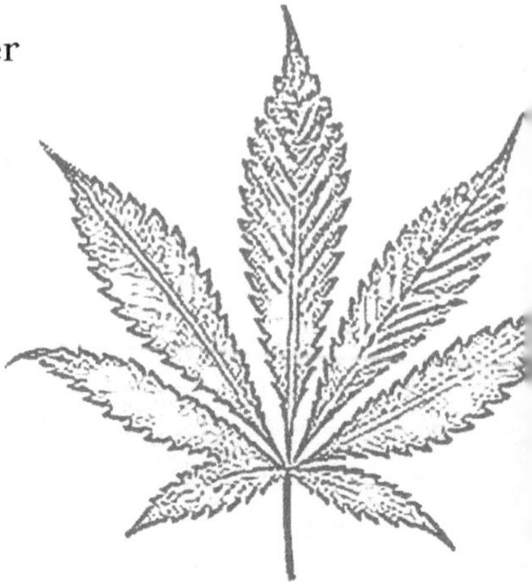

The 1994 *High Times* Cannabis Cup winner, Jack Herer was released as a seed variety and developed by cannabis seed bank Sensi Seeds, in Amsterdam. The variety was named in honor of Jack Herer (1939–2010), noted cannabis activist and author of the classic hemp history, *The Emperor Wears No Clothes* (Ah Ha Publishing, 1985). The Jack Herer variety was selected by Dutch company Bedrocan as a herbal cannabis product, available from Dutch pharmacies with a doctor's prescription.

A Jack Herer seed typically produces one of four different phenotypes: three narrow-leafleted and a single broader-leafleted. The Bedrocan Jack is the "Lemon" phenotype. When cultivated indoors, Jack can produce quite large flower clusters—in excess of seven grams. In many aspects, Jack Herer is the antithesis of the stereotypical stoner marijuana variety, since its effects are so upbeat and functional.

Medical Uses

Great for low-dose daytime medical regimens, both smoked and vaporized. Provides excellent distraction from pain and nausea.

Notes

One of the most popular varieties with patients throughout the world, Jack Herer is a true elite cannabis genetic. It is likely the most popular daytime cannabis variety. It requires extra protection from heat to keep its citrus components from harm, and also makes excellent extractions. As an alternative to smoking, the Dutch government encouraged the development of a tea often prepared with the Bedrocan Jack. The recipe calls for:

- one gram of Jack Herer
- one quart (roughly one liter) of water
- a saucepan and lid
- a strainer
- coffee creamer or whole milk

The creamer is a crucial ingredient, since it serves as an emulsifier and helps keeps the cannabinoids suspended in the water, preventing them from precipitating out of the solution. The tea is prepared by boiling water in a pan. Add the cannabis, reduce heat, and simmer covered for 15 minutes. Do not continue to boil. Afterward, strain the tea into a container. Immediately add creamer and mix thoroughly. Mint, lemon, or honey can also improve the taste a bit. A standard dose in the Netherlands is one cup, and the tea keeps refrigerated for three to five days. Cannabis tea, because it doesn't heat the cannabis to temperatures at which its THC acid is converted to free THC, is less psychoactive. While psychoactivity is reduced with cannabis tea, the tea can still pack a wallop. Don't drink it like regular tea—but like medicine.

TYPE: Narrow-leafleted hybrid *indica*.

SPECIES: *Cannabis indica var. indica* × *var. afghanica*

BREEDING DATE: 1994, released in 1995.

GENETICS: This variety was bred from Sensi Seeds and Dutch cannabis stalwarts: Northern Lights #5, Haze, and Skunk #1, though unconfirmed by Sensi. The phenotype more strongly resembles Shiva Skunk (NL#5 × Skunk), likely Jack Herer's parent.

SIMILAR VARIETIES: Jack Flash, Shiva Skunk.

AVAILABILITY: Jack Herer is available from many sources, as both Sensi Seeds and cuttings. It is widely cultivated in every medical cannabis jurisdiction in the United States.

EASE OF CULTIVATION: Jack Herer is not the easiest strain for a novice, though many have mastered it. Managing the growth of phenotypes indoors can require thought.

AROMA: The different phenotypes range from citrusy to a sweet skunk. The citrus comes in part from its high expression of terpinolene.

TASTE: The citrus phenotype is extremely well received for its sour fruit flavor.

POTENCY: High—regularly over 20 percent THC.

DURATION OF EFFECTS: Medium.

PSYCHOACTIVITY: Jack Herer produces strong upbeat reactions, with clear, clean cerebral effects from high terpinolene and low myrcene content that can border on electric.

ANALGESIA: Good for daytime pain treatment at moderate doses.

MUSCLE RELAXATION: This variety is a bit energetic to be considered relaxing, but is rarely jittery.

DISSOCIATION: At higher doses, Jack Herer phenotypes will cheerfully convey you to Mars.

STIMULANT: The persistent "up" effect of this variety is euphoric. Overmedication with Jack Herer *sativa* phenotypes can cause trigger anxiety in the susceptible.

SEDATION: While not sedating, Jack Herer won't interfere with relaxation.

LA CONFIDENTIAL

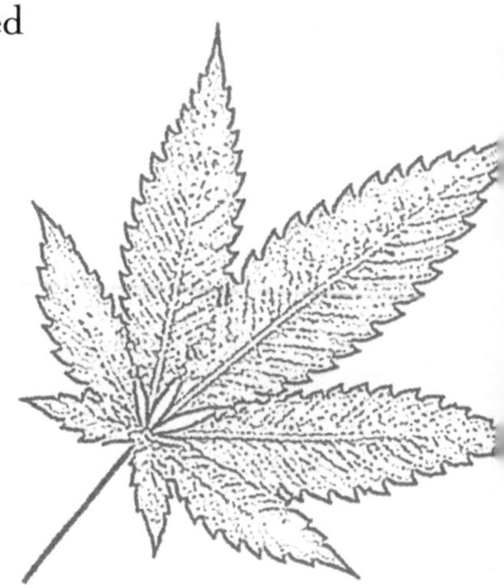

Don and Aaron, two friends from Los Angeles, moved to Amsterdam in the early 2000s to start a seed bank and develop medical varieties from the elite kush clones of Southern California. With them Don and Aaron brought many of LA's finest, including the Affie, several cuts of OG Kush, Master Kush, Bubba Kush, etc. It was a brilliant idea at precisely the right time. The California medical cannabis scene was starting to generate buzz for its extraordinary genetics. Dispensaries in West Hollywood were getting $125 for an eighth (3.5 grams) of their best Pure Kush. It was a bubble, and a relatively short-lived one.

But the hype of that bubble survived the crash. And the varieties that became famous stayed famous, partially thanks to hip-hop anthems which sang the praises of OG (see pages 152–55) and Sour Diesel (see pages 166–67). Don and Aaron's first big project was to try to re-create the Affie for the seed market, at a time when it was the toughest clone variety to acquire in Los Angeles. The result was an Affie × Afghani cross called LA Confidential. In 2004, they took third place in the *indica* division of the *High Times* Cannabis Cup. It was the highest award received by a new seed company in many years. The following year they took second place in the Indica Cup with LA Con.

Medical Uses

LA Confidential is a great pain medicine, as good as any cannabis variety gets. Patients report that it is also effective for calming flare-ups of Crohn's disease and irritable bowel syndrome. Low doses of LA Con are used to treat anxiety and slightly higher doses can help agoraphobia. It is also used for seizure disorders and migraines, because of its high myrcene and linalool content.

Notes

The medicinal uses of the elite indicas such as LA Con extend beyond their strong psychoactivity. Most of these elite genetics produce significant amounts of multiple terpenes, which increases these varieties' ranges of efficacy. Patients using these high-terpenoid elite genetics also report less THC tolerance buildup.

For many years, Dutch-developed cannabis genetics were the top of the cannabis potency heap. Since the mid-2000s, ultra-potent meds have been developed in the U.S. and Canada too. Well-cultivated LA Confidential is nearly indistinguishable from the Affie, down to the purple tinges that encircle both varieties' buds like halos. When Don and Aaron took the Affie to Amsterdam in 2004, it was selling wholesale in Los Angeles for $6,400 per pound (0.5 kilogram).

Today, Don and Aaron's DNA Genetics has won a prize in every *High Times* Cannabis Cup since they first entered LA Confidential. They have won several prizes for hashish, which is rarely awarded to foreigners. Ten years after they left Los Angeles, they introduced seeds of the actual LA Affie.

TYPE: Pure broad-leafleted *indica* cross.

SPECIES: *Cannabis indica ssp. afghanica.*

BREEDING DATE: 2003.

GENETICS: The Affie × Afghani.

SIMILAR VARIETIES: Afghan (see pages 118–19), Afghani, Bubba Kush (see pages 126–127), Hindu Kush (see pages 140–141), Master Kush, Purple Master.

AVAILABILITY: Seed from DNA Genetics, cuttings around California and Colorado.

EASE OF CULTIVATION: According to the breeders at DNA Genetics, there are two phenotypes of LA Confidential when grown from seed. The preferred phenotype has a much stronger aroma and is slightly taller. LA Confidential benefits from the "ScrOG" (Screen of Green) growing approach, which employs net mesh to control the height and shape of the flowering plants.

AROMA: Pure coffee and spice from linalool and perhaps humulene.

TASTE: Sandalwood incense and a sour citrus hint.

POTENCY: Over 22 percent THC.

DURATION OF EFFECTS: Three to four hours.

PSYCHOACTIVITY: LA Confidential is intense with a profound introspective effect. For its level of potency, the psychoactive effects remain relatively clear.

ANALGESIA: Excellent.

MUSCLE RELAXATION: Very good.

DISSOCIATION: Little, except at high doses.

STIMULANT: A touch of raciness, but subtle.

SEDATION: Strong.

MALAWI GOLD

Malawi is small landlocked country in southeastern Africa, nicknamed "The Warm Heart of Africa." For those familiar with Malawi Gold, a cannabis variety cultivated there for centuries, it's easy to imagine that the exceptional quality of their landrace cannabis inspired this sobriquet. Malawi Gold is of significant medicinal interest because it produces a portion of its THC as its rarer cousin: THCV. THCV is currently being studied for potential treatment for a range of liver diseases, and also for treating inflammation-related obesity. In Malawi, the variety is grown across the country and is the nation's third biggest export.

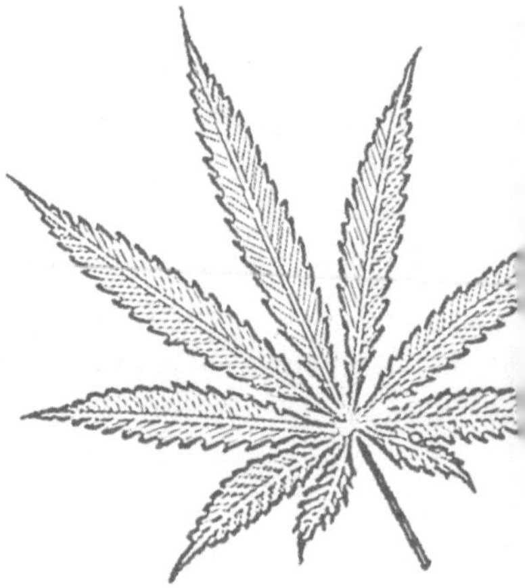

Medical Uses

THCV varieties are likely to become candidates for treating migraines, obesity, and metabolic disorders. They often act and wear off more quickly than THC or CBD varieties.

Notes

Landrace varieties are widely, and discreetly, traded among aficionados the world over. They are crucial to medical cannabis research, and they bring much-needed genetic diversity to our very inbred cannabis gene pool. Nepal, Kashmir, Brazil, China, and Korea all produce landrace varieties that may provide the next generation of medical cannabis. THCV, found in Malawi Gold, is so rarely present in cannabis that a 2013 survey of California dispensaries could not find a single medical cannabis variety containing it. One collective in Santa Cruz, WAAM, cultivates a cross of Malawi Gold for its very private community of severely ill patients.

The reason that THCV meds are scarce has more to do with the evolving progress of cannabis laboratories in California. The THCV varieties are out there, but have yet to been found by the laboratories, many of whom do not currently even test for THCV. But the push to bring THCV and other rare cannabinoids to patients is so resolute that by 2014, THCV varieties could be as easy to find as CBD varieties today—meaning challenging, but not impossible.

TYPE: African narrow-leafleted.

SPECIES: *Cannabis indica var. africana.*

BREEDING DATE: Grown in Malawi since the fifteenth century, likely brought there from India by slave traders.

GENETICS: Pure African landrace.

SIMILAR VARIETIES: Durban Poison (South Africa), Piggs Peak Swazi, Malagasy Black, Nigerian—as it seems that each country in Africa has its own cannabis varieties.

AVAILABILITY: Rare.

EASE OF CULTIVATION: Cultivation is challenging since the plant is acclimatized to the tropics and grows too tall, too fast, and too long for indoor cultivation.

AROMA: Fruit and almonds from pinene, beta-caryophyllene, and humulene.

TASTE: Sweet with a slight pineapple aftertaste.

POTENCY: Like many landraces, Malawi Gold rarely exceeds 12 percent in total cannabinoid content. But all raw potency numbers are deceptive, because they can convey very little of the actual quality of the medicinal effect. Any patient that has tried Malawi Gold can attest that its potency exceeds its test numbers.

DURATION OF EFFECTS: Relatively short, possibly due to its THCV content. Malawi Gold is excellent for intermittent use for symptom relief.

PSYCHOACTIVITY: Malawi Gold is electric and energetic with a quick onset. At higher doses, it produces mild visual tricks. Malawi Gold's "high" is often described as a "glow."

ANALGESIA: Light numbing of extremities, face, and mouth.

MUSCLE RELAXATION: Moderate to low.

DISSOCIATION: Very high. Patients with post-traumatic stress disorder report that THCV meds are effective.

STIMULANT: Malawi Gold is highly stimulating, but can provoke anxiety for some patients. What Malawi does not stimulate is appetite for food. THCV strains induce the "anti-munchies," which can make them the savior for those driven ravenous by cannabis.

SEDATION: Very little.

NEVILLE'S HAZE, also known as NEVIL'S HAZE

In the early 1980s, David Watson, hoping for a more cannabis-tolerant venue for his work, moved to the Netherlands with some original Haze seeds, as well as some other varieties from California. There, Watson established "Cultivator's Choice" Seeds. Some of Watson's California seeds (including Skunk #1 and Haze) were sold for breeding purposes to another expatriate in the Netherlands, Neville Schoenmaker, an Australian bird breeder who had founded the Seed Bank, one of Amsterdam's first seed companies.

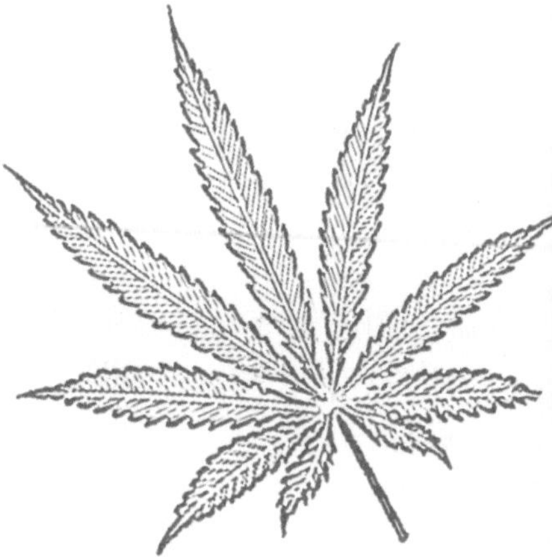

Medical Uses

Neville's Haze may be a better daytime med than Jack Herer, but Neville's is much more difficult to find and even more challenging to find well cultivated. At low doses, Neville's sharpens focus with minimal psychoactivity. At the moderate doses required for treating pain, Neville's psychoactivity can prove distracting if the patient is not acclimated. Patients report that small doses of Neville's can be effective for treating anxiety and depression, because of its mood elevation effects. Some phenotypes of Neville's can contain up to 1 percent CBD, which mellows some of the adverse effects of THC.

Neville began to breed Watson's original Hazes to tame their immense size and lengthy flowering cycles. Neville is supposed to have crossbred some his Northern Lights Afghan to tame the Haze. The result was Neville's Haze, the first in a long line of Dutch Haze varieties. Though rare today, Neville's Haze is both a snapshot of our past and a promise for the future. Varieties like Neville's Haze represent excellent prospects for next-generation micro-dose cannabis therapy.

Notes

A little Neville's Haze can spoil most patients, as do the rare varieties derived from tropical narrow-leafleted genetics.

TYPE: Nearly pure narrow-leafleted tropical *sativa*.

SPECIES: *Cannabis indica ssp. indica* × *afghanica* (90:10).

BREEDING DATE: mid-1980s.

GENETICS: Haze with a shot of Northern Lights.

SIMILAR VARIETIES: Haze (see pages 138–39), Thai Haze, Thai Haze × Skunk, and many contemporary Dutch Hazes. Special mention must go to Super Silver Haze (SSH), bred by Scott Blakey in the mid-1990s for Green House Seeds. SSH won back-to-back *High Times* Cannabis Cups. It is a very robust cross of Haze into Northern Lights and Skunk. SSH kept the bushier build of the Northern Lights, but delivered all the narrow-leafleted *sativa* effects. Super Silver Haze is among the most commonly available Haze crosses and a well-cultivated crop in world-class medical cannabis.

AVAILABILITY: Accessible fom Mr. Nice and Green House seed banks, with occasional cuttings around California.

EASE OF CULTIVATION: Growing Neville's Haze is very challenging and a long road with up to 16 weeks of flowering indoors. Some contend that often this variety requires 22 weeks of flowering, which seems mildly sadistic or masochistic depending on vantage point. The energy costs of cultivating this plant under indoor electrical lighting are excessive. In a controlled greenhouse environment, it is possible.

AROMA: Anise and cheese. When smoked, Neville's Haze is easily recognizable and not acrid.

TASTE: Spice, licorice, and chocolate.

POTENCY: Can easily exceed 21 percent THC with often over 1 percent CBD.

DURATION OF EFFECTS: Quick but smooth elevating onset, followed by a long slow guide over the next couple of hours.

PSYCHOACTIVITY: At small doses, Neville's Haze is like coffee, but without the jitters. It produces focus layered upon focus. At moderate doses, the high comes on. As the dose is raised, Neville's psychoactivity approaches psychedelic, especially when its flowers are at peak maturity.

ANALGESIA: Excellent at moderate to higher doses.

MUSCLE RELAXATION: More numbing than relaxing.

DISSOCIATION: Mild at moderate dose. At high doses, prepare to disappear into the stratosphere.

STIMULANT: Extremely clear stimulating effect and psychedelic at high doses.

SEDATION: Rare.

NORTHERN LIGHTS #5 X HAZE

A few years back a straw poll was taken of staff at Sensi Seeds in Amsterdam: Which was the most potent variety of cannabis that Sensi had ever developed? The response was nearly unanimous: Northern Lights #5 × Haze. The legendary Haze and Skunk #1 are both well represented in this small strain guide, but Northern Lights (NL) has wrought an enormous legacy in modern cannabis.

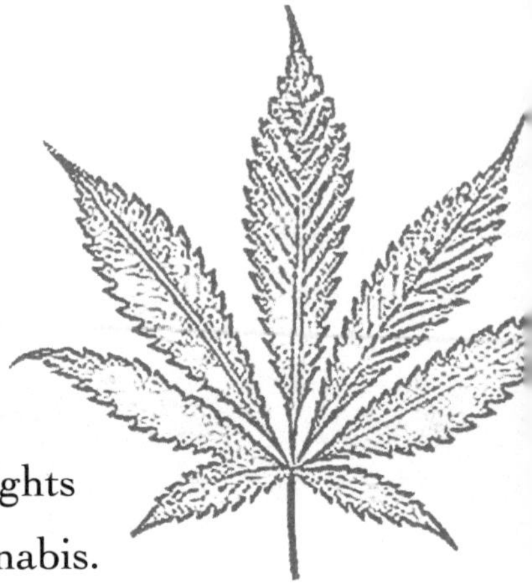

Northern Lights originated in the United States. There are supposedly 11 different phenotypes. NL #1 is a broad-leafleted cannabis plant nearly perfect for indoor cultivation, as it's tough with huge, wide leaves and amazing resin production. Even when cultivated by a beginner, it can produce a good harvest of high-quality cannabis. Of all the phenotypes however, Northern Lights #5 is the most admired for its potency. NL#5 has the distinct cocoa/blueberry musk aroma that is unique to the NL family. When NL#5 and Haze were crossed, the vigor between their two gene pools was extraordinary. The product: NL#5 × Haze has developed a fearsome reputation as being "too much" for most cannabis smokers. Still, it is respected for its peculiar form of potency.

Medical Uses

For years, NL#5 x Haze was considered to be more of an ordeal than a medicine. But low doses and micro-doses make this variety much more patient-friendly. At match-head-sized doses, this variety is still very potent, but not as likely to provoke anxiety. Its ability to provide distraction from pain appears to increase with these little doses. It's still too racy to allow patients to sleep, but is useful for daytime pain management without drowsiness.

Notes

In the decades since this variety appeared, many more potent cannabis products have been introduced. NL#5 × Haze is no longer a credible candidate for the "scariest cannabis on earth," if it ever was. A researcher has indicated that this variety produces a lot of beta-caryophyllene terpenes and this may trigger anxiety and panic in susceptible individuals. This variety seems the perfect candidate for crossing with a high-CBD variety, in hopes of getting it to calm down a bit. On some level, NL#5 × Haze is like a bronco that has rarely been ridden; it doesn't know how to do much beyond thrash about.

The majority of people who don't smoke cannabis are often concerned that "pot today is dangerous" because of varieties like this one, even when its reputation is overstated and overblown.

Understanding the underlying mechanism of what makes this variety the wrong choice for some patients is an important question, and the answer can assist us in developing better cannabis varieties in the near future.

TYPE: Hybrid.

SPECIES: Narrow-leafleted drug × broad-leafleted drug.

BREEDING DATE: circa 1980s.

GENETICS: Northern Lights #5 × Haze is a narrow-leafleted (70 percent) hybrid.

SIMILAR VARIETIES: Haze Skunk, Thai Haze × Skunk #1 (see pages 164–65), NL#5 × Skunk #1.

AVAILABILITY: Sensi Seeds and cuttings.

EASE OF CULTIVATION: Challenging for novices.

AROMA: Cocoa and spice with a hint of skunk. Heavy myrcene, pinene, and beta-caryophyllene expression.

TASTE: Like sweet incense with that special Northern Lights funk.

POTENCY: Around 20 percent THC, but there is something in this variety that makes that number a poor guide to its actual potency.

DURATION OF EFFECTS: Long and intense.

PSYCHOACTIVITY: Although racy and psychedelic, these attributes become much less intimidating at lower doses. Northern Lights #5 × Haze is definitely not for introducing someone to medical cannabis.

ANALGESIA: Numbing and distracting.

MUSCLE RELAXATION: Not much.

DISSOCIATION: Strong with flashes of occasional disorientation and panic.

STIMULANT: Very racy. Never share with an unsuspecting patient.

SEDATION: Many state that it is "impossible to sleep" while under the effects of this variety.

OG KUSH

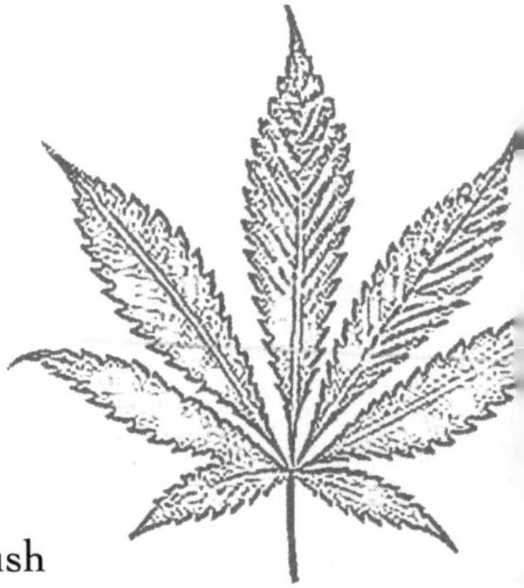

OG Kush is the most popular cannabis strain among medical patients in Southern California. It is also considered by testing labs to be the most potent cannabis variety currently available on the U.S. West Coast, and novice patients should exercise caution when medicating with OG Kush. The strain is noted for its outstanding flavor when smoked or vaporized. OG Kush is the highest priced cannabis available in the U.S., with prices reaching a peak of $35 per gram in 2011.

Medical Uses

OG Kush is preferred by patients looking for the strongest overall effects. It is very popular with chronic and neuropathic pain patients. OG Kush is tricky to dose because of its potency. Because of the wide range of terpenes that OG Kush produces, and the synergy of its terpenes with the variety's high level of THC, OG Kush is a very potent cannabis medicine. Many patients feel that it is more difficult to build a tolerance to OG Kush than other cannabis varieties, although this contention remains unproven.

Notes

With such popularity, OG Kush is surrounded by more accreted myth than any other cannabis variety. Being able to recite OG Kush lineage is *de rigeur* for California cannabis cognoscenti—and everyone tells a different version of the tale. However, while it is claimed that there are many different "cuts" of OG Kush, very little is known about any true genetic differences between them.

In California, OG Kush rules the medical cannabis scene. It's easy to understand its popularity since the strain has it all: potency, good looks, and an incredible smell and flavor. Its unique scent is the key characteristic of properly dried and cured OG Kush. The aroma can be distinguished from other kush genetics, since OG exhibits none of the vanilla aroma of a Pure Kush or sandalwood incense notes of a Bubba Kush (see pages 126–27).

The neon-green flower also has a characteristic "OG" appearance, where its bracts exhibit a rose-shaped structure—and an orange pistil intermittently appears throughout the bracts. The flowers should be covered with trichomes with prominent glandular heads, lending the buds a sparkly sheen and an overall "candied" look. The buds do not contain large stems. OG Kush is incredibly potent, stimulating, "heady," uplifting, and euphoric—with absolutely jaw-dropping psychoactivity. The result is one of the strongest and exhilarating range of effects available from contemporary cannabis. Because of its popularity and high value, fake and poor-quality OG Kush is common.

TYPE: Hybrid.

SPECIES: *Cannabis indica ssp. kafiristanica/ssp. indica hybrid.* Afghan, Nepali, and Thai landraces have likely contributed genetic characteristics to this quintessential hybrid.

BREEDING DATE: Uncertain. Depending on which origin story is to be believed, OG Kush first appears in 1978 in Los Angeles, or 1985 in Colorado, or 1991 on the East Coast.

GENETICS: The earliest OG Kush growers in Los Angeles claim that the strain originated from a cross of Northern Lights (see pages 150–51) with Mexican commercial marijuana bagseed. Another popular origin legend has OG Kush descended from Chemdawg (see pages 128–29), a Montana/Colorado variety. The story goes that, in 1993, a cultivator in the foothills of the Sierra Mountains in northern California got the Chemdawg cut. One of the growers with whom he shared Chemdawg lived on the ocean in Sunset Beach, California. The Sunset Beach breeder crossed Chemdawg into his "secret ingredient" male: a Lemon Thai x Old World Paki Kush. The resulting cross became legendary in Los Angeles connoisseur circles in the mid-'90s. Someone told the breeder the reason his kush was so good had to be that it was "mountain grown." The breeder famously replied, "Nah, bro, it's ocean grown." The Ocean Grown tag stuck and was soon shortened to OG Kush.

According to some reports, the OG breeder moved to New Zealand in early 1996. Before leaving the U.S., however, he gave OG cuts to a number of friends. He also sold some seeds, one of which produced the noted San Fernando Valley cut which displays more *sativa* narrow-leafleted characteristics. Elsewhere, a cutting of the original OG Kush became the Larry OG cut that is popular in Orange County today. The following list describes a number of popular OG cuts that are currently available in the western U.S.

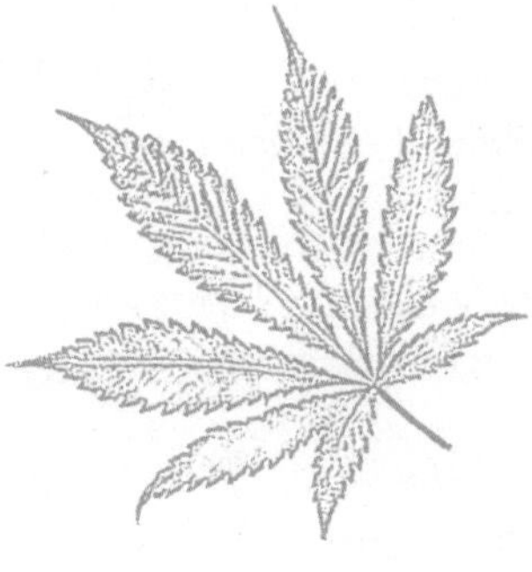

Ghost OG Associated with a well-known member of the Overgrow online cannabis community, Ghost resembles the earliest OG Kush cuts in its intense citrus/pine aroma and exceptional potency.

Abusive OG This cut is noted for its potency and is more *indica* in effect than classic OG.

Diablo OG Very fast onset effects and "face-numbing" analgesia characterize this cut, which is associated with the Reseda Discount Center dispensary in the San Fernando Valley area of Los Angeles.

HA OG Kush This cut supposedly originated in the Tahoe area and is associated with the Hells Angels Motorcycle Club. It was one of the earliest cuts to appear in Orange County south of Los Angeles and is produced by the same cultivators responsible for the Larry OG. It exhibits extraordinary trichome production, which extends from its flowers onto the edges of the surrounding water leaves.

Skywalker OG This became very popular from 2008 to 2010. It is a distinctly *sativa*-dominant OG cut with an intense psychedelic psychoactivity.

Purple OG Kush So-called for its distinctive purple stems, this OG Kush cut was popular in the Santa Barbara area. It is prized by connoisseurs as the greatest of all OG cuts.

Soul Assassin OG A cut that has long been associated with the band Cypress Hill. It is prized for its flavor and the special headiness of its psychoactivity.

Tahoe OG A cut sourced by the breeder known as Swerve of The Cali Connection seed company.

Blood OG This is an outlier version of OG Kush that was supposedly bred in Florida. It is not implausible that crosses with Afghan, Nepali, and Thai genetics independent of Californian efforts, could have produced a variety that resembles classic OG Kush.

SIMILAR VARIETIES: Pure Kush, Orange Master Kush, Kosher Kush (DNA Genetics).

AVAILABILITY: OG Kush is typically only available in the form of cuttings, although DNA Genetics

The Quest for the Truth about Cannabis

David Watson and Robert Connell Clarke are naturalists in the nineteenth-century tradition who set out to understand a facet of the world that nobody understood from a modern scientific perspective: the world of cannabis. The same passion overtook Ethan Russo, Mel Frank, Jorge Cervantes, Jack Herer, Arno Hazekamp, Martin Lee, and Fred Gardner. And countless others. There are so many myths about cannabis that the desire for veracity gnawed on these individuals until they had to ignore the risks and learn the truth. Many of them are still searching for large parts of that truth. Cannabis prohibition rests on a lie, surrounded by other lies. These lies form the fabric of what eventually constitutes the official truth about cannabis. Nobody knows where OG Kush came from. Is it Thai? Hawaiian? Nepalese? Afghan? No one knows. Prohibition has ensured that the secrets of its origins remain secret. For now. Eventually the DNA within cannabis varieties such as OG Kush will be examined and its patterns will yield secrets about the variety, where it came from, and what makes it so special.

in the Netherlands and Cali Connection in the United States are beginning to offer seed versions.

EASE OF CULTIVATION: Difficult. The plant tends to grow quickly and tall, has little pest resistance, and has a reputation as a picky feeder.

AROMA: Intense, distinctive citrus and fuel aroma with clear naphtha, orange, balsamic, pine, and earth notes. OG Kush exhibits a wide variety of aromas depending on the cultivation method and curing technique. Poorly cured OG smells like roses and lawn clippings. It can take a month of careful humidity and temperature-controlled curing to bring out the best aroma from a crop of OG Kush. Its immense terpene entourage combines limonene, beta-caryophyllene, myrcene, linalool, and alpha-humulene.

TASTE: When smoked, OG Kush offers a sweet, floral hashish exhalation with a tart citrusy undertone. When vaporized, it has an orange blossom floral taste and intense hash oil aftertaste. Exhalation of well-cultivated OG can produce a strong mentholated sensation.

POTENCY: Well-cultivated OG Kush consistently tests at over 20 percent THC with less than 1 percent CBD, while outliers may achieve 25 percent THC. Caution when initially dosing with OG Kush is strongly advised. It can cause disorientation, anxiety, and postural hypotension in novice patients.

DURATION OF EFFECTS: One to three hours when smoked.

PSYCHOACTIVITY: When smoked, OG Kush's massive THC content causes its initial onset to be accompanied by considerable dissociation, cerebral pressure, and inability to concentrate. OG Kush delivers a broad entourage of terpene effects from its high titers of limonene and myrcene. This spike subsides after 10 to 20 seconds, transitioning into a very intense psychoactivity. Patients generally report strong heady and stony sensations, with significant amounts of euphoria and mood elevation. Although generally stimulating, high-THC content often results in disorientation, "couchlock," and lethargy. Finally, there is not much loss of peripheral vision perception.

ANALGESIA: High analgesia offering both an excellent distraction and a numbing, soothing body effect.

MUSCLE RELAXATION: Medium.

DISSOCIATION: High.

STIMULANT: Moderate, although the initial onset of a low dose of OG Kush can be quite stimulating.

SEDATION: Low at onset, though as THC metabolites build up, OG Kush can be effective for insomnia.

TRIVIA: While popular with patients, OG Kush has achieved mythic status amongst the hip-hop music community and has been praised by Snoop Dogg, Dr. Dre, Cypress Hill, and Madlib, among others. A decade ago, OG Kush commanded up to $8,000 per pound (**0.5** kilogram) on the illicit market. Even today, it is typically the highest priced indoor cultivated cannabis variety, although it may eventually cede this economic distinction to even more labor-intensive, tropical, narrow-leafleted varieties, which possess extremely long flowering times.

PINCHER CREEK, also known as **CUSH**

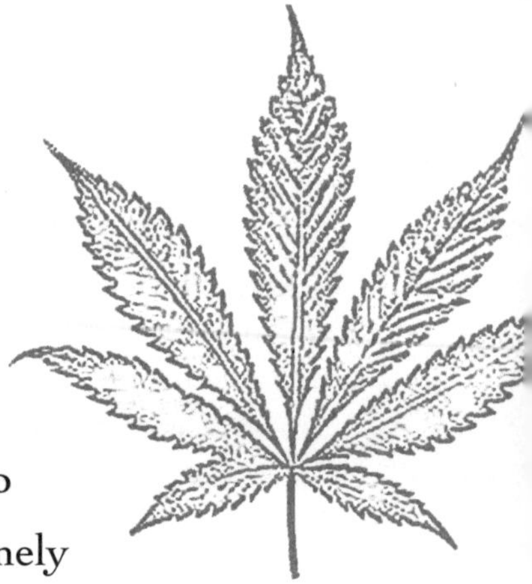

Pincher Creek is a very interesting medical cannabis variety first bred in Pincher Creek, Alberta, Canada, in the late 1980s. Though bred from commonly available varieties—Skunk and Afghani—the result was quite unique, a very fast flowering strain with a unique chemistry and range of effects. When it was brought to Southern California in the late 1990s, it became extremely popular within the creative community for its purported ability to encourage associative thought, composition, and improvization.

Medical Uses

Pincher Creek is the Swiss Army knife of medical cannabis; it can be employed to assist with a wide range of medical conditions. From migraine to nausea, from pain to spasticity, there is likely an effective dose of this variety that will be effective. The key to using Pincher Creek effectively is to select a normal dose, then cut that by half and proceed. With this variety, the "less is more" approach has worked for many patients.

Pincher Creek is one of the most popular medical cannabis varieties for its ability to distract from pain while relaxing the patient without sedation. Patients have successfully used the variety's ability to stimulate "out of the box" thinking as a springboard for exploring new approaches to wellness and living with chronic illness.

Notes

For patients who may have had unpleasant cannabis experiences in the past, Pincher Creek is a good variety for reintroducing cannabis. Obviously considerable thought should be given to whether the patient can potentially benefit from medical cannabis—but if so, this variety is a comfortable place to begin. Pincher Creek was the variety that inspired the concept of micro-dosing cannabis, which is employing a dose at the threshold of psychoactivity, typically around the equivalent of a two- to four-milligram dose of THC. This approach requires starting with a match-head-sized piece of cannabis, then increasing that dose only after real self-assessment identifies any potential benefits that could be gained. But as cannabis is nontoxic, patients use too much, too often. This approach to dosing cannabis is imprecise. The micro-dose method puts the patient back in control of the dose, rather than under the dose's control.

TYPE: 50/50 hybrid of broad-leafleted and narrow-leafleted varieties.

SPECIES: *Cannabis indica var. afghanica* × *var. indica.*

BREEDING DATE: circa 1989.

GENETICS: Sweet Afghani × Skunk #1.

SIMILAR VARIETIES: Green Skunk, Green Ribbon, Green Crack.

AVAILABILITY: Pincher Creek is available as a cutting on the U.S. West Coast.

EASE OF CULTIVATION: One of the fastest-flowering varieties of cannabis, typically finishing after six to seven weeks of flowering. Pincher Creek is a great yielder, but needs a experienced hand to make it flourish.

AROMA: Complex with notes of fruit, basil, caramel, and skunk from its wide range of terpenes—predominately the rare terpene ocimene, plus myrcene, pinene, and limonene. These terpenes are responsible for a broad synergistic "entourage effect" with THC, where terpenes interact with each other and cannabinoids, pharmacologically. Pincher Creek shares this ability to trigger an entourage effect with OG Kush, but few other cannabis varieties.

TASTE: Bananas, honey, and citrus.

POTENCY: Very potent, but a truly excellent choice for micro-dose regimens. Pincher Creek typically produces 1 percent CBG, which is a potent analgesic.

DURATION OF EFFECTS: Short—90 minutes.

PSYCHOACTIVITY: Remarkable. Pincher Creek's psychoactivity varies dramatically with dose. At higher doses, many patients find it very insightful and transcendent. At minimal dose, it is relaxing like a glass of wine. At in-between doses, Pincher Creek can be used for increasing concentration, providing distraction from pain, lowering dose requirements for conventional prescription pain medication.

ANALGESIA: Very good, especially at low to moderate dose.

MUSCLE RELAXATION: Good with little sedation.

DISSOCIATION: Typically only at higher doses.

STIMULANT: Mild.

SEDATION: Minimal, except after prolonged moderate doses.

PURPLE URKLE

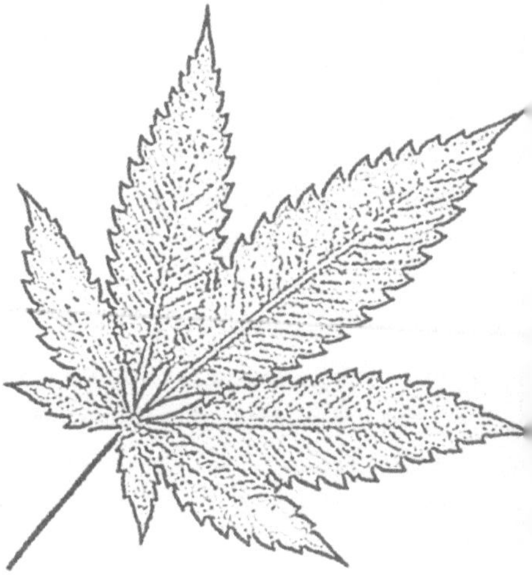

Purple Urkle is low-yielding variety of purple, broad-leafleted cannabis that is prized for its high THC content, pleasant flavor and aroma, and its calming effects. Purple Urkle is considered the definitive sedative, broad-leafleted *indica* and is a favorite with insomniacs. Purple *indicas* such as Purple Urkle and Granddaddy Purple are solid choices for bed rest or recovery from illness.

Notes

It would appear that Purple Urkle takes its name from Steve Urkel, a fictional character on the American TV comedy *Family Matters*. The character's name was appropriated from a real-life writer and director, Steve Erkel. As such, it was one of earliest cannabis varieties to be named after a celebrity. The Cannabis Buyer's Club of West Hollywood (CBCWH), where Purple Urkle is said to have originated, was one of the earliest medical cannabis facilities in California. In 1996, it was also one of the first cannabis clubs in California to be raided and closed by local authorities. Although the City of West Hollywood supplied the building to CBCWH, the federal government seized the building. As a result of this action, there was little to no municipal cooperation with medical cannabis dispensaries in California for the next 15 years.

Medical Uses

Purple indicas such as Purple Urkle and Granddaddy Purple are solid choices for bed rest or recovery from illness. These varieties are too potent to be functional. Because of its high THC content, Purple Urkle is a good choice for post-traumatic stress disorder. Purples are also popular for chemotherapy-induced nausea and discomfort, including neuropathy. And Purple Urkle was considered an effective remedy for HIV neuropathic pain when it first appeared in West Hollywood. For help with insomnia, it is recommended to smoke or vaporize Purple Urkle no closer than one hour before bedtime, which will enable THC metabolites to work their sedative magic.

TYPE: Broad-leafleted *indica* (100 percent).

SPECIES: *Cannabis indica var. afghanica.*

BREEDING DATE: Purple Urkle was first bred circa 1996 in West Hollywood, California, with its ancestors in Mendocino from the early 1980s. Although it was developed in Southern California, Purple Urkle achieved its popularity with patients in the East Bay communities of Berkeley and Oakland, where purple cannabis varieties are highly prized.

GENETICS: Unknown, but likely a descendent of Purple Afghan. Certainly a cousin to Grape Ape and Granddaddy Purple. Purple Urkle is said to have been bred at the Cannabis Buyer's Club of West Hollywood.

SIMILAR VARIETIES: Granddaddy Purple (see pages 134–35), Girl Scout Cookies, Mendo Purps, Grape Ape.

AVAILABILITY: Clone only in dispensaries in California, Colorado, and Washington.

EASE OF CULTIVATION: Not a big producer, but reliable source of very high-potency flowers.

AROMA: Grape, pepper, and spice, with a hint of skunk. Purple varieties typically produce smaller amounts of aromatic terpenes than other cannabis varieties, so it is important to protect them from heat and oxidation.

TASTE: Spicy and hashy with a hint of wine. It is this combination of spice and fruit that has made Urkle a popular choice with patients.

POTENCY: Properly cultivated Purple Urkle often approaches 24 percent THC. It contains virtually no CBD or other cannabinoids. Its sedative qualities likely stem from its myrcene/caryophyllene content with a touch of ocimene.

DURATION OF EFFECTS: Ninety minutes followed by several hours of slow fade afterward.

PSYCHOACTIVITY: Purple Urkle is a quintessential couchlocker that "leaves you where it found you." It produces a pure *indica* "stone," rather than a "high," and rarely causes anxiety at reasonable dosages. Caution should be observed when trying Purple Urkle, since it is far too sedative to be functional. Purple Urkle is an outstanding choice for use while recovering from a medical procedure.

ANALGESIA: Excellent and profound distraction from pain at the normal cannabis "sweet spot" of dose.

MUSCLE RELAXATION: Profound. Some patients liken Purple Urkle's effects to a sensation of being "deboned."

DISSOCIATION: Mild, though when in its grip, patients tend to get lost in slowly drifting thoughts accompanied by intermittent forgetfulness.

STIMULANT: Purple Urkle only produces the smallest amount of stimulation, and exclusively during the first few minutes of its initial onset.

SEDATION: The number one medical cannabis chemotype for insomnia and rest.

S.A.G.E.

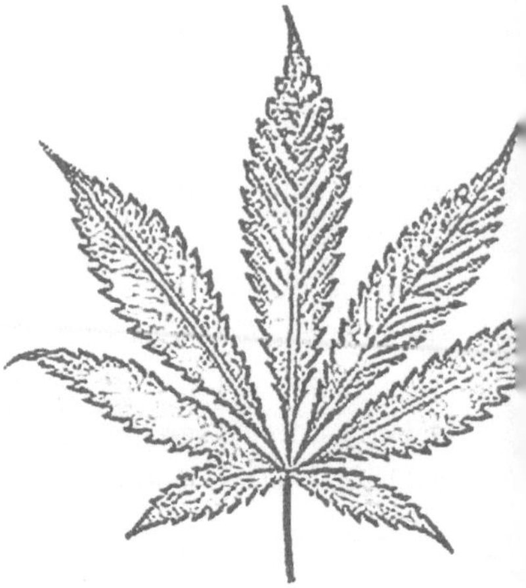

S.A.G.E. means Sativa Afghani Genetic Equilibrium. S.A.G.E.took 2nd place in the *High Times* Cannabis Cup in 2001. S.A.G.E. hashish won the Cup in 2000. S.A.G.E has also been the parent of several excellent crosses, including S.A.G.E. 'n' Sour and Zeta. An outstanding example of contemporary cannabis breeding, it shares many of the best qualities of Haze, but also carries the burden of Haze's 12-week flowering cycle. And like Haze, S.A.G.E. makes excellent breeding stock for new varieties.

Medical Uses

S.A.G.E. is an effective variety for daytime use, where its combination of stimulation and analgesia can be effective for a wide range of patients. Its high-THC psychoactivity can make some patients anxious, so caution is advised to carefully manage dose.

Notes

The founder of TH Seeds, New Yorker Adam Dunn, moved to Amsterdam in the late 1980s and began working at the Hash, Marihuana, and Hemp Museum. The museum was a magnet for many second-generation breeders in the Dutch cannabis scene and inspired Adam to form his first seed company, CIA (Cannabis in Amsterdam). Adam and CIA helped organize many of the early *High Times* Cannabis Cups, beginning with the fifth cup in 1992. In less than a decade, Adam would win the Cannabis Cup for his creation: S.A.G.E.

While the Haze × Afghan parentage of S.A.G.E is widely accepted, some growers claim that S.A.G.E. exhibits many characteristics of Big Sur Holy Weed, a much-loved rare cannabis variety from the central coast of California that was popular in the late 1970s. The legend of the Holy Weed is elaborate, with claims of a clandestine breeding project conducted by American-born Buddhist monks living above Big Sur. Holy Weed was said to be extremely resistant to the mold infestations caused by the early morning dew common along the coast. Some claim that Holy Weed was bred from Afghan stock; others claim that it originated in the highlands of Mexico.

TYPE: Broad-leafleted hybrid.

SPECIES: *Cannabis indica ssp. indica × cannabis indica ssp. afghanica.*

BREEDING DATE: 1999.

GENETICS: Haze × Afghan, although claims of Big Sur Holy Weed ancestry are rumored.

SIMILAR VARIETIES: Sage 'n' Sour, Zeta, Super Silver Haze.

AVAILABILITY: Bred and distributed by T H Seeds in Amsterdam.

EASE OF CULTIVATION: Because S.A.G.E. tends to grow tall, it might be challenging for a first-time indoor cultivation project. Like many varieties, S.A.G.E. is best grown in soil, rather than hydroponically. Unlike Haze varieties, S.A.G.E. is a big producer and can deliver big yields of large flowers.

AROMA: Sweet sandalwood and cocoa with a hint of mint.

TASTE: Spicy with hints of pepper and menthol. Much more mentholated than Haze varieties.

POTENCY: Moderate potency between 15 and 18 percent THC. S.A.G.E is often used for making hashish, and has won several Cannabis Cups in the hash category.

DURATION OF EFFECTS: Long-lasting.

PSYCHOACTIVITY: S.A.G.E. is a classic THC-dominant variety with a stimulating, cerebral psychoactivity. Like many pure-THC varieties, S.A.G.E can cause reddened eyes and dry mouth at increased dosages.

ANALGESIA: Effective analgesia at low dose.

MUSCLE RELAXATION: Mild.

DISSOCIATION: At higher doses, S.A.G.E. can make the user very forgetful and spacey.

STIMULANT: Moderately stimulating.

SEDATION: Very little.

SENSI STAR

Developed in the Netherlands by Luc Krol of Paradise Seeds in the early 1990s, Sensi Star has excelled in many cannabis competitions, including winning the *High Times* Cannabis Cup for best *indica* in 1999. Sensi Star has become a cult variety in California and Colorado, with devotees quickly snatching up each available batch.

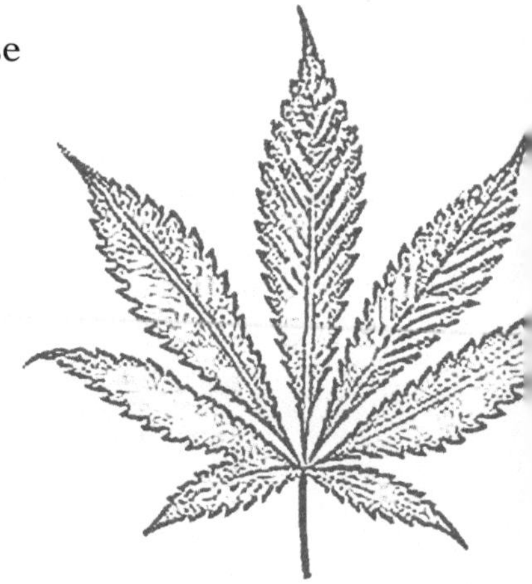

Notes

Sensi Star has developed a reputation as a truly classic cannabis variety with unique psychoactivity that can impress the most jaded cannabis patient. In the past few years, Paradise Seeds has replaced their Sensi Star with a new "feminized" version. Feminized seeds are produced by manipulating a female cannabis plant to produce male flowers, which is achieved by exposing the plant to stress. When a female plant is self-pollinated through this technique, it will produce seed that, when germinated, generates a much higher ratio of female to male offspring. Unfortunately, these feminized seed offspring will have a tendency to develop male flowers and subsequently pollinate the next crop, when in fact no fertilization is desired.

Medical Uses

Patients consider Sensi Star to be one of the most consistently effective medical cannabis varieties. Patients report that the *indica* phenotype of Sensi Star is effective for relieving symptoms of gastrointestinal disorders such as Crohn's Disease. The *indica* pheno is also good for relief from occasional insomnia.

TYPE: Sensi Star has both a *sativa*-dominant narrow-leafleted phenotype and a broad-leafleted *indica* phenotype. The two types exhibit differing effects, with the *indica* variety being more commonly available.

SPECIES: *Cannabis indica ssp. afghanica × cannabis indica ssp. indica.*

BREEDING DATE: Introduced in 1994.

GENETICS: Unknown, although Sensi Star is rumored to be descended from Big Sur Holy Weed, a legendary California variety. Another version of the story claims that Sensi Star was a cutting that Luc Krol received from Neville Schoenmaker.

SIMILAR VARIETIES: S.A.G.E. (see pages 160–61),White Widow (see pages 172–73).

AVAILABILITY: Available from Paradise Seeds in the Netherlands.

EASE OF CULTIVATION: Sensi Star is easy to grow and a good producer. The downside is that Sensi Star can be an extremely smelly plant, not remotely suitable for discreet cultivation.

AROMA: The *sativa* Sensi Star has a distinct citrus-skunk aroma. The Sensi Star *indica* pheno has a mint/metallic/skunk smell that is quite unique and extremely stinky.

TASTE: The *sativa* phenotype is mild tasting with notes of citrus. The *indica* phenotype has a distinct lemon/menthol tang with a slightly metallic aftertaste that is surprisingly palatable. When smoked, Sensi Star dilates the bronchial passages, imparting a feeling of rapid lung expansion, which can result in coughing.

POTENCY: High, a "one-hitter quitter" for many patients. The *indica* phenotype can approach 20 percent THC.

DURATION OF EFFECTS: The *indica* phenotype produces a deep, long-lasting effect for hours that often results in sleep or a nap. The *sativa* version produces a more cerebral psychoactivity that is more appropriate for daytime use, but similarly very long-lasting.

PSYCHOACTIVITY: The *indica* version is very stony with a tendency toward lethargy. The *sativa* phenotype is much more energetic, upbeat, and notable for inducing mild visual psychedelia. The *sativa* phenotype can trigger anxiety and even mild paranoia in susceptible patients. Neither phenotype produces a particularly functional psychoactivity, so complex tasks might suffer while using Sensi Star. Overall, Sensi Star's psychoactivity exceeds even what would normally be expected from a high-THC variety. This is likely due to Sensi Star's terpene content.

ANALGESIA: Very considerable for both the *indica* and *sativa* phenotypes, with the *indica* often characterized as producing a numbing effect.

MUSCLE RELAXATION: The *indica* version will turn most patients into a Slinky. Very relaxing.

DISSOCIATION: Both the *indica* and *sativa* phenotypes drop patients into a cocoon of daydreaming and drifting thoughts. Music is extremely enjoyable under the influence of Sensi Star.

STIMULANT: Mildly stimulating onset that quickly retreats into a floating relaxation.

SEDATION: The *indica* phenotype is notorious for its "couchlock" effect that tends to leave you where the cannabis found you.

SKUNK #1, also known as THE PURE

Skunk #1 is an infamous marijuana strain that contributed to one of the first modern cannabis medicines. Without Skunk #1 and its creator, there might not have been a modern cannabis medicine revolution. David Watson developed Skunk #1 in California in the late 1970s. In the 1980s, he brought Skunk #1 to the Netherlands, where it helped shape the early Dutch cannabis scene.

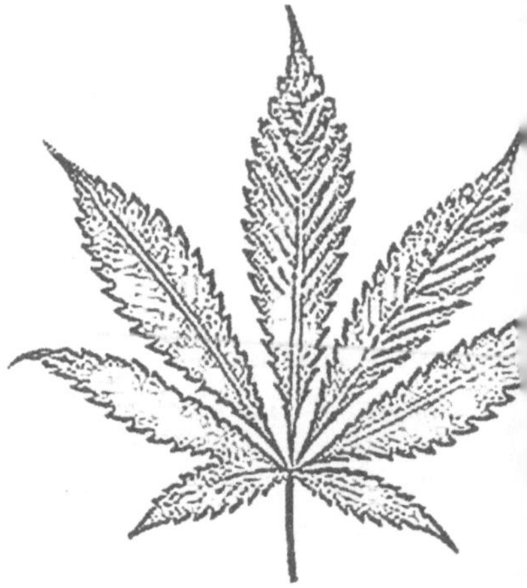

This variety leveraged the earliest Afghan genetics into a plant which kept the best characteristics of tropical sativas without the impracticalities, such as their post-Christmas harvest. Today, in the U.K. and elsewhere, the name Skunk is synonymous with high-potency drug cannabis. When GW Pharmaceuticals partnered with David Watson's Hortapharm company in the late 1990s, GW acquired the right to use Skunk in its new cannabis medicinal extractions. GW has shown off its new Skunk acquisition at several lectures in Britain. Sensi Seeds seed bank also holds a trademark on Skunk #1 and sells a variety.

Medical Uses

Useful across a range of indications benefiting from its high THC and myrcene combination, Skunk has been used by patients to treat everything from headache to severe chemo-induced nausea.

Notes

The circle of cannabis breeders around David Watson's development of Skunk #1 had an enormous impact on modern medical cannabis in the U.S., Canada, and Europe. He was part of a group of California breeders that produced or encouraged the development of many key varieties of contemporary cannabis. These pioneers include Mendocino Joe of Romulan fame, James Goodwin, Robert Connell Clarke, Ed Rosenthal, Jerry Kamstra, and many others. All of these were the best and the brightest. Remember that their feats of cannabis breeding derring-do were accomplished while cannabis was reeling from the first salvos of the Richard Nixon/Gerald Ford War on Drugs.

David Watson fled to Europe after some difficulties in California, bringing with him Skunk and Haze seeds, which were fortunate to have survived his ordeal. The Netherlands proved to be a much more conducive place to conduct cannabis research as President Ronald Reagan came into the White House.

TYPE: Hybrid.

SPECIES: *Cannabis indica ssp. afghanica* × *Cannabis indica ssp. indica.*

BREEDING DATE: mid-1970s.

GENETICS: Colombian Gold × Acapulco Gold × Afghan.

SIMILAR VARIETIES: Island Sweet Skunk, Sensi Skunk. There are two approaches to breeding Skunk cannabis: the sweet school epitomized by Island Sweet Skunk versus the "roadkill" school promoted by Scott Blakey of Mr. Nice. Patients seem evenly divided in their preference, but many consider the sweeter skunks to have a more refined psychoactivity.

AVAILABILITY: It is questionable whether Skunk #1 is still available outside of GW Pharmaceuticals' secure greenhouse on Porton Down, or David Watson's freezer. Recently, breeder Scott Blakey of Mr. Nice Seedbank and Research has worked to re-create a more pungent Skunk. Dutch Passion also has their version, SK1.

EASE OF CULTIVATION: Good for novices. The best phenotypes are ready for harvest around 60 days into flowering.

AROMA: The original Skunk #1 was said to be sweet, while other Skunk varieties were pungent and almost offensive. It sounds disgusting, but it's this aroma that propelled contemporary cannabis in the West. Interesting how an offensive odor like skunk can be recontextualized when it becomes associated with a new outcome such as intense psychoactivity.

TASTE: Skunk #1 tastes better than one might expect, given its name. It offers a smooth, expansive smoke, not harsh and with a sweet aftertaste.

POTENCY: High potency often approaching 20 percent THC.

DURATION OF EFFECTS: Long-lasting.

PSYCHOACTIVITY: Potent, but well tolerated by nearly all patients. Skunk's particular effects differ from the edgier Haze psychoactivity from the same period.

ANALGESIA: Skunk #1 is an excellent distraction from pain, though not as narcotic as some Afghan-dominant varieties.

MUSCLE RELAXATION: Excellent. Patients with spasticity report good relief from Skunk varieties.

DISSOCIATION: Not much.

STIMULANT: Initially, but never jittery.

SEDATION: At higher doses.

SOUR DIESEL, also known as SOUR D

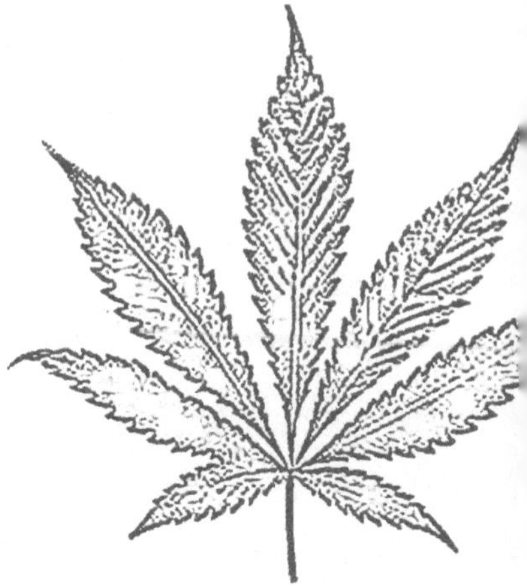

Sour Diesel is part of a unique class of cannabis varieties with a particularly stimulating medicinal effect, sometimes characterized as a cross between cannabis and caffeine. These are hybrids that produce a distinct aroma of fuel and citrus. They may carry a gene from a group of cannabis landraces from Nepal, Kashmir, and eastern Pakistan that also smell strongly of fuel. To the uninitiated, Sour Diesel's effects and their associated cautions might sound somewhat ominous.

Medical Uses

Sour Diesel is an excellent choice for patients avoiding potential sedation. When well tolerated by the patient, it provides excellent daytime distraction from pain and discomfort. Sour Diesel is also effective for reducing the amount of other prescription pain medications. It can also be an excellent mood elevator for many patients. Special caution should be observed however to ensure that patients with schizophrenia or bipolar disorder avoid this variety, since Sour Diesel's ability to stimulate can disorientate these patients to the point of crisis.

With care and intelligent, thoughtful dosing, Sour Diesel is an excellent medical cannabis variety. In 2004, Sour Diesel was perhaps the highest-priced cannabis in the world, fetching $1,000 per ounce on Wall Street, in the days when the price of gold was under $400.

Notes

Sour Diesel is associated with a group of cannabis genetics that are claimed to come from a single East Coast breeding collective. Its seeds are said to have been plucked from a single bag of legendary cannabis sold at a Grateful Dead concert in Indiana in July 1990. The cannabis genetics that are related to that single bag are said to include Chemdawg (see pages 128–29), Sour Diesel, OG Kush (see pages 152–55), Headband, and several other popular medical cannabis varieties. If true, this treasure trove of bagseed deserves a Cannabis Mother Lode Prize. With the exception of OG Kush, all of the varieties in this family are highly stimulating. Mistakenly, dispensary staff and patients often characterize Sour Diesel's stimulating effect as a *sativa* effect. Sour Diesel does not deliver an effect remotely similar to a true Haze (see pages 138–39) or Trainwreck (see pages 170–71). It is better to call this a "diesel" effect, to distinguish it and avoid confusion. Many patients that don't tolerate Diesels tend to avoid all sativas because of this common confusion.

TYPE: Broad-leafleted hybrid.

SPECIES: *Cannabis indica var. kafiristanica* x *var. afghanica.*

BREEDING DATE: mid-1990s.

GENETICS: [(Chem '91 × Massachusetts Super Skunk) × Northern Lights)] × (Northern Lights/ Shiva × Hawaiian).

SIMILAR VARIETIES: East Coast Sour Diesel, New York City Diesel, Chemdawg, Headband, Chem 4, AlienDawg.

AVAILABILITY: Cutting only.

EASE OF CULTIVATION: Sour Diesel is a huge producer when cultivated with skill, but can take up to 14 weeks to flower. Mentoring by an experienced cultivator is highly recommended for best results.

AROMA: Fuel with a squirt of citrus sitting atop a bed of classic skunk.

TASTE: Sour hashish.

POTENCY: Subjectively extremely high because of the intensity of the psychoactivity from a profusion of beta-caryophyllene. In the laboratory, Sour Diesel often approaches 24 percent THC.

DURATION OF EFFECTS: 90 minutes and counting down, somewhat akin to a rocket burn.

PSYCHOACTIVITY: Sour Diesel is extremely stimulating and often feels "racy." It is absolutely not recommended for patients suffering from anxiety issues, except at micro-dose level and then with caution. Susceptible patients can often have panic attacks with this variety. However, Sour Diesel may be very stimulating, but that does not equate to cognitive enhancement. Think of it as speeding everything up, but losing track of details as they whiz by.

ANALGESIA: Numbing. Sour Diesel's mental stimulation helps distract from discomfort.

MUSCLE RELAXATION: Surprisingly relaxing, given the intensity of its effects.

DISSOCIATION: Little, except at high doses where the patient can become withdrawn from overstimulation.

STIMULANT: Very high.

SEDATION: Varieties like Sour Diesel go up, but ultimately crash—so there is only sedation at the bitter end.

STRAWBERRY COUGH

If laughter is the best medicine, then Strawberry Cough will cure what ails you. Strawberry Fields was an East Coast strain that had a great strawberry aroma and not much else. Kyle Kushman, a talented cannabis breeder, discovered that the owner of the Strawberry Fields variety had crossed it with Haze—and Kushman knew a winner when he saw it. The Haze cross was christened Strawberry Cough and is an outstanding narrow-leafleted hybrid.

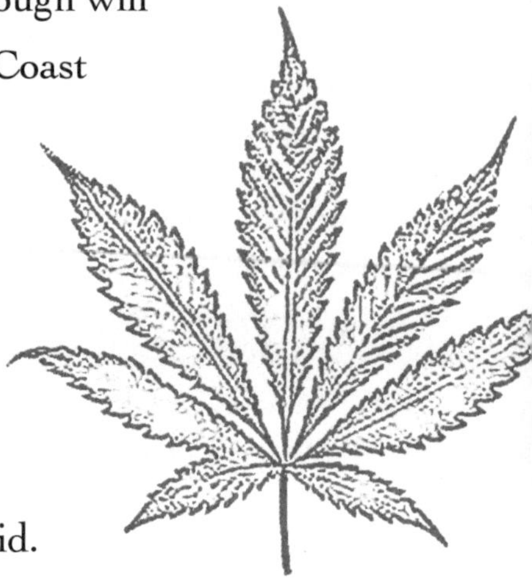

Medical Uses

Mood, mood, mood. Strawberry Cough is great for intractable and frustrating illnesses and symptoms. It is an excellent medicine for novice or older patients, provided that they have the tiniest appreciation for humor and absurdity. Some patients are just too dour for this medicine, though these cases are very rare. This variety can be very useful for helping a patient regain a reasonable perspective after being battered by discomfort. It makes a serious case for a cannabis variety as a possible antidepressant, especially at low doses.

Strawberry Cough is one of the few varieties of cannabis that is nearly impossible not to enjoy. It is a classic "giggle weed" like Trainwreck (see pages 170–71), but it makes everything seem even sillier. Strawberry Cough is an easy variety to find in U.S. dispensaries, but really good batches are considerably harder to source.

Notes

Strawberry Cough was the variety of cannabis cultivated by Michael Caine's character in the science fiction film, *Children of Men*. The "Cough" in its name comes from its thick, expansive smoke. Strawberry Cough is a good candidate for future development, since there is obviously something very special and interesting tucked away in its chemistry. It will be interesting to see if there are any rare cannabinoids or terpenoids hiding in it. Many of these newer cannabis varieties have not been extensively studied, though that is changing very quickly. Kyle Kushman, the strain's discoverer, has also pioneered a growing approach called Veganics, which avoids all animal products as plant nutrients. The results of this regimen look very promising.

TYPE: Narrow-leafleted hybrid.

SPECIES: *Cannabis indica ssp. indica.*

BREEDING DATE: Early 2000s.

GENETICS: Strawberry Fields × Haze.

SIMILAR VARIETIES: Hawaiian Timewarp, Timewreck, Sweet Tooth, Lemon Thai, Lemon Haze.

AVAILABILITY: Available as a seed from Dutch Passion; cuttings found widely in the U.S.

EASE OF CULTIVATION: Strawberry Cough is a great strain for beginners growing outdoors with conscientious and preventative pest management. Caterpillars just love this variety and their arrival must be anticipated. Indoors, it's manageable, but not for beginners. It requires a careful cure to protect and bring out the aroma.

AROMA: This variety should smell unmistakably of strawberries. Don't trust any batch that does not! Strawberry Cough's smoke is considered less offensive to nonsmokers than other varieties. Heat kills the aroma of this variety very, very quickly, so store it carefully.

TASTE: Spicy with just a hint of fruit, like a rum-soaked cigar. Strawberry Cough is great when vaporized because its strawberry taste survives intact.

POTENCY: This variety is quite potent, yet oddly gentle. Some batches have tested at over 19 percent THC. Even at this level, Strawberry Cough is rarely overwhelming.

DURATION OF EFFECTS: Moderate.

PSYCHOACTIVITY: Its psychoactive effects are clear as a bell, and it is a genuine smile-inducer. One of the happiest feelings in the cannabis sensorium is found with Strawberry Cough. This variety is recommended for those struggling with their illness, since it can lift crushed spirits. There's no crash either—just a gentle glide back to Earth.

ANALGESIA: Mild numbing.

MUSCLE RELAXATION: Good, and seemingly amplified by the mood elevation. It is difficult to remain tense while suffused with joy.

DISSOCIATION: At higher doses, Strawberry Cough will cause you to drift away like a helium balloon.

STIMULANT: Gentle but pervasive.

SEDATION: Very little, but it won't interfere with needed rest.

TRAINWRECK

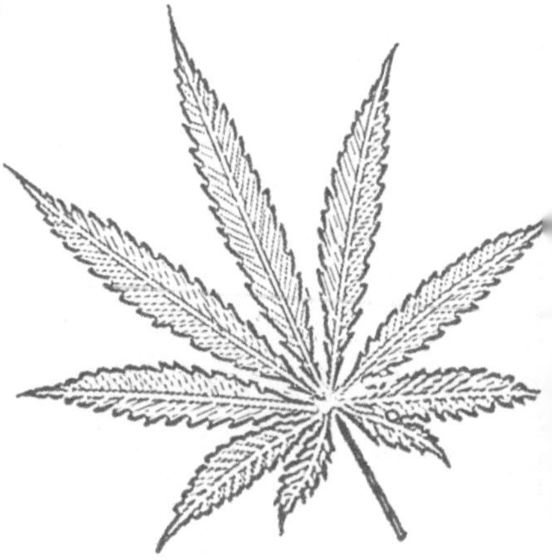

Before the storm of kush varieties hit Los Angeles in the mid-2000s, Trainwreck was tied with OG Kush (see pages 152–55) as the most valued cutting-only variety, commanding up to $80 for one-eighth of an ounce (3.5 grams) at some West Hollywood dispensaries. The reason? Trainwreck is an outstanding narrow-leafleted variety that reeks of spruce and lemon, delivering a clean, energetic psychoactivity with extraordinary mood elevation. That's a complex way to say that Trainwreck is "giggle weed," with the ability to make nearly anything appear absurd and often hilarious.

Medical Uses

Cannabis varieties that provide high medicinal value and THC content with minimal impairment are rare, and Trainwreck sits at the top of the short list. This variety has proved popular with many doctors and medical students who occasionally use medical cannabis. It is excellent for attention deficit/hyperactivity disorder, because it encourages hyperfocus. At higher doses, time seems to pass quickly when engaged in a task. High-quality Trainwreck also has very little "crash" as its effects wear off.

Notes

Trainwreck is an exemplar of medical cannabis, but with a ridiculous name. Many origin tales have sprung up around Trainwreck: In one example, the plant was found growing near the site of a Humboldt County train disaster. In another scenario, Trainwreck was on its way to Oregon with its breeder (who was returning to the U.S. after years of work in the mountains of Mexico) when his train crashed in Northern California. However the simplest explanation is that one of the first individuals who tried it hadn't smoked anything but broad-leafleted indicas for a long time, wasn't picking up on its more cerebral psychoactivity, and had no idea how high he was. When he figured out that he'd smoked too much and became dizzy and extremely disoriented, he might have remarked, "It felt like I'd been in a train wreck or something." High-quality Trainwreck will be very light green with a hint of gold. The variety is extremely frosty, meaning that it is almost encrusted with trichomes. The buds are rarely large, but its bracts are quite big. It is a notoriously low yielder, which is why some greedy fools attempted to "improve" Trainwreck by crossing it with Big Bud. Not surprisingly, the results looked like a bigger-budded Trainwreck, but the joy conveyed with the original's effects were lost—and a odd, skunky, sulfurous note inserted into its aroma. Good Trainwreck typically has small flower clusters.

TYPE: Nearly narrow-leafleted variety.

SPECIES: *Cannabis indica ssp. indica.*

BREEDING DATE: The first plant is believed to have been found in Arcata, California, by Eric Heimstadt around 2000. It was originally called the E-32 cut.

GENETICS: Thai × Mexican.

SIMILAR VARIETIES: Sno-Cap, Lemon Thai, Acapulco Gold.

AVAILABILITY: Clones only.

EASE OF CULTIVATION: Trainwreck flowers very quickly (60 days) for a narrow-leafleted variety.

AROMA: Citrus in a mountain forest from terpinolene, myrcene and ocimene, with a dash of limonene and pinene.

TASTE: Tart and very aromatic.

POTENCY: Up to 18 percent THC.

DURATION OF EFFECTS: Medium—around 90 minutes.

PSYCHOACTIVITY: Trainwreck demonstrates an extremely quick onset and very cerebral effects. Its pinene content reduces memory impairment resulting from THC. This variety displays very energetic and task-oriented psychoactive effects—a classic "let's clean up the place" result.

ANALGESIA: Moderate. Trainwreck is a great example of a variety providing distraction rather than relief from pain. However, both approaches can be effective in managing discomfort.

MUSCLE RELAXATION: Low.

DISSOCIATION: Low, except at high doses.

STIMULANT: Excellent stimulation makes this a top choice for daytime use. Overdoing Trainwreck can cause anxiety and dose control is highly recommended for novices. It is not as speedy as Diesel varieties.

SEDATION: Little.

WHITE WIDOW

White Widow was the first of the White family of cannabis varieties claimed by Scott Blakey. At that time, he was at Green House Seeds in Amsterdam, before he had left (with some acrimony) to found Mr. Nice. White Widow is a very potent cross of a Brazilian *sativa* with a South Indian hybrid of Afghan and Indian genetics. It won the 1995 *High Times* Cannabis Cup and its successors became known as the White family of cannabis genetics, going on to capture several more Cannabis Cups.

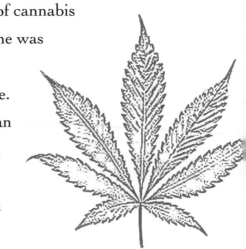

Medical Uses

White Widow is a good choice for neuropathy and nausea. Its strong *indica* nature enforces relaxation, rather than simply extending an invitation. High-myrcene varieties are great for encouraging rest and recuperation.

White Widow was one of the first cannabis varieties to be marketed worldwide within the cannabis cultivation community. That marketing push established White Widow as a brand and it remains one of the best-known varieties in modern cannabis culture.

Notes

Cannabis breeding for seed banks is an agricultural blood sport. Individuals that become breeders of great cannabis are rare and prized, and when they don't feel understood or appreciated they can bolt. This is what happened with Scott Blakey at Green House Seeds. After creating White Widow, he left Green House and started Mr. Nice with new partners that included Neville Shoenmaker and Howard Marks.

White Widow is an excellent variety of medical cannabis with great lineage, but its popularity has diminished from when it first appeared (in 1995) to today. This shift is an excellent example of how changing tastes in cannabis can impact the reputation of once noteworthy varieties. Part of this revisionism is simply fashion. Any criticism of White Widow as being a somewhat generic, high-THC med could be turned on its head a few years from now when it is rediscovered and embraced for its simplicity and economy of chemistry. Recently, Scott Blakey has revisited his White stable of cannabis genetics and tested some new crosses. It will be interesting to see how these new versions are received.

TYPE: Broad-leafleted hybrid.

SPECIES: *Cannabis indica var. braziliana × afghanica.*

BREEDING DATE: circa 1994.

GENETICS: Afghani male from Kerala, India × Brazilian *sativa* mother.

SIMILAR VARIETIES: White Rhino, Great White Shark.

AVAILABILITY: White Widow is available from Green House Seeds and Black Widow, a cross of similar parents, can be obtained from Mr. Nice. Cuttings are widely available.

EASE OF CULTIVATION: Moderate. Cultivation of White Widow has been attempted by many novice patient cultivators with mixed success. It is best to seek some experienced guidance with the variety.

AROMA: Sweet skunk with balsam and pineapple. This variety really needs to be well flushed and cured to hit the fragrant mark. Indifferently cultivated and cured White Widow can smell more like potatoes than cannabis.

TASTE: This strain offers a sweet, hashy flavor when perfectly cultivated—but this is difficult to achieve. White Widow is one of the few cannabis varieties with humulene, one of the primary terpenes found in hops. It is a powerful flavoring agent and is easy to taste in White Widow.

POTENCY: Hard-hitting with quick *sativa* onset, followed by a strong *indica* body high. White Widow often tops 20 percent THC. It has a myrcene-dominant terpene entourage with limonene, pinenes, and beta-caryophyllene.

DURATION OF EFFECTS: Long.

PSYCHOACTIVITY: Excellent, cerebral psychoactivity which quickly morphs into body effects.

ANALGESIA: Good pain reliever from its high-THC and myrcene content.

MUSCLE RELAXATION: Moderate.

DISSOCIATION: Moderate at higher dosages.

STIMULANT: Low stimulation, though initial onset is heady.

SEDATION: White Widow's myrcene content encourages sleep. This can be an issue when using this variety during the day. It is also good for reducing nausea and symptoms of anxiety.

Medical Uses of Cannabis

Medical cannabis can address the symptoms of many ailments. It is rarely a cure, but supplementation of the endocannabinoid system with judicious amounts of plant cannabinoids may reduce the incidence of some diseases and prevent others. The key to the successful use of cannabis as a medicine is to select the proper dose and frequency. The ailments that follow have been selected because cannabis has been used, or has been shown to be effective, for symptomatic relief. Potentially unfounded claims of efficacy are also addressed throughout.

4

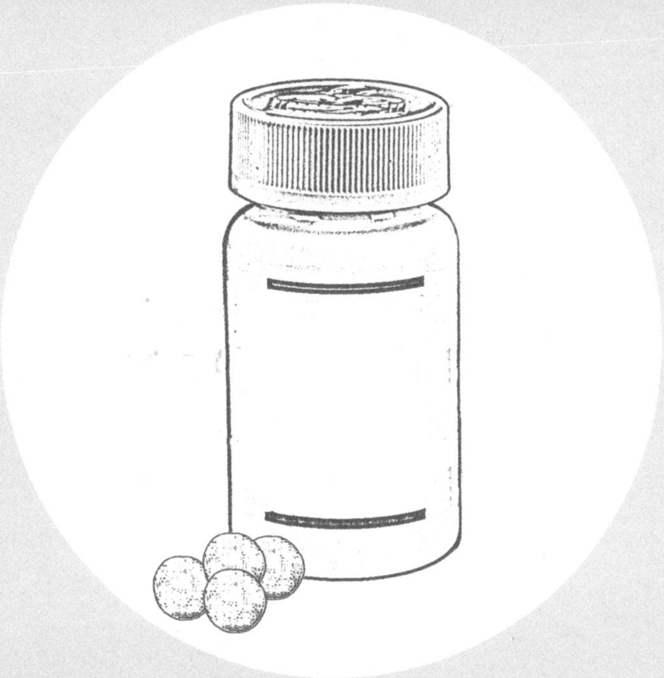

ALZHEIMER'S DISEASE

Alzheimer's disease is an age-related brain disease often associated with profound cognitive decline. Recent research suggests that key aspects of the disease may be tightly intertwined with the body's endocannabinoid system. In the near future, preventive measures for Alzheimer's could foreseeably target parts of the endocannabinoid system and some treatments for Alzheimer's could be cannabinoid-based.[1]

Historical Uses

In 1890, Sir John Russell Reynolds, MD, physician to Queen Victoria, published an account of using cannabis to treat senile dementia in the British medical journal *The Lancet*. Reynolds described using a *Cannabis indica* extract.

He wrote: "In senile insomnia, with wandering; where an elderly person probably with brain-softening, in the 'delirium form' (Durand-Fardel) is fidgety at night, goes to bed, gets up again, and fusses over his clothes and his drawers . . . but may be quite rational during the day, with its stimuli and real occupations. In this class of case I have found nothing comparable in utility to a moderate dose of Indian hemp-viz., one-quarter to one-third of a grain of the extract, given at bedtime. It has been absolutely successful for months, and indeed years, without any increase of the dose."[2] Reynolds's account is a classic example of using cannabis to calm and mildly sedate a patient with Alzheimer's-like dementia.

Description

Alzheimer's disease is a form of dementia that worsens over time, interfering with memory, thinking, and behavior. In Alzheimer's disease, deposits of a protein plaque called beta-amyloid build up between nerve cells, while tangled fibers of another protein called tau accumulate within the brain cells. Scientists believe that this combination of plaques and tangles interferes with communication among nerve cells, eventually killing the adjacent cells.

EFFECTIVENESS—Today, herbal cannabis is still primarily used to calm agitated Alzheimer's patients, encourage sleep, and increase appetite. Future treatments employing cannabinoids may address the actual mechanism and progression of the disease, by harnessing the anti-inflammatory and neuroprotective effects of cannabis and cannabinoids. The body's own endocannabinoids are intimately involved in signaling between nerve cells. It may be that plant cannabinoids, including THC and CBD, may slow the buildup of plaques and tangles, or reduce the inflammatory response to their buildup.

PROPOSED MECHANISM—Typically, the mild sedating effects of cannabis calm the agitated Alzheimer's patient. But plant cannabinoids are also anti-inflammatory and neuroprotective. Inflammation plays a critical role in the progression of Alzheimer's disease. The anti-inflammatory and antioxidant properties of THC, CBD, other cannabinoids, and their analogs may have future therapeutic potential in Alzheimer's treatment. Targeting the body's own endocannabinoid system may offer the potential to stimulate neuroprotective mechanisms while dampening neuro-inflammation caused by the buildup of amyloid proteins in the brain.

DOSAGE—Dosage of THC for calming and sedation of Alzheimer's patients is akin to dosing for insomnia: 5 to 10 milligrams from a high-myrcene variety of cannabis, taken orally. Care must be observed with higher doses of neutral psychoactive cannabinoids, such as THC, since they could potentially cause severe agitation and disorientation. For CBD's anti-inflammatory effects in other illnesses, CBD dosage typically begins at 160 milligrams in most studies and has gone as high as 600 milligrams. It is unknown whether THC or CBD can slow down the progression of the disease.

Methods of Ingestion

ORAL—Oral cannabis preparations are an excellent choice for Alzheimer's, since the effects are long lasting and easily incorporated into a palatable and appealing form for the patient. Care should be observed not to leave the oral preparations accessible where they could be mistakenly eaten by the patient as a snack.

VAPORIZATION AND SMOKING—Vaporized and smoked cannabis are not recommended for Alzheimer's patients without direct supervision, because of safety concerns.

INDICATED CHEMOTYPES—For oral administration, primarily high-THC varieties of cannabis are indicated, if sedation and calming are the desired outcome. High-myrcene varieties may be very helpful for their additional sedative effects and synergy with the cannabinoids. For neuro-protective effects, high-CBD varieties are worth consideration. Propyl variations of cannabinoids such as THCV and CBDV are promising, but studies have not been completed with Alzheimer's patients.

POPULAR VARIETIES—Purple and Afghani broad-leafleted varieties, such as Purple Urkle, Grand Daddy Purple, Bubba Kush, and Hash Plant are recommended for their calming effects. High-CBD varieties, such as Cannatonic and Harlequin, may be of use for their anti-inflammatory effects.

ANXIETY DISORDERS

For thousands of years, cannabis has been used to address symptoms associated with anxiety.[3] However caution is definitely advised here, since there is considerable evidence that large doses of cannabis can trigger anxiety and even paranoia in susceptible individuals.[4] Additionally, studies have shown that female patients diagnosed with social anxiety disorders may be more prone to developing cannabis dependency.[5]

Historical Uses

In Indian medicine it has been claimed that *bhang*, the milk-based cannabis drink, "begets joy and destroys every anxiety." The oral use of cannabis as a medicine to treat anxiety appears in the *Atharvaveda*, a core Vedic text dating to around 2000 BCE.[6] Cannabis traditionally grown as a field crop for the production of hashish in the Middle East and Central Asia has much more CBD than cannabis grown indoors. Patients have long reported that CBD is very effective for reducing the likelihood of cannabis-induced anxiety. Studies in Brazil and elsewhere have confirmed this assertion. The high CBD content of hash plants from Lebanon and Afghanistan made traditional hashish much less likely to trigger anxiety in users than contemporary cannabis cultivars containing little, if any, CBD.

Description

Anxiety disorders include generalized anxiety disorder, obsessive-compulsive disorder (OCD), panic disorder, and post-traumatic stress disorder. Commonalities include worry, rumination, fear, apprehension, and physical tension. Anxiety is also a feature of other psychiatric conditions: depression, bipolar disorder, and schizophrenia.

EFFECTIVENESS—Cannabis is widely used to mitigate the symptoms of anxiety. But cannabis can reduce or increase anxiety depending on the variety, its chemistry and dose, the mind-set of the user, and the setting in which the cannabis is used. Understanding these variables increases the likelihood of relieving the symptoms of anxiety disorders. Cannabis has been described as "biphasic and bidirectional," meaning that it can cause relaxation in some cases, anxiety in others.[7]

PROPOSED MECHANISM—The density of the CB1 cannabinoid receptors found in the brain's amygdala, hippocampus, and anterior cingulate cortex indicates that the endocannabinoid system regulates anxiety, since these structures regulate anxiety and related conditions.

DOSAGE—Both THC and CBD are effective for relieving symptoms of anxiety. However, there is an argument that it may be more effective to use these cannabinoids separately, rather than together, for treating anxiety. THC dosage for anxiety is successful at between 1 and 3 milligrams, while CBD dosage ranges between 2.5 and 10 milligrams. Some studies on humans have used enormous doses of CBD to treat anxiety, but the side effects of such doses include cognitive impairment characterized as "mental sedation." Linalool, the terpene found in a few cannabis varieties and the herb lavender, has been shown to be quite effective for relieving anxiety. CBD dosage for panic disorders and phobias has ranged in studies, reaching up to 600 milligrams—but such high doses have been characterized as causing significant mental sedation, and given the relative scarcity of CBD, may not be practical. It is safe to assume that doses of up to 50 milligrams of CBD (as the sole cannabinoid) can be well tolerated by most patients. However, if long-term usage of cannabinoids is considered, then its dose should be monitored to avoid tolerance effects. Drug holidays are recommended, as appropriate.

Methods of Ingestion

ORAL—Both sublingual and swallowed THC cannabis is effective for anxiety. Special caution should be taken with successive doses of oral THC cannabis to avoid an additive overdose, since this can be anxiety-provoking. CBD cannabis is effective orally and sublingually. Combinations of low-dose oral THC and CBD appear to be mildly synergistic in some patients, which can be slightly anxiety-provoking. If using oral THC and CBD together for anxiety, it is recommended that you reduce the dose of each. Cultivars that contain THCV and CBDV may increase anxiety.

VAPORIZATION AND SMOKING—Smoking and vaping medical cannabis for anxiety is particularly effective, since the patient quickly learns precisely to titrate the proper dose. It's important with vaporization to start with a very small dose of herbal cannabis, typically the size of a match head, and then completely vaporize the active ingredients of the dose.

INDICATED CHEMOTYPES—Nearly any type of cannabis can be used to relieve anxiety, even the most typically anxiogenic varieties such as the Diesels and Hazes, provided that the dose is tightly constrained. This micro-dose approach enables the use of cannabis varieties that are less sedating. For phobias, avoid any strains that are high in pinene, since one's fears may benefit from THC's ability to interfere with memory and recall, and pinene tends to counter the memory effect. CBD varieties appear to be extremely effective for social anxiety and possibly phobias and panic disorders.

POPULAR VARIETIES—Low doses of Bubba Kush are recommended. Any purple indica is suggested, so long as its dose is controlled to avoid sedation.

ARTHRITIS

Arthritis appears to be one of the earliest illnesses for which cannabis was employed as a treatment. Studies have shown that THC in cannabis can reduce arthritis pain. Separately and together, THC and CBD reduce the cytokine activity that is believed to be responsible for the deterioration of joint tissues in arthritis.

Historical Uses

Cannabis has been used for the treatment of arthritis and rheumatoid diseases since around 2500 BCE, when it was first recommended in Shen-Nung's classic Chinese pharmacopeia. The herbalist and author Vivian Crawford notes in her history of medicinal cannabis use in England that Pedanius Dioscorides recommended cannabis for restoring "the softness of joints" in his *De Materia Medica* (50 and 70 CE), which was later cited by William Turner in his noted herbal of 1551. However, the cannabis type used for this sixteenth-century medicine was likely a fiber variety of hemp, rather than a drug variety, since there is no mention at all of psychoactivity. While hemp varieties have no THC, they often contain significant amounts of CBD, which is an effective anti-inflammatory. Crawford also notes that cannabis was featured in the famous Culpeper herbal of 1653 as a treatment for "the hard humors of knots in the joints."[8]

Description

Arthritis covers a wide range of inflammatory conditions, but typically refers to two forms of joint inflammation. Rheumatoid arthritis (RA) is an autoimmune disease, characterized by serious inflammation of a joint's interior lining. RA can cause chronic severe pain, permanent joint damage, and disability. Osteoarthritis (OA), arthritis of the bones, is characterized by loss of cartilage in the joints, typically the hands, hips, knees, and spine. Common OA symptoms include pain, stiffness, loss of motion, and deformation of the joints.

EFFECTIVENESS—Cannabis treatment is moderately effective in treating pain for most patients, but the psychoactivity of drug varieties may not be all that well tolerated by older, cannabis-naive arthritis patients.

PROPOSED MECHANISM—The ability of cannabis medicines to distract from arthritis pain is well established. Plant cannabinoids also elicit a range of anti-inflammatory responses. It has been established that the endocannabinoid system and its receptors are found in the synovial membrane of joints. It is also believed that cannabinoids may play a role in protecting cartilage in the joints. THC has been cited as having twice as much anti-inflammatory activity as hydrocortisone.[9] The two primary cannabinoid receptors within the body are the CB1 and CB2 receptors. CB1 is primarily in the nervous system and stimulation of this receptor is responsible for the psychoactive effects of cannabis. The CB2 receptor is primarily found on immune cells. Endocannabinoids produced by numerous cell types in the body react with both CB1 and CB2, thereby regulating a number of important functions. CB2 activation is linked to modulation of both immune and inflammatory response. The protective anti-inflammatory effects of CB2 stimulation have been noted in animal models of arthritis. The powerful anti-inflammatory effects of the cannabinoids THC and CBD may prove useful in controlling the secretions of pro-inflammatory factors secreted by cells associated with the tissue damage that occurs in several forms of arthritis.

DOSAGE—Dosage of THC for arthritis pain should follow the "sweet spot" model for cannabis-induced distraction from pain. Start with 5 milligrams of THC and slowly increase the size of subsequent doses until pain relief peaks. For anti-inflammatory effects with THC and CBD, dosage recommendations are still being developed. Caution is advised when using large doses of cannabinoids, since receptor downregulation (tolerance) to the effects of cannabis may develop and potentially interfere with its medicinal efficacy.

Methods of Ingestion

ORAL—Oral cannabis preparations are an excellent choice for arthritis pain, since their effects are long lasting. Oral cannabis may be used as an anti-inflammatory on its own or in combination with other medications.

VAPORIZATION AND SMOKING—Both vaporized and smoked cannabis are effective for arthritis pain.

TOPICAL—There are some preliminary indications that topical application of cannabinoids for arthritis could be effective, but research in this area is ongoing.

INDICATED CHEMOTYPES—For oral administration, both THC and CBD varieties of cannabis are indicated, depending on patient needs. THC is a powerful anti-inflammatory agent.[10] Cannabis varieties high in terpenes—myrcene, limonene, and/or linalool—may add synergistic effects that help with arthritis. It may be that chemotypes high in the cannabinoid CBC (cannabichromene), which is noted for its anti-inflammatory effects, may also prove useful with arthritis.

POPULAR VARIETIES—Mildly stimulating, high-THC varieties, such as Trainwreck and the high-CBG Pincher Creek, are popular for providing daytime pain distraction and anti-inflammatory effects. In tandem with THC varieties, high-CBD cannabis such as Cannatonic can be blended to increase anti-inflammatory effects.

ASTHMA

It is easy to understand how asthma treatment with cannabis was discovered, since cannabis smokers often notice the sensation of cannabis smoke expanding rapidly within the lungs.[11] Cannabis smoke can work as a bronchodilator to release bronchospasm associated with asthma. But while some evidence is promising for the use of cannabis with asthma, there is also contradictory evidence. In late 2013, the state of Michigan rejected asthma as a proposed additional qualifying medical condition for medical cannabis use within the state.

Historical Uses

An ancient Egyptian treatment for asthma was inhaling the vapors from herbs placed on heated bricks. Smoking medical plants as a treatment for asthma was somewhat common into the twentieth century, with the most popular being the Jimson weed cigarettes, Cigares de Joy.[12] Henry Hyde Salter, a nineteenth-century physician, wrote that cannabis was widely used in tincture form for asthma.[13] In the early twentieth century, it was believed that asthma was a psychological disorder and only in the 1960s was asthma discovered to be an inflammatory condition.

Description

Asthma is a common inflammatory condition of the airways characterized by bronchospasm and airflow obstruction. Both genetic predisposition and environmental factors play a role in asthma.

EFFECTIVENESS—As cited in a 2000 study in the journal *Nature*, cannabis and THC exert a strong bronchodilation effect on the airways when smoked or vaporized.[14] The overall effects of smoked cannabis on the lungs are decidedly mixed, with light and moderate use causing little to no damage to the lungs, while heavy use is thought to be associated with increased incidence of bronchitis. Because cannabis smoke shares many of the same constituents as tobacco smoke, physicians have long been concerned about the possible increased risk of pulmonary disease from smoked cannabis. Several studies of cannabis smokers have found damage to mucosal tissue lining the airways and evidence of inflammation.[15] However, meta-analysis of lung function and disease has not detected evidence of adverse effects of moderate cannabis use on lung function.[16] One interesting study hypothesized that, in the short term, cannabis smoking improved lung function by stretching the lungs, while, in the long term, it damaged the lungs through the exposure to smoke[17].

PROPOSED MECHANISM—As noted in the *Nature* study, both airway dilation and spasm response are controlled by the endocannabinoid system. In a noted study from 1975, Donald Tashkin at the University of California, Los Angeles, conducted an experiment on eight otherwise healthy patients with stable bronchial asthma. In one of the experiment's protocols, Tashkin had the participants exercise until they suffered an acute asthma bronchospasm. During the attack, the patients smoked either placebo marijuana or 2 percent THC marijuana. The group receiving the placebo took 30 to 60 minutes to recover from the bronchospasm. The group receiving the actual marijuana recovered "immediately," according to Tashkin.[18] Later studies confirmed the potent bronchodilatory effects of THC.[19]

DOSAGE—Tashkin effectively treated bronchospasm with cannabis containing 2 percent THC, only one-eighth as potent as today's average medical cannabis. The Tashkin study supports the idea that very little THC is required to dilate the airways. Later studies put the optimal inhaled dose of THC at only 200 micrograms. That would seem to indicate that an extremely small dose of a cannabis concentrate, high in THC, might be the optimal approach. Cannabis that contains bronchodilatory terpenes such as pinene are also recommended.

Methods of Ingestion

ORAL—Tinctures of cannabis were a popular asthma treatment in the nineteenth century. However, if swallowed they were likely to take too long to work to be of use for an acute asthma attack, because of the length of time required to metabolize a swallowed dose. A sublingual dose is likely more effective.

VAPORIZATION AND SMOKING—Some patients react to cannabis smoke and vapor with bronchospasms, so great care must be exercised. Start with a very small inhalation when stable, before a bronchospasm, to gauge how it might be tolerated. Additionally, it is important to use extremely clean cannabis with low microbial and mold/yeast counts, since these pathogens can irritate the airways or cause secondary lung infections.

INDICATED CHEMOTYPES—THC-dominant varieties high in pinene are suggested, as pinene is also a bronchodilator.

POPULAR VARIETIES—Trainwreck, Sno-Cap, Super Silver Haze, and any variety with high bronchodilatory terpene content. Look for varieties that smell like evergreen trees.

ATTENTION DEFICIT HYPERACTIVITY DISORDER

Cannabis has been shown in case studies to help some ADHD patients to focus on tasks. Patients consistently report that narrow-leafleted cannabis varieties can encourage hyperfocus. The use of cannabis to treat ADHD in younger patients remains controversial due to potential adverse effects of THC on developing brains. CBD and alternative cannabinoid treatment of ADHD has yet to be explored.

Historical Uses

ADHD treatment with cannabis has only emerged in the last decade as an alternative/adjunct to treatment with prescription stimulants and antidepressants.

Description

Attention deficit hyperactivity disorder, or ADHD, has three subtypes: Combined Type, Predominantly Inattentive Type, and Predominantly Hyperactive-Impulsive Type. The term ADD is often used to encompass all types of ADHD. The most common core features of ADHD are distractibility, hyperactivity, and poor impulse control. While these features are commonly found together, each case varies, with over one-third of patients exhibiting no hyperactivity. In brain scans of ADHD patients, the regions of the brain thought to be responsible for attention have reduced glucose uptake, which indicates a lower level of activity. ADHD is very likely caused by changes in neurotransmitter activity within the brain.

EFFECTIVENESS—Cannabis is moderately effective in treating ADHD,[20] though perhaps less successful than some prescription medication alternatives. Some patients report that cannabis also reduces the "jitters" of prescription stimulants used for ADHD treatment. As dosage guidance is developed based upon the terpene profiles associated with different varieties, the effectiveness of cannabis for ADHD should be improved. Caution must be observed when using cannabis with younger ADHD patients because of potential adverse effects. Some doctors assert that the use of THC cannabis makes treatment of ADHD with conventional prescription medications almost impossible.[21] However, this opinion does not appear to be widespread within the medical community. As science learns more about the endocannabinoid system and how it regulates neurotransmitter release within the brain, it is likely that an optimal cannabinoid medicine approach will emerge.

PROPOSED MECHANISM—Studies have indicated that a dysfunction in the dopamine neurotransmitter system may be the underlying mechanism of the ADHD family of conditions.[22] Dopamine receptors interact extensively with the endocannabinoid receptors in parts of the brain, including the striatum. There is also a profusion of cannabinoid receptors located within the limbic system of the brain, specifically the amygdala and hippocampus, which are strongly linked with attention deficit and many other neuropsychiatric disorders, including anxiety and phobias. CB1 receptors are significant in ADHD and are a therapeutic target of increasing interest. Cannabinoid medicines are likely to be developed to target the endocannabinoid system in the treatment of ADHD and related disorders.

DOSAGE—Typically, micro-doses under 2.5 milligrams of THC of relatively low-myrcene content cannabis varieties are used to encourage hyperfocus for up to 90 minutes. Often momentum established from 90 minutes of task focus can preclude the need for further cannabis doses. High-dosage regimens have been shown to be effective in at least one case study, but this approach raises the risk of cannabis dependency and tolerance to THC's effects.

Methods of Ingestion

ORAL—Sublingual ingestion works well for treating ADHD because of the relatively rapid uptake of cannabinoids into the bloodstream from beneath the tongue. The effects of swallowed oral cannabis tend to be too sedating.

VAPORIZATION AND SMOKING—It is easiest to titrate low doses with smoked cannabis. Vaporized cannabis is effective, but care should be observed to control dose and avoid overmedication.

INDICATED CHEMOTYPES—Narrow-leafleted THC varieties that are high in pinene and terpinolene, but without appreciable amounts of myrcene, are suggested. If hyperactivity is an issue, low doses of myrcene- and linalool-dominant cannabis varieties may be of medicinal value for their calming effects. Pure-CBD chemotypes may also be of interest for their proposed ability to help concentration and "clear the mind."

POPULAR VARIETIES—Patients often recommend Neville's Haze at low doses as the most effective variety. Stimulating varieties with low myrcene, such as Trainwreck, are advised, and any narrow-leafleted variety of Central/South American or South Asian genetics may be of interest. Hybrids such as Pincher Creek are also effective.

AUTISM SPECTRUM DISORDERS

Some physicians and parents have embraced cannabis as a treatment to calm severely agitated and violent autistic children. This use of oral cannabis to treat children and adolescents with autism remains controversial. In 2013, the American Academy of Pediatrics recommended that state legislatures issue tighter restrictions on the use of medical marijuana by children, primarily to counter a growing trend of parents using cannabis to treat their autistic-spectrum children. But everyone agrees that more research needs to be done on the uses of cannabis with autism spectrum disorders.

Historical Uses

Bernard Rimland, in the early 1960s, pioneered modern research into childhood neurobehavioral disorders, including autism. He later became an early advocate of the use of cannabis with autism spectrum disorders. According to Rimland's Autism Research Institute, cannabis has successfully reduced some autistic children's aggression, anxiety, panic disorders, tantrums, and self-injurious behavior. In the Internet age, parents of autism spectrum children have taken to the blogosphere to chronicle their experiences using cannabis medicines. In the summer 2010 issue of *O'Shaughnessy's*, Harvard professor Lester Grinspoon, MD, wrote an argument supporting future research into the uses of cannabis to treat autism spectrum children, but also supporting the rights of parents to try experimental treatments in the hopes of helping their severely ill children.[23]

Description

Autism is one of several conditions, including Asperger's syndrome, which compose the autism spectrum of pervasive developmental disorders. Conditions in this spectrum are complex neurobehavioral disorders characterized by impaired communication and social interaction. Autism may severely impede the development and use of language. Asperger's does not interfere with language, but shares the social interaction deficits associated with autism. There is evidence that autism spectrum disorders run in families.[24] There is also controversial evidence that exposure of pregnant women and infants to certain drugs and chemicals may increase the likelihood of these disorders developing.[25]

EFFECTIVENESS—More research is needed to support the initial anecdotal accounts of successful treatment of autism spectrum symptoms with cannabis. There have been few clinical trials or formal case studies, though there is one open-label study of synthetic THC (Marinol) in treating self-injurious behavior among developmentally disabled adolescents, some of whom were on the autism spectrum.[26] Most parental accounts of the successful use of cannabis claim that the medicine calms certain violently oppositional autistic children. It is currently unknown whether CBD or other cannabinoids are effective in treating the symptoms of autism spectrum disorders.

PROPOSED MECHANISM—Nearly all of the anecdotal accounts point to the calming influence of cannabis. This would support the use of cannabis as a mild sedative and tranquilizing agent. In 2013, evidence emerged that the endocannabinoid system of autistic children is significantly different to that of healthy children. Autistic individuals exhibit an average of five times the number of CB_2 receptors than healthy counterparts. This indicates that the endocannabinoid system may prove to be an important target for future treatments for autism. Also recent research points to variations in the gene responsible for the CB_1 receptor (CNR_1 gene) and CB_2 receptor (CNR_2 gene) being linked to several disturbances in the brain involving emotional and social processing, including autism. It may be that poor-functioning CB_2 receptors play a key role in autism and the body reacts to this dysfunction by drastically increasing the number of CB_2 receptors in response.

DOSAGE—Cannabis doses should be recommended by the patient's physician. The child's doctor should calculate the dose of cannabinoids and terpenes from analytical testing results for the individual patient based on the child's condition, response to other medication, age, and other pertinent factors. Information on the use of Marinol and other cannabis medicines by children and adolescents may provide some guidance.

Methods of Ingestion

ORAL—Because orally swallowed cannabis can have a profoundly psychoactive effect on a patient, great care should be taken to understand the dose that is being delivered in order to minimize adverse effects.

VAPORIZATION AND SMOKING—Smoking cannabis is not recommended for autism spectrum children, simply for the fact that it would upset child welfare authorities to an extraordinary degree. Vaporized cannabis for adolescent autism spectrum patients might be more successful under close medical supervision.

INDICATED CHEMOTYPES—High myrcene and linalool varieties containing THC and CBD for their anti-anxiety and neuroprotective effects. CBD is warranted for its neuroprotective effects.

POPULAR VARIETIES—Myrcene and linalool THC varieties are recommended, such as Bubba Kush and Grand Daddy Purple. Adding CBD can be accomplished through blending a pure-CBD variety such as Cannatonic 6 or ACDC with THC strains.

AUTOIMMUNE DISORDERS

The CB2 cannabinoid receptor is responsible for modulating the function of all immune system cells in the body.[27] The endocannabinoid system plays a key role in many autoimmune disorders, but using plant cannabinoids to treat these conditions is not well understood. Both naturally derived and synthetic cannabinoids demonstrate anti-inflammatory and immunosuppressive activity that may be of interest in the treatment of autoimmune disorders including multiple sclerosis, rheumatoid arthritis, diabetes, asthma, and septic shock.[28]

Description

Autoimmune disorders are conditions wherein an immune response wrongly targets healthy tissues. These disorders can sometimes be treated through immunosuppression.

EFFECTIVENESS—Medical cannabis is possibly effective in treating autoimmune disorders and promising research is ongoing.

PROPOSED MECHANISM—Cannabinoids in cannabis can lower the production of inflammatory protein interleukin-2, while raising the production of the anti-inflammatory protein interleukin-10.

DOSAGE—Doses of THC required to suppress immune response may be too high to avoid significant adverse levels of psychoactivity. It may be worth exploring a model that gradually increases THC dosage to assess immunosuppression levels, once the patient develops tolerance to the psychoactivity of THC. The issue of psychoactivity can be avoided by exploring non-psychoactive cannabinoids such as THCV and CBD.

Methods of Ingestion

ORAL—Swallowed and sublingual cannabinoids are effective for partial symptomatic relief of pain from autoimmune disorders including rheumatoid arthritis.

VAPORIZATION AND SMOKING—These methods can also be effective for symptomatic relief.

INDICATED CHEMOTYPES—For symptomatic relief of pain, use high-THC varieties with limonene and myrcene. For anti-inflammatory effects, use high-CBD and -THCV varieties.

POPULAR VARIETIES—For pain due to these disorders, OG, Bubba, and Master Kush varieties are suggested. A hybrid variety, Pincher Creek, is suggested for its additional CBG content. For inflammation, try high-CBD cannabis, such as Harlequin, Cannatonic, or Omrita RX.

CACHEXIA AND APPETITE DISORDERS

The ability of cannabis medicines to encourage appetite is part of popular culture: the "munchies." Cachexia was once the least controversial medicinal property of cannabis, but not always the best understood. Some forms of cachexia, especially ones associated with advanced cancer, may not respond to cannabis. The 2006 clinical study of cannabis with advanced cancer patients, conducted by the Cannabis in Cachexia Study Group, was discontinued when cannabis showed little advantage over the placebo, and produced more side effects. While this was only one study, it has been widely cited as evidence that cannabis is of little use in cancer cachexia, though this remains disputed.[29]

Historical Uses

Cannabis as an appetite stimulant is recognized in ancient Chinese and Indian medical traditions. Cannabis is cited in later Indian Ayurvedic medical texts as increasing the digestive fire.[30] It was also used in British nineteenth-century patent medicines intended to stimulate appetite. The modern medical marijuana movement began in the early 1980s, when it was noted that marijuana use increased the appetite of patients suffering from AIDS.

Description

Cachexia, also known as wasting syndrome, results in emaciation, weakness, and fatigue. It is currently characterized by skeletal muscle loss with or without the loss of fat tissue.[31] Cachexia is much more than loss of appetite, as body mass itself is lost and responsible for the drastic change in the appearance of patients with late-stage cancers and AIDS. In addition to affecting cancer and AIDS patients, cachexia is also common in patients with multiple sclerosis, chronic obstructive pulmonary disease, and tuberculosis. In 2013, there were no FDA-approved drugs for the treatment of cancer cachexia, although several candidate drugs are undergoing clinical trials. One key to successfully treating cachexia is to reverse the loss of muscle mass.

EFFECTIVENESS—Cannabis is effective in treating cachexia, but there are inconsistent results in clinical trials of THC and CBD in combination versus THC alone. At high doses, cannabis tolerance will develop, and the ability of cannabis to stimulate appetite will decline. A recent study from Israel indicated that a wide range of cancer patients reduced their weight loss when smoking cannabis as a palliative treatment during the eight-week study period. In fact, nearly all cancer and anticancer treatment related symptoms were improved among the study participants.[32] However, inhaled cannabis has shown less effectiveness in reviews of other studies.[33]

PROPOSED MECHANISM—The endocannabinoid system is the principal modulator of food intake.[34] Cannabinoids stimulate receptors in the hypothalamus and structures of the hindbrain responsible for appetite regulation. Additionally, phytocannabinoids modulate cytokine activity. Cytokines include signaling molecules, such as interleukin and interferon, which modulate immune system activity. It may be that the inflammatory response linked to cytokine activity is responsible for cachexia. The ability of cannabinoids to interfere with this inflammatory response is currently being studied.

DOSAGE—The "munchies" are a response to a large dose of cannabis, typically occurring 90 minutes after ingestion. This may be because larger doses of cannabis exceed the sweet spot of appetite stimulation, and the stimulation must wait for some of the dose to be metabolized. Appetite stimulation actually requires a very small dose of cannabis. Marinol, the synthetic prescription form of THC, is used to treat cachexia in small, sub-psychoactive doses of 2.5 milligrams before meals. Additionally, varieties of cannabis that are high in beta-caryophyllene should stimulate appetite and may beneficially interfere with the immunological responses underlying cachexia.

Methods of Ingestion

ORAL—Both sublingual and swallowed cannabis medicines are effective.

VAPORIZATION AND SMOKING—If there are no accompanying lung issues, cannabinoid inhalation can be very effective at quickly stimulating the appetite at low doses.

INDICATED CHEMOTYPES—Varieties that are high in beta-caryophyllene are recommended. THC-dominant varieties are most commonly used for appetite stimulation and cachexia treatment. Alternative cannabinoids such as CBD have shown mixed results. Tetrahydrocannabivarin (THCV) varieties will likely retard appetite. Cannabidivarin (CBDV) varieties are promising, but as yet unstudied. High-CBG (cannabigerol) varieties may also be of interest. GW Pharmaceuticals has applied for a patent to use CBG for simultaneous agonism of the CB1 and CB2 receptors in conditions such as cachexia.

POPULAR VARIETIES—Any THC-dominant variety with the distinct peppery aroma of beta-caryophyllene is recommended. The most famous of the peppery cannabis varieties is legendary Panama Red. Super Skunk is another peppery variety, as are many Mexican landraces.

CANCER

Cannabis medicines have been used successfully to treat nausea and vomiting resulting from cancer chemotherapy. They have also potentiated the effects of prescription opioid pain medications in treating cancer pain. They can stimulate appetite, encourage sleep, reduce anxiety and depression, and lift the spirits of patients undergoing cancer treatment, all of which can contribute significantly to quality of life for those living with cancer.[35] But cancer treatment also attracts dubious claimants who extend hope to those desperate for any optimism, resulting in claims of cancer cures—for which there is only promising anecdotal evidence. These overstated or outright false claims have recently extended to cannabis medicines and cancer.

Historical Uses

In the 1950s, Royal Brompton Hospital in London administered the "Brompton cocktail" for intractable cancer pain. This combination of morphine, cocaine, chloroform, and cannabis with cherry syrup was used for 70 years until it fell out of favor and was replaced by next-generation opioids. A tincture of cannabis BPC (British Pharmaceutical Codex) was a prescription pain medicine in the U.K. until 1971. And cannabis has been used to treat the side effects of cancer chemotherapy since the late 1970s, although it gained more widespread notice in the 1990s. Cannabis use among chemotherapy patients is widely responsible for medical cannabis laws being passed in many states.

In studies of cancer cells and some animal models, cannabinoids have been shown to inhibit tumor growth through a variety of mechanisms, though this antitumor activity has not yet been consistently demonstrated in human clinical trials. The effects include suppression of cancer cell signaling mechanisms, inhibition of both blood vessel growth to the tumor and cancer cell migration, and stimulation of programmed cell death in the cancer cell.[36]

While there is limited and widely circulated anecdotal evidence for the antitumor effect of cannabis medicines, there is not enough evidence to claim that cannabis is a broadly effective antitumor treatment. Given the complex variation between cancer types, it is likely that cannabinoids could inhibit one cancer, but promote the growth of another. What is also potentially significant in cell studies is the noted difference in dose response.

For example, at high doses, cannabinoids such as THC may inhibit or stop the growth of some tumors, but at low doses they appear to encourage the proliferation of the same tumors.[37] What can be noted is epidemiological evidence that cannabis use may provide a slight protective effect from developing some cancers, such as head, neck, and lung cancers.[38] By contrast, there are some studies that indicate that cannabis users have increased incidence of prostate, cervical, and brain cancers, though this evidence is far from conclusive.[39]

Description

"Cancer" describes more than 100 diseases in which abnormal cells divide uncontrollably and invade other types of cells. Cancer is not one disease and different forms require different treatments. Our understanding of cancer has progressed, but examining the molecular and genetic mechanisms underlying these diseases—and to the degree required to effect a cure—is an unbelievably complex task.

EFFECTIVENESS

Nausea and vomiting—Chemotherapy, especially with agents such as cisplatin, causes severe nausea and vomiting. Cannabis medicines have been shown to be as effective in relieving chemo-induced vomiting as many conventional antiemetics.[40] Additionally, the "set and setting" aspect of medical cannabis psychoactivity appears to increase the effectiveness for chemo-induced nausea, in that many younger cancer patients strongly embrace the belief that cannabis will be more effective because it is a botanical medicine. Since cannabis became popular for treating nausea and vomiting, a new class of antiemetic drug, Emend, was released in 2003. Some patients get more relief from nausea and vomiting from this medication than from using cannabis. Others prefer a combination of the two medicines.

Appetite stimulation—The endocannabinoid system regulates appetite. Conventional antiemetics prevent vomiting and nausea but do not increase appetite, while cannabis medicines can do both. Appetite stimulation was the first medical condition for which the FDA approved a cannabinoid medicine. Dronabinol (Marinol), synthetic THC in sesame oil, was approved to stimulate appetite in the treatment of cachexia in AIDS patients in 1992.[41] At the same time, and not coincidentally, the George H. W. Bush administration suspended new applications to the Compassionate Investigational New Drug program that provided herbal cannabis to a limited number of seriously ill patients. The U.S. government hoped that Marinol was the answer to the medical marijuana question. But Marinol turned out to be highly psychoactive even at low doses, which ensured that it would be poorly tolerated by a number of patients. And because Marinol was orally administered, absorption was quite variable among patients, which made dosage challenging. Many early Marinol patients quickly switched to herbal cannabis medicines in an attempt to minimize side effects and gain more precise control over dosage. A recent randomized placebo-controlled preliminary study of the effectiveness of Sativex for controlling chemotherapy-induced nausea and vomiting indicated that the THC:CBD spray was effective at daily doses of four sprays, a total of 10 milligrams of THC and CBD.[42]

Pain—Cannabis medicines are quite effective for reducing, and even preventing, some forms of cancer pain. Ten milligrams of THC was shown to be as effective as 60 milligrams of codeine over seven hours of treatment.[43] In animal models of chemotherapy-induced neuropathic pain, CBD (cannabidiol) has been shown to prevent neuropathy.[44] Sativex is currently in Phase III clinical trials for treating advanced cancer pain that is not responding to opioid pain treatment. In combination therapy, cannabis medicines have been shown to improve the pain relief of administered opioids.[45]

Sleep—Given their track record as soporifics, cannabis medicines might be expected to effectively encourage sleep in cancer patients, but research in this area has been disappointing.[46]

Anxiety and depression—Caution must be exercised when using cannabis to treat cancer-related anxiety and/or depression, since cannabis medicines high in THC are biphasic: at higher doses they can cause feelings associated with anxiety, but at lower doses they reduce anxiety. These effects extend to symptoms of depression.[47]

Mood elevation—Assessing the ability of cannabis medicines to lift the spirits of cancer patients is less evidence- than experience-based. Anyone who has worked with patients using cannabis while undergoing chemotherapy has heard numerous anecdotes about how the medicine can help patients get through rough stretches of chemotherapy. Part of this may be due to how THC interferes with memory creation.

Antitumor activity—Dr. Donald Abrams, a noted San Francisco oncologist, is asked constantly about the potential antitumor uses of cannabis medicines. His response is compassionate, but terse, as he feels that cannabis cures for cancer are far from proven. Dr. Manuel Guzman, a leading scientist conducting studies that test cannabinoid medicines on cancer cell lines, stated on the International Association for Cannabinoid Medicines website that, "Although it is possible—and of course, desirable—that cannabis preparations have exerted some antineoplastic activity in some particular cancer patients, the current anecdotal evidence reported on this issue is pretty poor, and, unfortunately, remains far from supporting that cannabinoids are efficacious anticancer drugs for large patient populations." An encouraging 2012 study led by Italian researchers Luciano De Petrocellis and Vincenzo Di Marzo clearly demonstrates that non-THC cannabinoids such as CBD were effective in treating certain prostate cancer lines. Evidence shows that the endocannabinoid system in the normal prostate is not functioning correctly in prostate cancer. The researchers in the Italian study strongly assert that cannabidiol should be further tested against prostate cancer lines.[48] Based on this research, Pál Pacher from the National Institutes of Health published a commentary which suggested that Sativex be tested as a potential treatment for prostate cancer.[49]

PROPOSED MECHANISM—As Abrams and Guzman note in *Integrative Oncology*, because cannabinoids have multiple mechanisms of actions with different receptors throughout the body, much more research must be conducted to fully understand these mechanisms. What is known is that at rational doses, cannabinoids have low toxicity and very little drug interaction with chemotherapy agents.

DOSAGE

This discussion of dosage uses the amount of THC as its general guideline for calculating cannabis dose. To use this section effectively, cannabis of known THC content is recommended. If lab-tested cannabis is not available, it might be helpful to note that the average potency of high-quality, seedless, dried cannabis flowers that have been cultivated indoors is typically between 15 and 17 percent THC.

Nausea and vomiting—Reducing vomiting brought on by chemotherapy requires a relatively high dose of THC. This dose is calculated using a body surface area (BSA) calculation, as is common in many cancer drug treatments. The dose by BSA is typically 5 milligrams per square meter. For example, for a six-foot (1.8-meter) male weighing 175 pounds (79 kilograms), the BSA formula would recommend an initial 10 milligram dose of THC, three hours before the chemotherapy session. If that dose proves ineffective, the dose can be slowly and incrementally increased up to a maximum of 15 milligrams per square meter, which, for our male subject, converts to a dose of up to 30 milligrams—an amount which most patients find to be extremely psychoactive, perhaps uncomfortably.

Appetite stimulation—Treatment of weak appetite typically requires a very small dose of THC, around 2.5 milligrams, which is commonly considered to be below the threshold of psychoactivity.

Pain—Understanding the "sweet spot" approach to cannabis dose and pain, most patients respond best at doses between 10 and 15 milligrams of THC every three to six hours.

Sleep—Normally between 2.5 and 7.5 milligrams of THC, one hour before bedtime.

Anxiety and depression—Small doses of THC between 2.5 and 5 milligrams. Care must be exercised not to induce anxiety with high doses of THC. CBD is most effective for reducing anxiety, especially that which is brought on by higher doses of THC.

Mood elevation—Very small doses under 2.5 milligrams of THC, at the threshold of psychoactivity.

Antitumor activity—Dose and choice of cannabinoid for treatment of tumors should be done under the supervision of an integrative oncology team.

Methods of Ingestion

ORAL—Sublingual and swallowed forms are quite effective, but sublingual has a quicker onset and is more predictable. Swallowed medicines tend to provide longer-lasting effects and seem to have some advantages for nausea and vomiting, provided they are taken three hours before a chemo session.

VAPORIZATION AND SMOKING—Vaporization is quite effective and titration of dose is easily achieved. In Israel, it is not uncommon to see patients vaporizing or even smoking cannabis during the chemotherapy session.

INDICATED CHEMOTYPES—Typically broad-leafleted varieties high in myrcene, limonene, and linalool are recommended. CBD chemotypes are also useful for anxiety.

POPULAR VARIETIES—Nearly all varieties of cannabis will address the adverse effects stemming from cancer treatments. In particular, Cannatonic for its CBD content; and OG Kush, Grand Daddy Purple, Pincher Creek, and Bubba Kush for their THC and terpene content.

CHRONIC FATIGUE SYNDROME

Chronic fatigue syndrome (CFS) describes a cluster of symptoms characterized by severe fatigue unrelieved by rest. Dozens of explanations have been proposed, ranging from environmental toxins to viruses, but no cause has been proven. CFS symptoms vary considerably among the affected population.

Description

The Centers for Disease Control and Prevention define CFS as "self-reported persistent or relapsing fatigue for at least six consecutive months." Sufferers must also experience four or more of the following symptoms: post-exertion malaise, impaired memory and concentration, unrefreshing sleep, muscle pain, joint pain, tender cervical or axillary lymph nodes, sore throat, and headache. The symptoms must have persisted or recurred during six or more consecutive months of illness and must not have predated the fatigue.[50]

EFFECTIVENESS—The effectiveness of cannabis for mitigation of chronic fatigue symptoms is reportedly mixed, and no formal studies of the use of cannabis medicines have been conducted.

PROPOSED MECHANISM—The underlying mechanism of CFS is not well understood. A 2008 paper discusses a potential connection between a key enzyme (which is overproduced in CFS) and exposure to organophosphate pesticides. The endocannabinoid link is tenuous, but exposure to these pesticides has also been shown to interfere with enzymes that the body uses to break down endocannabinoids.[51] Another hypothesis is that chronic fatigue is the result of oxidative stress. Oxidative stress refers to the toxic byproducts of reactive oxygen, which include peroxides and free radicals that attack and damage cellular components. It is thought that oxidative stress disrupts endocannabinoid signaling. Cannabis extracts containing CBD have been shown to be effective in reducing the symptoms directly linked to oxidative stress.[52] It may be possible that CBD also reduces the damage of oxidative stress, which in turn may underlie aspects of CFS.

DOSAGE—When using "pure" CBD varieties with trace amounts of THC, large doses can be tolerated. Doses of up to 50 milligrams of CBD are not uncommon, although lower doses may be effective.

Methods of Ingestion

ORAL—Oral CBD should be effective, but to avoid the first-pass liver metabolism, sublingual CBD should be considered. Avoid taking CBD too close to bedtime, as it has a mild stimulating effect.

VAPORIZATION AND SMOKING—Vaporized, CBD-rich cannabis flowers and concentrates are recommended.

INDICATED CHEMOTYPES—High-CBD varieties with CBD to THC ratios of at least three to one.

POPULAR VARIETIES—Cannatonic or Harlequin.

DIABETES

In 2012, the total healthcare costs for diagnosed diabetes in the U.S. reached $245 billion.[53] In the lead editorial of the July 2013 issue of the *American Journal of Medicine*, Dr. Joseph S. Alpert, its editor-in-chief and a professor of medicine at the University of Arizona, posed the question: "Is it possible that THC will be commonly prescribed in the future for patients with diabetes or metabolic syndrome… ?"[54] Alpert's editorial accompanied a new epidemiological study by University of Nebraska researchers, which indicated that current cannabis users had significantly healthier levels of insulin, as well as less insulin resistance than nonusers of cannabis.

Historical Uses

In 2000, Raphael Mechoulam (codiscoverer of THC) joined a group of Israeli immunologists to explore the use of cannabinoids as potential treatments for autoimmune disorders such as rheumatoid arthritis.[55] Preliminary success in their explorations encouraged the team to examine cannabinoid effectiveness in suppressing or modulating the immune response in the onset and progression of type 1 diabetes in a mouse model.[56] Since 2006, research studies have been conducted to determine how cannabinoids might be used to treat diabetes.[57] In the United Kingdom, GW Pharmaceuticals is conducting Phase 1 clinical trials with the cannabinoids THCV and CBD to treat fatty liver disease and high cholesterol in type 2 diabetes patients.

Healthy levels of insulin and insulin resistance translate into fewer instances of diabetes.[58] Diabetes and prediabetes affect over 100 million Americans, according to the Centers for Disease Control and Prevention.[59] Cannabis and cannabinoid medicines might eventually provide new treatments and prevention approaches for diabetes and related metabolic syndromes.

Description

Diabetes is a group of metabolic conditions in which the body does not produce enough insulin or has become resistant to its effects. Insulin is a hormone required to convert sugar, starches, and other food into energy. The two most common forms of diabetes are designated type 1 and type 2. Type 1 diabetes is typically diagnosed in children and young adults. In type 1 diabetes, the pancreas does not produce insulin. Type 2 diabetes is the much more common form, normally affects adults, and is associated with obesity. In type 2 diabetes, the body becomes resistant to the effects of insulin, which enables glucose to accumulate to dangerous levels within the body. High glucose levels damage vascular and other tissues, resulting in heart disease, stroke, blindness, and kidney and nerve damage. According to a National Institutes of Health review, diabetes is the leading cause of preventable blindness among adults.[60]

EFFECTIVENESS—The effectiveness of medical cannabis to address the underlying causes and complications of prediabetes and diabetes is still being researched but is very promising.

PROPOSED MECHANISM—The endocannabinoid system appears to play a key role in the development of diabetes and its complications. Diabetic complications that are linked to endocannabinoid system function include: blindness, atherosclerosis, kidney failure, heart disease, and neuropathic pain.[61] Plant cannabinoids with reduced or no psychoactivity—including CBD, CBDV, and THCV—may be of interest in maintaining pancreatic function and insulin resistance Recent research has proposed that CBD may prevent retinal damage associated with diabetes by acting as an antioxidant and enhancing the retina's own defenses against inflammation.[62] THCV may prove of interest since it is an antagonist of the CB1 cannabinoid receptor; CB1 antagonists such as rimonabant have shown some promise in obesity and other metabolic conditions related to diabetes in the ARPEGGIO clinical trial.[63]

DOSAGE—The suggested dose of medical cannabis for the treatment of prediabetes and diabetes will vary depending on the dominant cannabinoid (THC, CBD, THCV, CBDV, etc.) of the variety being used. More research will clarify the appropriate combination and dose of phytocannabinoids for addressing these conditions.

Methods of Ingestion

Both oral and vaporized use of high-CBD/CBDV/THCV cannabis varieties may eventually prove of interest in controlling metabolic illnesses such as diabetes.

POPULAR VARIETIES—South African varieties produce some THCV, particularly Durban Poison, which may be useful in treating some symptoms of diabetes and metabolic disorders. High-THCV cannabis is currently scarce in the U.S. High-CBD varieties such as Cannatonic and Harlequin are increasingly easy to find. CBDV cannabis is not readily available, but may actually exist in the U.S. and has yet to be identified simply because of the lack of lab testing for this particular cannabinoid.

FIBROMYALGIA

The cause of fibromyalgia remains unknown, but its prevalence reaches 3 percent of the population and seven times more women than men. Conventional pharmaceutical treatments target fibromyalgia symptom relief, but patient response is typically mixed and cannabis has become a common alternative.

Description

Fibromyalgia is a rheumatic disorder, such as arthritis. It is characterized by chronic pain throughout the body, heightened and painful response to pressure, insomnia, morning stiffness, and debilitating fatigue. A number of factors are involved, including nervous and endocrine system abnormalities, genetic factors, and social and environmental stressors.[64]

EFFECTIVENESS—The success of cannabis in treating fibromyalgia varies, but should provide at least mild reduction in symptomatic intensity, especially for pain and sleep issues.

PROPOSED MECHANISM—Fibromyalgia remains poorly understood. It may be the result of overall central sensitization to pain signaling, a defect in neurotransmitter release, or the obstruction of pathways that the body uses to inhibit pain signaling.[65] It has also been suggested that it may be the result of a dysfunction in the body's response to stress.[66] Another hypothesis has been proposed that the condition may be due to deficiency of endocannabinoids.[67] A small group of patients may be genetically predisposed to a defective endocannabinoid system wherein too much anandamide circulates through the body; this might be a key underlying factor.[68]

DOSAGE—Patients have reported initial doses equivalent to 4 milligrams of THC, the threshold of psychoactivity. The dose can also be raised to 10 milligrams of THC. By using THC and CBD cannabis medicines in combination, some of the side effects of THC may be mitigated. CBD in doses up to 10 milligrams might be used to restore endocannabinoid tone.

Methods of Ingestion

ORAL—Because oral cannabis delivers long-lasting relief, it is popular with fibromyalgia patients. Avoid overmedication, since it has been shown to increase pain in a University of California study.[69]

VAPORIZATION AND SMOKING—Vaporization is a good approach for controlling. Smoking remains the most common delivery method.

INDICATED CHEMOTYPES—Both THC and CBD chemotypes are recommended, and THC/CBD hybrids should be quite effective.

POPULAR VARIETIES—Harlequin is recommended for its CBD and THC content. Purple wide-leafleted varieties such as Grand Daddy Purple are suggested for their relaxing terpene content.

GASTROINTESTINAL DISORDERS

Popular wisdom states that the most common effect of cannabis on the gastrointestinal (GI) tract is the phenomenon known as the "munchies," a popular term for the food cravings that strike recreational cannabis users. The munchies are actually triggered in the brain, not the GI tract. But the munchies are about more than encouraging eating; they are a mechanism to encourage the consumption of rich, high-fat foods.[70] The body's endocannabinoids regulate not only all feeding behaviors, including infant suckling, but nearly all gut function. The regulatory functions of the GI tract are tightly linked to the endocannabinoid system. And the actions of the GI tract are primarily controlled by the enteric nervous system, a mesh of 100 million neurons located in the epithelium of the GI tract, which acts on its own to regulate gut function. Both CB1 and CB2 receptors are found on these enteric neurons. While it is suspected that endocannabinoid receptors are also located throughout other parts of the gut, the picture remains incomplete.

What is known is that the endocannabinoid system's role in GI function is merely a facet of its job in controlling energy balance and metabolism throughout the body. From feeding to insulin production to fat storage, endocannabinoids and their receptors are crucial to how the body acquires energy and uses it.

Description

The profusion of cannabinoid receptors located within the gastrointestinal system is a primary reason that cannabis has been used effectively for gastrointestinal disorders from vomiting and cramping to pain and inflammatory conditions. Cannabinoids interact with a range of gut receptors beyond just cannabinoid receptors, including TRPV1 receptors which are also the receptors for capsaicin, found in hot chili peppers. There are also more recently discovered receptors in the gut, which interact with cannabinoids, though their role is not well understood.

EFFECTIVENESS—Cannabinoids have been shown to be effective in treating chemotherapy-induced nausea and vomiting in over 40 studies.[71] Because of the widespread occurrence of cannabinoid

Historical Uses

Some of the earliest use of medical cannabis occurred in India in around 5000 BCE, where the plant was used to stimulate appetite and counter weight loss.[72] By 1900, cannabis was prescribed by physicians in North America and Europe to treat stomach pain, diarrhea, and gastrointestinal disorders.[73] In the early 1980s, a University of California professor studied the use of cannabis to treat chronic peptic ulcers; his subjects were the local population in a remote group of fishing villages on Cape Breton Island in Nova Scotia. The nearest health care facilities for these villages were 35 miles (56 kilometers) away and cannabis became a popular remedy for the gastric pain of the peptic ulcers, which were unusually prevalent within this region (37 percent of the population).[74] Contemporary cannabis medicine can be traced to the use of the plant to treat decreased appetite and vomiting among HIV/AIDS and cancer patients in the early 1980s. Contemporary Indian Ayurveda medicine recommends cannabis for irritable bowel syndrome, Crohn's disease, and chronic diarrhea.

receptors throughout the GI tract, it is not surprising that cannabis provides a range of effective treatments for GI disorders. As CB receptor mechanisms are better understood, there is considerable promise for cannabinoid-based treatments. But this system is complex, and therapies will have to be better understood in order to avoid the disappointment of rimonabant. Rimonabant was a diet drug that blocked the action of the CB1 receptor, in order to reduce appetite. It had the side effect of making some patients severely depressed, even suicidal. Rimonabant was withdrawn as a diet drug in 2008.

Cannabinoids may eventually provide treatments for colorectal cancer, since a range of these cannabinoids have shown promise in preliminary cell studies of several lines of these tumors.[75] Endocannabinoids have been shown to encourage cell death in some gastrointestinal cancer cells in laboratory studies.

Tolerance to cannabis has more side effects than just reduced psychoactivity. Studies in the 1970s showed that cannabis tolerance reduced THC's ability to slow down movement through the intestinal tract. This means chronic, high-dose use of medical cannabis will likely reduce the effectiveness of cannabis for treating the symptoms of bowel disorders. The latest research on the effectiveness of cannabis for treatment of GI disorders is contradictory. A recent study in Canada demonstrated that cannabis provided effective symptomatic relief for inflammatory bowel disease, but increased the likelihood of surgical interventions among Crohn's disease patients. While in Israel, a small study of Crohn's patients found that cannabis treatment resulted in complete remission of symptoms in over half of the participants.

PROPOSED MECHANISM—Endocannabinoid production levels increase in the brain between meals until they eventually trigger feeding, then quickly drop when feeding begins. Within the GI tract, CB1 receptors respond to endocannabinoid signaling to regulate a wide range of functions, including stomach acid secretion, stomach emptying, pyloric valve contraction between the stomach and small intestine, and the ability to move food along the digestive tract. Additionally, CB1 and CB2 receptors can reduce pain signaling in the viscera. The endocannabinoid system is apportioned throughout the GI system and involved in an extraordinary range of roles in the regulation of appetite, nausea, vomiting, gastric acid and enzyme secretion, gut motility, and intestinal inflammation. The production of CB2 receptors within the gut actually may be stimulated by probiotic acidophilus bacteria, and because of CB2's role in the gut's immune response, it may explain the mechanism by which probiotics seem to reduce some forms of intestinal inflammation.[76]

DOSAGE—Choosing an effective cannabis dose for GI disorders will be condition dependent. Appetite stimulation usually requires a very small dose, often below the threshold for psychoactivity at 2 to 4 milligrams. Chemotherapy nausea is at the other end of the scale, sometimes requiring THC doses in excess of 20 milligrams. Most GI disorders require a dose between these two, typically in the 5 to 7 milligram range. Recent animal research into the use of the non-psychoactive cannabinoid cannabigerol (CBG) appears quite promising for the treatment of inflammatory bowel disease (IBD) and ulcerative colitis. Varieties of cannabis are increasingly available with 1 to 2 percent CBG content and this content should be factored into dose calculations.

Methods of Ingestion

ORAL—Oral cannabis medicines can be very soothing to the gut, if properly prepared. Avoid strong spices and flavorings in cannabis edibles for these conditions.

VAPORIZATION AND SMOKING—Most patients smoke or vaporize cannabis for GI disorders.

INDICATED CHEMOTYPES—Most patients use *indica* varieties for GI disorders ranging from appetite stimulation to more serious immune disorders such as Crohn's disease. THC has been shown to reduce spasmodic activity in the intestines, so high-THC varieties can be quite effective. CBD varieties can calm gut cramping and inflammation. THCV cannabis varieties are likely to reduce appetite, since THCV is a cannabinoid receptor antagonist, though THCV varieties remain scarce in 2013. In Italy, recent research using mice provided evidence that the cannabinoid CBG may help reduce gastrointestinal inflammation. Varieties such as Pincher Creek typically contain an appreciable amount of CBG.

POPULAR VARIETIES—Purple wide-leafleted and Afghan varieties are popular with irritable bowel syndrome and Crohn's disease patients. OG Kush phenotypes with a citrus aroma, which produce limonene and THC, are popular with patients with gastroesophageal reflux disease and Crohn's. Beta-caryophyllene, found in varieties such as Panamanian- and Colombian-derived genetics, is synergistic with THC in protecting cells lining the GI tract.[77] South African varieties high in THCV should help stem unwanted "munchies," while any high-THC variety such as Pincher's Creek should encourage appetite and reduce nausea.

GERONTOLOGY

Cannabis medicines are increasingly used to address many medical issues facing older patients. Among this older population, the use of cannabis remains a controversial issue, partially because of divergent experiences with the drug. Among patients ages 54 to 59, almost 60 percent have used cannabis, while among individuals over 80 years of age, less than 10 percent have ever used cannabis.[78] In the U.S., the number of people over the age of 50 using cannabis daily has doubled from 2002 to 2012.[79]

Historical Uses

The use of cannabis to treat diseases and conditions of the elderly goes back as far as the nineteenth century when the noted physician John Reynolds used *Cannabis indica* extract to treat an older patient with dementia.[80] Reynolds was ahead of his time, as recent evidence shows that cannabis may slow or prevent some aspects of Alzheimer's disease and other forms of senile dementia (see pages 176–77).

The biggest problem facing seniors who wish to use medical cannabis is safe and reliable access to the medicine in states or countries lacking formal systems of access to medical cannabis. In 2009, for example, when the retirement community of Laguna Woods in southern California decided to allow a marijuana collective to be organized by 150 of its 18,000 residents, the foundation that ran the community banned outdoor cultivation of medical marijuana after a few plants were stolen. Increasingly, the desire of an aging baby boomer population to revisit cannabis for its medical, rather than recreational, value will likely be the source of friction in many communities.

Description

Many of the conditions for which cannabis medicines can be effective, from chronic arthritis pain to appetite stimulation to insomnia, are common among the elderly. Baby boomers who used cannabis recreationally in the 1960s are now returning to it as a medicine, many of them after decades of abstinence.

EFFECTIVENESS—One of the key issues for using cannabis effectively with older patients is education. Expectations must be set for an achievable outcome, along with a frank assessment of potential side effects and how they might be avoided. While there is no reason to overly dramatize the likelihood or severity of side effects from psychoactive cannabis medicines, the older patient should be prepared for some measure of side effects.

PROPOSED MECHANISM—Cannabis contains a variety of constituents that are pharmacologically interesting in the treatment of symptoms associated with aging, especially as many of these compounds are analgesic, anti-inflammatory, regulate appetite, and elevate mood.

DOSAGE—Dosage with cannabis-naive, older patients can be challenging and needs to be carefully and conservatively managed. Many of the psychoactive effects of cannabis medicines can be somewhat alarming to an older patient. Special care must be observed when using psychoactive cannabinoids since the side effects can be difficult to frame for these patients. What a regular medical cannabis user might consider "euphoria" is often described by older, cannabis-naive patients as "dizziness" or "vertigo." It is also important to avoid drug interactions with other medications which the elderly patient may be taking. Reduction in any opiate medication might be recommended, since cannabinoids tend to increase the effectiveness of opiates.

Methods of Ingestion

ORAL—Oral ingestion is likely the safest method, but establishing the minimum effective dose is important in order to avoid adverse effects of psychoactive cannabinoids. With THC-based medicines, start with dose of 2 to 2.5 milligrams, which is slightly below the threshold of psychoactivity. For the first few days, dose twice per day, at lunch and after dinner. Increase the cannabis dose by a few milligrams per day until a balance between medicinal effect and tolerable levels of psychoactivity are reached. Because there is a wide variation in response to oral cannabis, establishing proper dosage often requires trial and error. And it is always preferable to underdose than overdose.

VAPORIZATION AND SMOKING—Many older patients prefer the fast onset and ease of dose titration that accompanies vaporized and smoked cannabis. An understanding of how cannabis constituents are vaporized sequentially, according to the constituent's boiling point by the heat of the vaporizer, will help the patient achieve a complete and predictable dose of cannabis.

TOPICAL—For arthritis and skin conditions, THC, CBD, and combination creams are increasingly popular with patients.

INDICATED CHEMOTYPES—THC- and CBD-based varieties are recommended. Typically, relaxing myrcene-dominant varieties are better tolerated than stimulating beta-caryophyllene and limonene varieties.

POPULAR VARIETIES—Functional, wide-leafleted varieties with moderate THC levels, such as Bubba Kush, are easier to titrate for older patients when vaporized or smoked. High-myrcene, narrow-leafleted hybrids such as Trainwreck or Pincher Creek are also good for daytime pain, appetite stimulation, and mood elevation.

GLAUCOMA

Glaucoma is one of the medical conditions most often cited as being effectively treated by medical cannabis. While cannabinoid-based medicines continue to show promise as the basis of future glaucoma treatments, the use of THC and herbal cannabis is not widely accepted as effective for glaucoma. Cannabis is infrequently recommended by ophthalmologists for glaucoma treatment, but remains among the most common alternative treatments for the disease.

Historical Uses

In the 1970s, glaucoma became one of the first medical conditions to be cited as a justification for a compassionate exception to prevailing laws against cannabis use. Cannabis as a potential treatment for glaucoma was noted in a 1971 study, in which smoking cannabis lowered intraocular pressure (IOP) among the participants by 25 to 30 percent.[81] A 1984 study in California recruited 20 ophthalmologists to study the effect of oral and inhaled cannabis on IOP levels of glaucoma patients, but only nine patients were ultimately recruited into the study. The results of this study were published in 2002 and the results were mixed, with many of the patients complaining of unacceptable levels of psychoactivity from the oral THC administered during the study. Interestingly, the two patients with the best results took smaller doses than nearly all the participants who left the study because of side effects.[82]

Description

Glaucoma is a catchall term used to describe a group of diseases of that attack the optic nerve; it is the leading cause of blindness. High pressure of fluid within the eye typically, but not always, causes this nerve damage. Primary open-angle glaucoma, the most common form, has no noteworthy signs or symptoms, except gradual loss of vision. Pressure builds and damages the eyes because the fluid within the eye (called aqueous humor) does not properly move from behind the iris into a small chamber at the front of the eye, where it filters through a spongy tissue before passing into a larger channel and merges into the bloodstream.

EFFECTIVENESS—The American Glaucoma Society and the Canadian Ophthalmological Society released position papers in 2010 that were highly critical of the efficacy of medical cannabis for glaucoma treatment.[83] There are significant obstacles to overcome in developing effective cannabinoid medicines to reduce IOP and protecting neural tissue in the retina. THC is only effective at reducing IOP in glaucoma patients for three to four hours. There is evidence that, over time, patients build up a tolerance to the IOP-reducing effects of THC.

PROPOSED MECHANISM—Endocannabinoid receptors are located throughout the eye, including the retina, the cornea, and surrounding tissues. These receptors are also located within the trabecular meshwork, which drains the liquid intraocular aqueous humor from the eye. Glaucoma causes buildup of pressure in the aqueous humor that is thought to damage retinal nerve cells. As the endocannabinoid system within the eye has become better understood, additional therapeutic targets for cannabinoid medicines emerge. THC reduces IOP in glaucoma. CBD does not reduce pressure, but it does offer neuroprotective effects that may possibly protect retinal ganglia from injury by glaucoma.[84]

DOSAGE—THC has been shown to reduce intraocular pressure at doses of 5 milligrams, four times a day—though the ability of THC to reduce IOP may decline over treatment. The use of CBD or alternative cannabinoids to protect optic and retinal nerve tissue is still being studied. There have been suggestions that innovative delivery methods to target the cannabinoid receptors within the eye may be developed in the near future. These innovations rely on the use of "prodrugs," pharmacologically inactive substances that the body metabolizes into drugs.

Methods of Ingestion

ORAL—Orally administered THC is effective for short-term reduction of intraocular pressure due to glaucoma, but tolerance to the benefits of THC treatment typically builds over time.

VAPORIZATION AND SMOKING—Inhaled cannabis is effective for short-term reduction in pressure (three to four hours) due to glaucoma, but tolerance to THC's effects builds following sustained usage, reducing its efficacy.

TOPICAL—Although topical application to the eye, in the form of eyedrops, would be an optimal route of administration, cannabinoid molecules in such preparations are not well absorbed or distributed and therefore not very effective. Eventually, an eyedrop might be developed that employs an innovative prodrug that the eye metabolizes into a cannabinoid that reduces pressure within the eye.

INDICATED CHEMOTYPES—High-CBD cannabis is recommended for its potential neuroprotective effect on the optic nerve. Consistent and lasting reduction in interocular pressure is unlikely to be achieved with cannabis alone.

POPULAR VARIETIES—Cannatonic or other high-CBD varieties are suggested. High-THC varieties can provide short-term benefits as an adjunct therapy, but their use and efficacy should be discussed in depth with an ophthalmologist.

HEPATITIS C

In a major study of the impact of cannabis smoking on the progression of liver disease among hepatitis C/HIV coinfected patients, published in July 2013, researchers from McGill University in Canada found no link between cannabis use and liver fibrosis progression in hepatitis C. This result was surprising, since daily cannabis use had previously been associated with the progression of liver fibrosis in this population.[85] Earlier studies had shown that cannabis use among patients with the hepatitis C virus resulted in increased liver fibrosis and steatosis.[86]

Historical Uses

The first antiviral drugs began to emerge in the late 1970s. An early study of combination therapy on an emerging hepatitis variant took place in 1986, before hepatitis C had even been identified as the cause. The use of cannabis to combat the nausea and vomiting of such antiviral treatments had become more prevalent after the AIDS crisis of the early 1980s, when alternative approaches to deal with pharmaceutical side effects became crucial to compliance with these treatments.

The liver disease that accompanies the progression of hepatitis C viral infection typically occurs in a number of stages. The first, steatosis, is an accumulation of fat in the liver and is common in hepatitis C. Fibrosis is the replacement of damaged cells with scar tissue, which interferes with the organization and function of the liver. Steatosis can lead to fibrosis, which can then lead to cirrhosis of the liver, the final stage of liver disease where scarring severely impedes the liver's function to the point of failure.

Description

In the past, before the emergence of combination pharmaceutical therapies, hepatitis C often led to liver cancer. But now hepatitis C treatments often result in a cure. And different variants of the hepatitis C virus respond differently to these combination treatments. Despite these treatments, hepatitis C–related liver cirrhosis remains the primary indication for liver transplants.

EFFECTIVENESS—Cannabis is often used to lessen the side effects of pharmaceutical treatments for hepatitis C and helps with treatment compliance. Hepatitis C is treated with a long-term course of pharmaceuticals, often peginterferon and ribavirin. Other drugs that impede the ability of the virus to replicate are also employed. All of these drugs in combination therapy produce side effects, which frequently include nausea and vomiting. The use of cannabis to mitigate these side effects has become increasingly widespread.

PROPOSED MECHANISM—The use of cannabis to reduce pharmaceutical side effects such as nausea and vomiting is common. Recently, a better understanding of how the endocannabinoid system functions within the liver has led to the proposal of using CB1 receptor antagonists to blockade the endocannabinoid response within the liver. This blockade would reduce accumulation of fat in the liver and lessen insulin resistance. Cannabinoids such as THCV and CBD may be of value in blocking the CB1 receptors in the liver. Cannabinoids that activate CB2 receptors, such as CBD, may be of interest in helping to protect the liver from hepatitis C damage.[87] Recent research appears to indicate that a specific genetic variation in the CB2 receptor is linked to more severe liver inflammation and damage among HCV patients.

DOSAGE—Because of the complexity of endocannabinoid activity in the liver, dosage with cannabis medicines becomes a bit of balancing act. It is important to use the least amount of THC required to manage any side effects of combination drug therapy. Additionally, CB1 antagonists such as THCV and CBD may be helpful in protecting the liver from additional damage, and CBD may actually help repair the liver—although these approaches remain currently unproven in human subjects. Up to 25 milligrams of THC can be used to help reduce nausea and vomiting during cycles of combination therapy.

Methods of Ingestion

ORAL—For nausea and vomiting, oral cannabis medicines provide the longest sustained relief, provided that they can be kept down during acute nausea.

VAPORIZATION AND SMOKING—Vaporization and smoking can provide much faster relief that is easily dosed with a little experience.

INDICATED CHEMOTYPES—Hybrids are great for nausea, as are CBD hybrids specifically.

POPULAR VARIETIES—White Widow, Harlequin, Pincher Creek, and OG Kush.

HIV/AIDS

The modern medical cannabis movement leaped onto the national stage from its beginnings as a patients' rights issue during the HIV/AIDS crisis around San Francisco in the 1980s and 1990s. Medical cannabis was found to help the wasting syndrome that made early AIDS patients lose dangerous amounts of weight. Cannabis also relieved the nausea and appetite suppression side effects of AZT (azidothymidine), the first approved retroviral treatment for AIDS. The government attempted to suppress and ignore this medicinal use of cannabis to no avail, at which point AIDS activists took up the cause.

Description

Human immunodeficiency virus (HIV) caused the AIDS (acquired immunodeficiency syndrome) epidemic that began in the United States in 1981. Since then, around 1.7 million Americans have been infected with HIV, while 600,000 of those infected have subsequently died of AIDS-related illnesses. Today, over one million Americans are living with HIV/AIDS and it is believed that as many as 18 percent of people living with HIV remain undiagnosed. Approximately 55,000 people each year will contract HIV in the U.S.—a number that has remained steady for almost a decade.

EFFECTIVENESS—For the treatment of AIDS wasting syndrome, cannabis is effective orally and when smoked/vaporized. A 2007 Columbia University clinical study found that oral and smoked cannabis medicines significantly increased caloric intake by HIV/AIDS patients and stimulated appetite.[88]

One of the additional side effects of HIV/AIDS treatment is neuropathic pain. In 2007, Dr. Donald Abrams of San Francisco General Hospital conducted a small placebo-controlled study in which HIV patients with painful sensory neuropathy were given smoked cannabis or a smoked placebo. The study concluded that smoked cannabis was as effective as oral cannabinoids for neuropathic pain.[89]

A small study searching for potential negative immunological impact on HIV/AIDS patients using medical cannabis showed no additional impact on immune function while using cannabis. While cannabis is anti-inflammatory and can trigger cell death in specific immune cells, no risk associated with using cannabinoids in HIV/AIDS patients has been discovered. Additionally, drug interaction studies of THC and the combination protease inhibitors used to treat HIV infection found no impact on these protease inhibitors' efficacy.[90] Recent studies on the effects of THC on the immune function of rhesus monkeys with SIV (simian immunodeficiency virus) showed the monkey's mortality rate and viral load declined.[91] A 2013 Cochrane review questioned the efficacy of cannabis for HIV/AIDS, but encouraged research.

PROPOSED MECHANISM—Cannabinoids very effectively interact with both the receptors in the brainstem and the receptors within the enteric nervous system (ENS), which controls the gastrointestinal tract. The ENS manages the appetite, nausea, and vomiting responses triggered by HIV/AIDS and the treatments used to manage the illness.[92] Recently, cell studies have looked at the possibility that new drugs or combinations of plant-based cannabinoids—intended to target the CB2 receptor—could address severe symptoms of wasting and neuropathic pain in HIV/AIDS patients, but

Historical Uses

The history of using medical cannabis to fight the symptoms of AIDS and the side effects of the first drugs used to treat it occupies a significant role in the early modern medical cannabis movement.

When AIDS struck San Francisco in 1981, as recounted in Clint Werner's "Medical Marijuana and the AIDS Crisis," the disease affected some of the city's most prominent and noted gay rights activists, who became the first AIDS activists.[93] In post-1960s San Francisco, cannabis remained plentiful and soon the word spread that smoking or eating cannabis often resulted in the "munchies," which helped AIDS patients eat, reduced nausea, and resulted in weight gain. AIDS activists aligned with early medical cannabis activists to take on the U.S. government's insistence that cannabis had no medicinal value. Volunteers like "Brownie Mary" Rathbun would visit the San Francisco General Hospital's AIDS ward to distribute her homemade cannabis edibles to patients.

Dr. Donald Abrams, at the time the assistant director of the AIDS program at the hospital, saw firsthand how many of his patients benefited from using cannabis. In the early '90s, Abrams began a seven-year battle to get U.S. government approval to conduct a study with medical cannabis. In 1998, Abrams received permission to conduct the first government-approved study on cannabis and HIV treatment.

By the time Abrams's study was approved by the National Institute of Drug Abuse, 410,000 people had died of AIDS in the United States. California had formally embraced the medical marijuana movement with the 1996 passage of Proposition 215 legislation, authored by some the earliest medical cannabis activists, including Dennis Peron. Peron was the founder of San Francisco's first cannabis buyers' club, which he modeled upon the 1980s buyers' clubs that imported promising drugs from overseas to fight AIDS.[94]

without the psychoactivity associated with cannabinoids interacting with the CB1 receptor.[95]

DOSAGE—Appetite stimulation tends to occur at the lower end of the cannabis dosage scale, typically around 5 milligrams of THC, once before lunch and once before dinner. Many patients find the sweet spot dose is around 12.5 milligrams per day. Some patients find the need to increase this dose up to 20 milligrams of THC in order to stimulate their appetites, especially if accompanied by nausea from drug side effects. However, in studies with oral THC capsules (Marinol), only half of the patients could tolerate a 20 milligram per day regimen before side effects forced them to scale back their dose. Many patients will settle into a routine of approximately 10 to 12.5 milligrams twice daily. Cannabis psychoactivity typically declines when a dose is maintained, so cannabis-naive patients may find that side effects diminish within a few days.

Care should be taken to monitor any CBD content in the chosen cannabis medicine, since CBD is thought to be slight antagonistic at the CB1 receptor, meaning that it could reduce appetite. Additional study is warranted in order to confirm whether CBD interferes with THC's ability to stimulate the appetite.[96]

Methods of Ingestion

ORAL—The oral use of cannabis by HIV/AIDS patients goes back to the early 1980s. Cannabis was infused into sweets such as brownies, cookies, and candy in the hopes of appealing to those with no appetite. Cannabis-infused lollipops can be quite effective for patients having difficulty with solid food, with the added benefit of more rapid cannabinoid absorption through the tissues of the mouth. Oral cannabis is quite effective for stimulating appetite, increasing the quality of rest and sleep, and long-lasting analgesia in HIV/AIDS patients.

VAPORIZATION AND SMOKING—Patients report that smoked and vaporized herbal cannabis is effective in treating the neuropathic pain associated with HIV/AIDS and its pharmaceutical treatments.

INDICATED CHEMOTYPES—Nausea and appetite stimulation are typically addressed with conventional high-THC cannabis. Neuropathy responds well to high-CBD chemotypes, which can be alternated with high-THC varieties to seek a wide range of effects. High-CBD varieties are also effective for reducing symptoms of stress and anxiety.

POPULAR VARIETIES—For nausea and appetite stimulation, ultra-high-THC varieties such as OG and Banana Kush and robust hybrids such as Green Skunk are recommended. Afghan varieties are noted for their tendency to trigger the "munchies." Blue Dream, with its appealing aroma and high potency, is another good choice for nausea. Indian landraces are also of potential interest, since the cannabis has been used for digestive disorders in the Ayurvedic medical tradition for centuries.

INSOMNIA AND SLEEP DISORDERS

Cannabis and its extracts have been successfully used to treat a range of sleep disorders, including insomnia, sleep disruption, and sleep apnea. A primary reason for this is that most cannabis medicines are mildly sedative. However, studies have shown that successful treatment of sleep disorders with cannabis medicines may be dose-dependent and affected by the THC/CBD ratio of the cannabis medicine.

Description

Insomnia is the inability to fall asleep or maintain sleep. Sleep disorders often attend many medical conditions, especially pain syndromes.

EFFECTIVENESS—In clinical studies of pain syndromes, cannabis and its extracts have been found to help a majority of patients achieve restful sleep without residual grogginess the following morning. Long-term studies of up to four years have shown no tolerance buildup when using cannabis as a sleep aid.

PROPOSED MECHANISM—Sleep laboratory studies have shown that different cannabinoids vary in their ability to sedate or stimulate. THC produces residual sedation, while CBD is wake-promoting. However, CBD is effective for reducing anxiety, which can make it easier to fall asleep. CBN, produced as THC oxidizes over time, has been shown to be synergistically sedative when combined with THC. It is likely that the essential oils unique to each cannabis variety can also affect cannabis' ability to sedate. Therefore, highly stimulating *sativa* cannabis varieties are not recommended.

DOSAGE—As noted, insomnia and sleep disorders are conditions for which the cannabinoid profile of the medicine, along with the timing and size of the dose, are critical to a successful outcome. Nearly all recreational users of cannabis note the residual sedative properties of cannabis that occur 90 minutes after dosing, as the drug's initial stimulation gives way to sleepiness. THC appears to be initially stimulating while its metabolites are more sedative, which means that patients should smoke or vaporize cannabis about an hour before bedtime to let these sedative THC metabolites accumulate. If the patient awakens in the middle of the night, a dose of oral cannabis can be more effective in keeping the patient asleep. However, overmedicating with cannabis can produce intense psychoactivity, which makes falling asleep difficult and can interfere with normal sleep cycles. Moderate to low dosage is recommended.

Methods of Ingestion

ORAL—If the patient is waking in the middle of the night, oral cannabis—with its longer-lasting effects—may be more appropriate. Care must be taken not to overmedicate the patient, since the

Historical Uses

The Indian Ayurvedic medical tradition recognizes the sleep-inducing qualities of cannabis, in which it is characterized as *nidrajanan* (sleep-inducing). This ancient tradition is reflected in a 1991 survey of Indian cannabis users in the city of Varanasi, where 90 percent of the participants found cannabis effective for sleep. Historically, the use of cannabis to treat sleep disorders has been closely associated with its ability to reduce pain and discomfort. William O'Shaughnessy, an Irish physician working in colonial India in the nineteenth century, noted the effectiveness of cannabis as a sedative for the treatment of pain and rheumatism. After THC was first isolated in 1964, early studies showed that THC reduced the time required for patients to fall asleep, suppressed deep sleep, and sometimes produced hangover-like symptoms. In the late 1990s, a review was published that claimed that THC adversely altered brain wave patterns during sleep studies and left most patients with hangover effects (e.g., headaches, exhaustion).[97] However, this was strongly contradicted in a 2007 review on the use of Sativex to treat sleep disorders caused by multiple sclerosis or arthritis pain; Sativex was shown to be highly effective in treating pain-induced insomnia in 13 different studies. In 2011, a Dutch pharmaceutical company introduced a medicine that was high in the cannabis essential oil called myrcene. Myrcene is found in *indica* varieties of cannabis and has been shown to be sedative when combined with THC.

stimulating and psychoactive effects of high doses of cannabis may awaken the patient and make sleep impossible.

SUBLINGUAL—Sublingual cannabis preparations such as Sativex have been shown to be effective for insomnia and other sleep disorders. Sativex is a 50/50 blend of THC and CBD, and the CBD limits THC's psychoactivity, which can reduce side effects in novice patients.

VAPORIZATION AND SMOKING—For most patients, vaporized or smoked cannabis is quite effective for insomnia when taken one hour before bedtime.

INDICATED CHEMOTYPES—Heavier *indica* varieties, such as purples and Afghan/Pakistani true kush, are appropriate for their sedative and analgesic effects.

POPULAR VARIETIES—Purple cannabis varieties are consistently cited as being most effective for sleep disorders. This is likely because these cannabis varieties are high in myrcene and linalool. These varieties include Grape Ape, Lavender, Purple Urkle, Grand Daddy Purple, and Purple Kush.

MIGRAINE AND HEADACHE

Cannabis medicines have been used, primarily orally, to treat migraine and other forms of headache for 1,500 years. Dr. Ethan Russo hypothesized that some forms of migraine may result from an endocannabinoid deficiency. Because the symptoms of other serious ailments can be misinterpreted as migraine, patients should always consult a physician for proper diagnosis and treatment of severe headaches.

Description

Migraine is a class of severe headache with two primary variants: common migraine headache occurring with nausea, vomiting, and sensitivity to sensory stimuli; and classical migraine headache preceded by an aura of warning symptoms—for example, visual disturbances. Less common migraines include ocular, abdominal, and chronic migraines. Cluster and thunderclap headaches, while severe in intensity, are not considered migraine. Common tension headaches affect up to 80 percent of the population. The causes of tension headaches can include lack of sleep, poor posture, and emotional stress.

EFFECTIVENESS—Cannabis is effective as prophylaxis for reducing the frequency of migraine in many patients. It is also successful in treating the symptoms of many common tension headaches. Because of potential serious adverse effects when using cannabis with adolescents and children, caution is advised before using cannabis to treat the headaches of younger patients.

PROPOSED MECHANISM—Current thinking about migraine views the headache as a series of steps. The patient encounters a migraine generator or trigger: bright light, hunger, chemicals in a certain food, hormones, and so on. This trigger initiates a chemical reaction within the brain, one that may normally stimulate the release of endocannabinoids to restore equilibrium. For some unknown reason, migraineurs don't always release these endocannabinoids and this absence may be indicative of an endocannabinoid deficiency. Without endocannabinoids to normalize communication, the trigger causes pain-sensing cells in the brain stem to release neuropeptides, which sensitize other pain-sensing cells into releasing more neuropeptides, starting a cascade. This flood of chemicals causes abnormal dilation of blood vessels on the brain's surface. This jump in pressure increases swelling in the surrounding tissue, causing pain levels to skyrocket.

DOSAGE—There are two approaches to cannabis dosage for migraine: prophylactic and symptomatic. Prophylaxis is intended to reduce the frequency and intensity of the headaches. The symptomatic approach relieves the pain and nausea associated with migraine after its onset.

Historical Uses

As noted by Russo in his excellent historical review,[98] cannabis has been used for the prevention and relief of migraine headaches for over a thousand years in Chinese, Indian, Egyptian, Greek, Roman, and Islamic medicine. The earliest reference to cannabis in migraine treatment dates from ninth-century Persia and recommends inserting cannabis juice into the patient's nose, thus avoiding its rejection by vomiting. As cited by William Dymock, a later Persian source additionally claimed that cannabis was good for "deterging (washing) the brain."[99] A twelfth-century herbalist and abbess, Hildegard von Bingen, wrote of cannabis in her *Physica*, "Whoever has an empty brain and head pains may eat it and the head pains will be reduced. Though he who is healthy and full of brains should not be harmed by it—He who has an empty brain shall be caused pain by indulging in hemp. A healthy head and a full brain will not be harmed."[100] Extracts of *Cannabis indica* for oral administration were available from most apothecaries in the West, beginning in the 1840s. Oral cannabis extracts became Western medicine's drug of choice for migraine from the mid-nineteenth century until the early 1940s. From the 1870s onward, prestigious medical journals including *The Lancet*, the *Journal of the American Medical Association*, and *Merck's Archive* all printed articles recommending cannabis in migraine treatment. The 1912 *Merck Manual* entry on migraine gives cannabis as the sole medicinal option. A 1919 Eli Lilly catalogue lists, "Cannabis Indica, Extract" as a treatment for migraine and neuralgia at doses up to 1 gram. By the 1930s, physicians began to complain about the wide variance in potency found in pharmaceutical cannabis extracts. This inconsistent level of quality and the first marijuana laws encouraged the ultimate removal of cannabis from the Western pharmacopeia in 1941. The final appearance of cannabis as an established treatment for migraine in the West appears in a 1942 issue of the *Journal of the American Medical Association*.[101] Over the next 50 years of prohibition, most Western physicians forgot that cannabis had ever been used to treat migraine. In China, India, and Southeast Asia, despite prohibition in the West, cannabis remained a common treatment for migraine headaches. In the 1990s, Russo attempted to gain permission from the National Institutes of Health (NIH) to conduct clinical trials with cannabis on migraine patients. Although NIH and the FDA approved Dr. Russo's research protocol, the National Institutes of Drug Abuse blocked the study. In 2004, Russo published a hypothesis that a deficiency of endocannabinoids in some patients underlies the pathophysiology of migraine, fibromyalgia, and irritable bowel syndrome, thus coining the term Clinical Endocannabinoid Deficiency (CECD).[102] THC seems to be the primary anti-migraine agent in cannabis, although other phytocannabinoids may be of use.

Prophylaxis is intended to supplement endogenous cannabinoids with its equivalents from the cannabis plant. Patients take a small daily dose of cannabis, often below 2.5 milligrams of THC or its equivalent, which produces little or no intoxication. This prophylactic dose appears to be most effective if taken upon rising or during the midafternoon, depending on whether the patient has noted a pattern for the occurrence of headaches. Symptomatic relief is most effective when taken early in the migraine's progression. Sublingual administration, smoking, or vaporizing of up to 10 milligrams of THC can be helpful if the patient is already vomiting. With a migraine that has progressed in severity, doses of up to 25 milligrams of THC can be effective for helping to sedate the patient and reducing extreme nausea. The addition of CBD to the THC dose can reduce the intensity of THC psychoactivity. Remember that cannabis dosage has a "sweet spot" for pain relief, so caution must be observed to avoid overmedication.

Dosage for common tension headaches should also follow the "sweet spot" approach. For tension headaches, 2.5 to 5 milligrams of THC should be effective. An additional 2.5 milligrams of CBD can help. Interestingly, CBD when dosed alone can result in mild headache.

Methods of Ingestion

ORAL—Patients report that small doses of oral cannabis can be quite effective in reducing migraine occurrence. These oral doses can be administered sublingually for faster onset, or swallowed for slower release of THC. Caution must be exercised with oral cannabis to avoid overdose. If using an edible from a cannabis dispensary, choose one that provides less than 5 milligrams of bioavailable THC and start by eating half.

VAPORIZATION AND SMOKING—Both vaporized and smoked cannabis are effective for migraine treatment, especially early in the course of the headache. Patients with classical migraine have found that administering cannabis at the onset of the migraine's aura phase can halt the headache's progression.

INDICATED CHEMOTYPES—For oral administration, any THC-rich strain of cannabis is indicated. For smoking or vaping, stimulating *sativa* chemotypes are more appropriate at the early onset or aura phase of the migraine. After migraine onset, heavier *indica* strains, such as purples and true kush varietals, seem effective for their combination of sedative and analgesic effects.

POPULAR VARIETIES—For low-dose migraine prophylaxis, try Hazes. For acute pain and nausea, Purple Urkle, Grand Daddy Purple, Purple Kush, and MK Ultra are preferred.

MULTIPLE SCLEROSIS AND MOVEMENT DISORDERS

Spasticity is defined as uncomfortable and painful muscle spasms and stiffness. It is associated with a range of movement disorders and diseases including multiple sclerosis (MS), cerebral palsy, amyotrophic lateral sclerosis (ALS), and spinal cord injuries.[103] Spasticity often increases in severity as the disorder progresses. It is believed that the increasing severity of spasticity symptoms over time may stem from a malfunction of the stretch reflex, resulting in excessive and cumulative muscle contractions.[104]

Cannabis is a common alternative treatment for spasticity, and predates our understanding of how the body's endocannabinoid system regulates the neural signaling that goes awry in spasticity and its underlying disorders.

Description

Nerves descend from the brain and spinal cord to the periphery, where they control muscular movement. Multiple sclerosis is an inflammatory neurodegenerative disease of the brain's white matter, where the immune system attacks the myelin sheath surrounding these descending nerves. When myelin is damaged, the signals from one damaged nerve conduct to other nearby damaged nerves. This cross-transmission overexcites the nerves, releasing excessive amounts of the neurotransmitter glutamate. Glutamate is responsible for propagating certain excitatory signals along nerve pathways. Release of excessive glutamate in multiple sclerosis can be toxic to nerve cells. Multiple sclerosis symptoms include muscle spasms and pain, tremors, visual impairment, weakness, loss of bladder control, and cognitive and speech impairment. Spasticity is defined as an involuntary limb function that results from damage to the motor nerves responsible for controlling voluntary movement. Spasticity manifests as muscle spasms, rapid muscle contractions, and increased muscle tone. The severity of symptoms ranges from mild discomfort to disabling stiffness and cramping

EFFECTIVENESS—THC-dominant cannabis medicines are effective in dealing with pain and spasticity, though with some limitations. A 2013 animal study with CBD hints at significant therapeutic potential. A recent placebo-controlled study of 30 MS patients at the University of California Center for Medicinal Cannabis Research (CMCR) examined the effectiveness of smoked cannabis on MS pain and spasticity.[105] Sixty percent of the participants were also taking antispasticity medications and 70 percent were undergoing disease-modifying treatments such as interferon. They continued these treatments during the study. Nearly 80 percent of the participants had used cannabis previously and 30 percent had used it in the last year. Two-thirds of the participants required mobility aids such as a cane or wheelchair. The patients divided into two treatment groups, and were given either 4 percent THC cannabis or a placebo to smoke. The first treatment phase lasted three days, then 11 days off, and then the participants switched over.

They were measured for spasticity, pain, ability to walk, and were given cognitive tests. The results showed a significant reduction in spasticity when cannabis was administered, as compared with the placebo. Pain was reduced by an average of 50 percent in the cannabis-treated group. The primary limitation of the CMCR study was its lack of cannabis-naive participants.

Previous studies on spasticity with orally administered cannabinoid medicines produced mixed results, where significant reductions in spasticity were noted only on subjective scales.[106] Orally administered cannabinoids also tend to reduce multiple sclerosis pain less effectively than smoked or sublingual cannabis medicines.[107] While many MS patients report symptomatic relief of pain and spasticity from cannabis administration, this relief ranges from subtle to significant and is inconsistent among patients.

PROPOSED MECHANISM—A 2011 paper by David Baker and scientists from Blizard Institute at Queen Mary, University of London, examines the biological mechanisms of spasticity and how cannabis medicines provide symptomatic relief. Since endocannabinoids regulate neurotransmission, cannabis-based medicines can mimic endocannabinoids and regulate the dysfunctional neurotransmission that underlies spasticity. There is also interest in how cannabinoid medicines might limit the progression of these diseases by limiting the excessive glutamate release over time, possibly reducing the accumulation of neural damage.[108]

DOSAGE—Moderate doses, equivalent to 2.5 to 10 milligrams of THC, seem effective for spasticity and chronic pain. Neuropathy from these conditions likely responds to much lower doses, under 2.5 milligrams.

Methods of Ingestion

ORAL—Sublingual cannabis medicines appear to be more effective in treating spasticity than swallowed oral cannabis medicines.

VAPORIZATION AND SMOKING—The significance of the CMCR study is that it showed objective improvement in MS-induced spasticity when smoking cannabis.

INDICATED CHEMOTYPES—Experience with MS and spasticity patients in California dispensaries indicates that blending different THC-dominant chemotypes yields the best relief from spasticity and pain. The logic of this approach seems valid in that, through blending different types of cannabis, a greater entourage effect of terpenoids and minor cannabinoids is created.

POPULAR VARIETIES—Blue Dream, Bubba Kush, Pincher Creek, Trainwreck, and OG Kush are the most common varieties used for blending.

NAUSEA AND VOMITING

Despite 40 years of research supporting its efficacy, even among very young patients, cannabis and cannabinoids remain lightning rod treatments for nausea and vomiting. In a 2012 issue of the *Journal of the National Comprehensive Cancer Network*, a respected pharmacist wrote, "Although patients may like to pursue this treatment option in states that have approved the use of marijuana for medical purposes, its use remains legally and therapeutically controversial."[109] In some cases, cannabis use has been linked to the rare cannabinoid hyperemesis syndrome, in which the drug causes severe nausea and vomiting.

Historical Uses

In the mid-1970s, the inability to control nausea and vomiting among chemotherapy patients encouraged oncologists to explore the use of cannabis and its derivatives. In 1975, a study in the *New England Journal of Medicine* found that THC effectively reduced vomiting during treatments within a study group of patients receiving seven different antitumor drugs.[110] This study was prompted by anecdotal accounts that smoking cannabis had reduced nausea and vomiting associated with chemotherapy. By the mid-1990s, the Federal Drug Administration approved THC that was synthesized, as opposed to extracted from cannabis, as an approved prescription medicine to treat nausea and vomiting in patients undergoing chemotherapy. A purely synthetic cannabinoid, nabilone, was also developed and is sold as Cesamet.

Description

Many opponents of medical marijuana have been converted by a cancer diagnosis accompanied by chemotherapy and radiation treatments. A majority of oncologists in the U.S., polled in a survey in early 1990s, recommended cannabis to at least one of their patients undergoing chemotherapy, long before state medical cannabis laws became widespread.[111]

EFFECTIVENESS—Through 2006, over 30 studies have been conducted on the use of cannabinoids to effectively treat nausea and vomiting.[112] Recently the use of CBD, the non-psychoactive cannabinoid, has been shown in animal models to be extremely effective as both an antinausea and antiemetic.[113] In 2013, an animal study was published that indicated that the non-psychoactive, acidic form of THC, THCA, as found in raw cannabis flowers, might be a more potent alternative to THC.[114]

PROPOSED MECHANISM—A major breakthrough in understanding the mechanism underlying nausea and vomiting was the discovery that blockading a specific brain receptor in the 5-HT, or serotonin family of receptors, could suppress vomiting induced by the chemotherapy agent cisplatin. However, these 5-HT antagonist drugs are not effective at reducing the sensation of nausea, and they do not effectively minimize delayed nausea and vomiting, which are commonly associated with this widespread form of chemotherapy. This delayed nausea and vomiting has proven to be particularly distressing to chemotherapy patients. Fortunately, cannabinoids are effective.[115]

CANNABINOID HYPEREMESIS SYNDROME—In 2004, J. H. Allen, an Australian physician, coined the term cannabinoid hyperemesis to describe a syndrome of vomiting and abdominal pain where, oddly, the symptoms are relieved by taking hot showers. Allen described this syndrome in nine patients, all long-term cannabis users.[116] The symptoms abated once the patients stopped using cannabis. A 2012 review by the Mayo Clinic found almost 100 cases of cannabinoid hyperemesis in the literature.[117] Nearly all cannabinoid hyperemesis patients are under 50 and exhibit symptoms in the morning. The Mayo researchers hypothesize that cannabis impairs regulation of body temperature and the relief from taking hot showers is linked to temperature regulation. More in-depth study of cannabinoid hyperemesis needs to be conducted.

DOSAGE—For many patients undergoing chemotherapy, dosage for nausea and vomiting tends toward the higher end of the range. Typically, it's recommended to build up to the effective dose of THC, in order to allow the patient to become accustomed to the psychoactivity. If using THCA or CBD, a larger dose can be used, since unwanted psychoactivity will not be an issue. A basic dose of 5 milligrams of THC, scaled up to 15 milligrams over a week before chemo begins, is often an effective approach.

Methods of Ingestion

ORAL—Oral and sublingual cannabis are both quite effective, with oral providing the longer-lasting effects.

VAPORIZATION AND SMOKING—Vaporization and smoking allow for convenient titration and absorption of the dose.

INDICATED CHEMOTYPES—Nearly all THC and CBD chemotypes will be effective.

POPULAR VARIETIES—For treating nausea, OG Kush and Bubba Kush are currently the most popular cannabis varieties in California, along with Blue Dream.

NEUROPATHY

Conventional pharmaceutical treatments for neuropathic pain are not effective for every patient and adverse effects from these medications can prove problematic. Several small clinical studies have shown that cannabis acts as a moderately effective analgesic for intractable neuropathy.

Description

Neuropathy typically occurs from damage to nerves within the peripheral nervous system (the nervous system not including the brain and spinal cord). Often, neuropathy is felt in the hands and feet as pain, burning, tingling, and numbness. There are two primary classifications of neuropathy: mononeuropathy, involving a single nerve as in carpal tunnel syndrome; or polyneuropathy, which involves a range of peripheral nerves such as in diabetic or HIV neuropathy. Thirty percent of neuropathies are from diabetes and another 30 percent are of unknown cause. Multiple sclerosis, chemotherapy, and HIV treatments can lead to nerve damage, which it turn can result in neuropathy. Two clinical features of neuropathic pain are allodynia (perception of pain in the absence of painful stimuli, merely pressure or temperature chance), hyperalgesia (an exaggerated response to painful stimuli), or a group of painful sensations called dyesthesias ("pins and needles," electric shock, cold, burning, and even numbness).

Historical Uses

A noted early example of the use of cannabis to treat neuropathy was a case report by Dr. Martin H. Lynch from the mid-nineteenth century. Lynch treated a woman suffering from severe shooting pains around one eye socket and the side of her head with a "tincture of Indian Hemp." The result was remarkable, with the neuralgia symptoms disappearing within 48 hours. In his published case report, Lynch noted another study that appeared in the *Dublin Medical Press* issue of March 1843 in which Sir James Murray treated a case of neuralgia in the arm with 10 drops of *Cannabis indica* tincture.[118]

EFFECTIVENESS—Cannabis is an effective treatment for a variety of neuropathies. A recent review by Dr. Igor Grant, director of the Center for Medicinal Cannabis Research at the University of California, compared the effectiveness of cannabis against tricyclic antidepressants, gabapentin, anticonvulsants, and selective serotonin reuptake inhibitors. Cannabis was not quite as effective as tricyclics at reducing neuropathy, but more effective than the other types of drug intervention.[119] An early study by Dr. Donald Abrams indicated similar results in HIV-associated neuropathy.[120] Sativex, the prescription cannabis extract spray applied to the oral mucosal tissue of the mouth, contains both THC and CBD cannabis extracts and, over a two-year period, has been shown to be an effective treatment for neuropathy due to multiple sclerosis.[121] A 2014 study showed that CBD reduced chemotherapy-induced neuropathy. Another 2014 study with Sativex showed the THC/CBD combination was effective for treatment-resistant neuropathy.

PROPOSED MECHANISM—Communication of pain throughout the body is mediated by endocannabinoids interacting with cannabinoid and other receptor-based signaling systems. Plant cannabinoids also interact with these receptors, enabling the analgesic effects of cannabis on several kinds of pain, including neuropathy.

DOSAGE—The key to effectively treating neuropathies with cannabis medicines is finding the correct dosage. The dosage should be effective as an analgesic, yet not cause unwanted adverse effects such as excessive levels of psychoactivity, sedation, or dizziness.[122] A randomized, controlled trial with small, smoked doses of 9 percent THC cannabis demonstrated effective pain relief below the typical threshold of psychoactivity.[123] The results of this trial are of particular interest because it highlights the unexpected medical effectiveness of cannabis dosages which are far below that which is commonly consumed within the medical cannabis community. In the aforementioned study led by Mark A. Ware, a single inhalation of smoked cannabis (25 milligrams of cannabis with 9.4 percent THC by dry weight) decreased pain intensity in post-traumatic or post-surgery-induced neuropathic pain, as measured by a numeric rating scale. This translates to a dose of less than 2 milligrams of THC. If doses this low prove effective in future studies, concern about the adverse effects of cannabis as a medicine may decrease.

Methods of Ingestion

ORAL—Oral and sublingual/buccal cannabis medicines are effective for relief of neuropathic symptoms. Sativex has been tested extensively for the treatment of neuropathies, with significant success. Conventional cannabis edibles are widely used to treat neuropathy among patients frequenting California cannabis dispensaries. The advantage to swallowed cannabis medicines is that they can provide four to six hours of relief.

VAPORIZATION AND SMOKING—Vaporization and smoking are both effective for treating neuropathy, and have the advantage of rapid onset and ease of dose titration.12

INDICATED CHEMOTYPES—Both THC and CBD chemotypes are effective for treating neuropathy. Cannabis chemotypes that produce small amounts of CBG may also increase the medicine's analgesic effect.

POPULAR VARIETIES—Pincher Creek, Bubba Kush, Harlequin, Cannatonic.

PAIN

Today, pain is the most common symptom for which patients report using medical cannabis. The key to effectively using cannabis for pain is finding the optimal dose. Since the body uses its endocannabinoid system to modulate overall pain levels and signaling, dose becomes crucial to remain in the "sweet spot" of sustained pain relief. It may be that some painful conditions, including fibromyalgia and migraine, may actually be linked to a deficiency of endocannabinoids.[124] In such a situation, cannabis is used like a vitamin to supplement this deficiency and restore balance—a novel treatment approach.

Description

There are different types of common pain. Acute pain typically persists until the painful stimulus is removed or physical damage has healed. Chronic pain is pain that lasts for more than three months, as found with conditions such as cancer or arthritis. Neuropathic pain is caused by damage to nerve tissues, often in the extremities from conditions such as diabetes or as a side effect of drugs, including chemotherapy agents. Neuropathy often produces a "pins and needles" or burning sensation. Pruritus, a severe itching, has many similarities to pain and can be closely associated with neuropathic pain, although pain inhibits itching.

EFFECTIVENESS—Most studies on the use of cannabinoids for treating chronic pain have been encouraging, while the use of cannabinoids to treat acute pain has proven less successful in trials. Because of the widespread use of opioid pain medications, cannabinoids have been investigated for treating forms of pain that do not always respond to opiates. Dr. Sunil K. Aggarwal conducted a survey of patients treated for chronic pain.[125] Allowed to use herbal cannabis to treat their symptoms, these patients amassed over 200 years of medical cannabis experience. They were treating a wide number of chronic pain conditions including myofascial pain, neuropathic pain, back pain, osteoarthritic pain, central pain syndrome, fibromyalgia, and visceral pain. Cannabinoids are effective at relieving these types of pain, so long as an effective dose range can be established.[126]

As noted by Russo and Hohmann, cannabinoids can provide an adjunct therapy for opioid pain medications, and indeed they tend to reduce the amount of opioid medication required, even restoring opioid pain relief after that ability has been lost.[127] Cannabinoids can also lessen the buildup of tolerance to opioids and may reduce the severity of opioid withdrawal. Cannabinoids, particularly the combination of THC and CBD,

Historical Uses

Hua Tho, a second-century Chinese physician, invented *mafeisan*, "hemp boiling powder," which dissolved in wine. It was the first recorded general anesthesia employed during a surgical procedure. In the ninth century, the Persian physician Shapur ibn Sahl would pack the nose of migraine sufferers with juice from cannabis flowers to treat their severe headache pain. In the Middle East cannabis was used to treat a variety of forms of pain, including several neuropathic varieties. By the nineteenth century, physicians had discovered that cannabis could also be used to relieve neuropathic pain, which was otherwise difficult to treat.

In 1887, Hobart Amory Hare, a professor of medicine at Jefferson Medical College in Philadelphia, published a long article in the *Therapeutic Gazette* about the advantage of cannabis over opium for treating pain.[128] Hare thought that cannabis held this advantage because it did not produce the sedation or nausea of opium. He also noted that cannabis was effective because it sometimes appeared to make pain gently fade into the distance. In the last decade, the THC/CBD oral spray Sativex has been approved in Canada for neuropathic pain associated with multiple sclerosis and intractable cancer pain.

appear particularly effective for intractable pain conditions, including those associated with multiple sclerosis and cancer. The cannabinoid CBG is a stronger analgesic than THC. THCV, which is not as psychoactive as THC, has also been shown in animal models to reduce intense pain.[129] Recent data from animal studies indicate that THC reduces gastrointestinal bleeding and even hemorrhages caused by nonsteroidal, anti-inflammatory drugs used to control pain.[130]

PROPOSED MECHANISM—Cannabinoids relieve pain through a variety of mechanisms, including producing analgesic and anti-inflammatory effects, through the modulation of neurotransmitter release, and by stimulating the release of the body's own opioids. The endocannabinoid system helps to modulate pain signaling throughout the nervous system. Endocannabinoids are released in response to discomfort, reducing sensitivity to pain. Endocannabinoids also reduce the wind-up phenomena, which occurs when pain appears to increase in intensity as the pain stimulus is repeated, and allodynia, the sensation of pain from stimuli that are normally not considered painful. Cannabinoids quell the transmission of ascending (toward the spine and brain) pain signals. They also modulate pain signaling in the descending pain pathway from the brain/spine to the affected region. Endocannabinoids and possibly their deficiency are involved in painful syndromes such as fibromyalgia and migraines, which might be addressed through low-dose cannabis prophylaxis.

DOSAGE—In a University of California study in San Diego, it was noted that smoked cannabis appears to have a "sweet spot" dose for optimal pain relief.[131] In this study, participants were injected with a small amount of capsaicin to produce the pain model. After this injection, participants then were given different doses of smoked cannabis to relieve the pain. The low dose had little to no effect; the medium dose significantly reduced the pain; and the high dose significantly increased the pain. A study of Sativex cannabinoid spray on intractable cancer pain showed that it was most effective at lower and medium doses, which would seem to support the hypothesis that higher doses of cannabinoids do not necessarily provide increased pain relief.[132]

Methods of Ingestion

ORAL—Both sublingual and swallowed forms of cannabis are effective. Oral cannabis may be more useful for treating chronic pain conditions, which do not benefit from the rapid spike in blood serum cannabinoids that occurs with smoked or vaporized cannabis. Using oral cannabis containing both THC and CBD prolongs the effects of THC while reducing some of its side effects, including anxiety and rapid heartbeat. The inclusion of CBD can make the use of cannabis considerably easier on cannabis-naive patients, for whom the psychoactivity of THC may be problematic.

VAPORIZATION AND SMOKING—Many chronic pain conditions can benefit from the rapid onset of smoked or vaporized cannabis. Another advantage of inhaled cannabis is the ease by which a dose can be titrated without exceeding the sweet spot.

TOPICAL—Topical, high-THC cannabis is useful for pain-related conditions such as itching, skin inflammation, and dermatitis. These topical preparations may also be synergistic with capsaicin-based ointments used for muscle pain. CBD-rich cannabis medicines are also extremely effective for skin inflammation. Combinations of THC and CBD hold even more promise. Hemp oil creams infused with CBD and THC are increasingly popular among West Coast patients because they are non-psychoactive but effective.

INDICATED CHEMOTYPES—Most chemotypes are effective for chronic pain, with high-CBD varieties particularly so for neuropathic pain. Cannabis that is high in both THC and CBD may be more helpful for intractable and chronic pain syndromes. Cannabis chemotypes that produce high levels of myrcene and linalool provide additional pain relief in synergy with THC. Beta-caryophyllene is also a powerful anti-inflammatory and is synergistic with THC in protecting the stomach from nonsteroidal anti-inflammatory drugs used for pain management.[133]

POPULAR VARIETIES—The choice depends on whether a patient needs a more stimulating option for use during the day, or a more sedating variety to assist with recovery and sleep. Afghan, which is high in both myrcene and THC, provides significant pain relief and more relaxation than many stimulating varieties. While Trainwreck is a classic stimulating variety, it also contains a significant concentration of myrcene and is popular for daytime pain relief. Purple cannabis often contains considerable linalool and THC levels. For intractable pain, CBD/THC varieties such as Harlequin are quite effective. If psychoactivity is not appropriate, extremely low-THC/high-CBD varieties such as Cannatonic or AC/DC can be effectual for inflammatory pain.

PARKINSON'S DISEASE

Parkinson's disease is most common among older people, with the majority of sufferers age 50 and above. Along with other neurodegenerative disorders, such as Huntington's disease, it provides promising therapeutic targets for cannabinoid medicines, especially since the treatment options for these serious conditions are somewhat limited.

Description

Parkinson's disease (PD) is a progressive neurodegenerative disease caused by the loss of neurons that produce the neurotransmitter dopamine within a small region in the midbrain called the substantia nigra. Reduced levels of dopamine interfere with coordination and motor function. The precise reason that these dopamine-producing neurons are lost in PD is still unknown although inflammation, along with environmental and hereditary factors, are thought to be partially responsible.[134] The classic symptoms of PD are muscular rigidity, tremors, and slowness of movement. These symptoms are the result of decreased stimulation of the brain's motor cortex caused by the insufficient formation and action of dopamine. The principal drug treatments for PD are levodopa and carbidopa. Levodopa is converted to dopamine in the brain and carbidopa prevents levodopa from being broken down before it reaches the brain. The use of levodopa can result in a severe side effect: another movement disorder called dyskinesia, which produces unusual or uncontrolled movements of the mouth, tongue, face, head, neck, arms, and legs.

Historical Uses

Parkinson's disease was first described as a neurological syndrome by James Parkinson in 1817, although descriptions that match Parkinson's disease appear in traditional Indian medical texts from 1000 BCE.[135] William Gowers, a nineteenth-century British neurologist, used cannabis in combination with opium to treat Parkinson's disease and stated, "I have several times seen a very distinct improvement for a considerable time under their use."[136]

EFFECTIVENESS—The effectiveness of medical cannabis in treating Parkinson's disease is somewhat inconclusive, although observational studies and surveys appear promising. In 2004, a survey at the Prague Movement Disorder Center indicated that more than half of the PD patients who tried cannabis noticed subjective improvement.[137] In 2013, at the 17th International Congress of Parkinson's Disease and Movement Disorders, Israeli researchers presented an observational study of 17 PD patients currently using cannabis to control motor symptoms. The effects of cannabis on these patients' PD symptoms were evaluated with the Unified Parkinson's Disease Rating Scale (UPDRS). The patients' non-motor symptoms and cannabis side effects were also evaluated. There was an overall 30 percent improvement in the patients' average UPDRS score. Analysis of different motor symptoms revealed significant improvement for tremors, rigidity, and slowness of movement. Cannabis smoking had no effect on the patients' posture. In addition, there was a significant improvement in pain scores after smoking cannabis. Patients reported drowsiness as a primary side effect.[138] Recent evidence indicates that other cannabinoids may be of more value than THC in PD treatment. THCV, found in some southern African and central Asian cannabis, has been shown to provide neuroprotection and symptom relief in animal models of PD.[139] THCV cannabis is still extremely rare in the U.S., though that situation will likely improve over the next few years. With the additional neuroprotective characteristics associated with CBD, there is discussion of potential combination therapy of these two cannabinoids as a treatment to interfere with the progression of PD.[140]

PROPOSED MECHANISM—The endocannabinoid system changes observed in Parkinson's disease are currently thought to occur both in compensation to the disease and also as part of its pathology. The endocannabinoids released in the early phases of PD, as compensation to maintain control of locomotion, may actually end up impairing locomotion in later phases of the disease. The use of cannabinoids in PD may require a better understanding of how cannabinoid medicines can boost the production (or prevent the degradation) of endocannabinoids in the early stages of PD, then how different cannabinoid medicines might curb the production (or accelerate their degradation) of endocannabinoids in later stages of the disease.[141]

DOSAGE—Care should be observed with cannabis dosage for PD, since little clinical research on this particular topic has been conducted.

Methods of Ingestion

Currently, smoked and sublingual cannabis are the primary delivery methods for PD; these methods appear promising.

INDICATED CHEMOTYPES—High-CBD and -THCV varieties are indicated for their potential neuroprotective properties. THC varieties are favored for pain relief.

POPULAR VARIETIES—South African cannabis varieties, such as Durban Poison and Swazi Skunk, have elevated THCV and may be useful for some minor symptomatic relief of some symptoms of PD.

POST-TRAUMATIC STRESS DISORDER

During the Vietnam War, U.S. soldiers often smoked Southeast Asian cannabis to deal with the horrors of combat. After returning home from the war, many veterans continued to use cannabis to deal with the post-traumatic stress of their experience in Vietnam.[142] Data from the National Comorbidity Study demonstrated that adults suffering from PTSD were three times more likely to have cannabis dependence as compared with those without PTSD.[143] Recent research underscores a strong connection between the endocannabinoid system and how the brain processes traumatic memories.

Historical Uses

"In war, there are no unwounded soldiers." — Jose Narosky. Cristobal Acosta, a Portuguese doctor and botanist, traveled to India as a soldier in the sixteenth century. He studied the use of medicinal plants in India and first noted the use of cannabis in the form of the traditional Indian preparation, *bhang*, for "battle fatigue"in his text, "On the Drugs and Medicines from the East Indies." [144] Acosta noted that soldiers used cannabis for different symptoms of PTSD: "Some to forget their worries and sleep without thoughts; others to enjoy in their sleep a variety of dreams and delusions; others become drunk and act like clowns." This account is extraordinary in its anecdotal appraisal of the efficacy of cannabis for PTSD almost 500 years ago.

In 2012, a petition with over 8,000 signatures from a veterans' group was submitted to the White House asking to legalize the use of cannabis for PTSD. The director of the Office of National Drug Control Policy denied the petition. Yet just one year earlier, on April 28, 2011, the U.S. Food and Drug Administration accepted a protocol design from the Multidisciplinary Association for Psychedelic Studies for their study of cannabis as a treatment for symptoms of PTSD in war veterans.

Description

Post-traumatic stress disorder is typically triggered by exposure to an extreme traumatic stress, involving direct experience of death or serious harm, actual or threatened. The response to this stress usually involves an intense experience of terror or helplessness. The classic symptoms of PTSD include repetitive and intense recollections of the original event, often from flashbacks or nightmares. PTSD often leads to emotional distancing, avoidance, and intense arousal or rage. Traumatic experiences that can lead to PTSD symptoms include combat, natural disasters, sexual abuse, traffic accidents, and violent crime. It is estimated that over 10 percent of the U.S. population will experience some PTSD symptoms during the course of their lives.[145]

EFFECTIVENESS—Cannabis is effective in treating PTSD symptoms, often in combination with selective serotonin reuptake inhibitor medications. In 2012, a fascinating case report emerged of a 19-year-old male German patient with a spectrum of severe PTSD symptoms—including intense flashbacks, panic attacks, and self-mutilation—who successfully self-medicated with hashish. This case study led researchers from Hannover Medical School and Harvard Medical School to publish a comprehensive review of the potential for cannabis as a breakthrough treatment for PTSD. Their properly understated conclusion: "Findings from studies suggest that by altering fear conditioning, memory systems, general CNS [central nervous system] arousal, mood, and sleep, exogenous cannabinoids may hold potential for the treatment of people with PTSD."[146]

PROPOSED MECHANISM—The amygdala is a small almond-shaped portion of the brain associated with emotional memory and fear conditioning. PTSD changes the structure and function of the amygdala.[147] The endocannabinoid system is associated with the extinction of aversive memories, such as those associated with the amygdala.[148] The ability of phytocannabinoids to interfere with memory processing has been known for decades. A recent brain-scanning study indicated that abnormal endocannabinoid signaling in the brain is strongly implicated in PTSD patients.[149]

DOSAGE—Dosage of THC and CBD for symptoms of PTSD needs to be refined and better understood. The efficacy of cannabis to treat PTSD appears to be dose dependent. Care should be observed to avoid varieties of cannabis that are high in pinene, since this terpene may reduce the ability of cannabinoids to extinguish aversive memories.

Methods of Ingestion

ORAL—Oral cannabis is excellent for reducing dreaming, including the nightmares that plague some PTSD sufferers.

VAPORIZATION AND SMOKING—Vaporizing and smoking are by far the most common delivery methods preferred by PTSD patients.

INDICATED CHEMOTYPES—High-CBD and -THC varieties, especially with terpenes such as linalool and limonene.

POPULAR VARIETIES—Cannatonic, Bubba Kush, and OG Kush.

SCHIZOPHRENIA

Cannabis and its potential link to psychosis has been a hot-button topic for the last two decades. Cannabis produces cannabinoids that mimic endocannabinoids, which the body uses to regulate neural signaling throughout the brain. And the endocannabinoid system is widely distributed throughout parts of the brain responsible for regulating mental health. Therefore, it should not be surprising that a plant cannabinoid such as THC might be capable of interfering with brain function to a degree that could mimic psychosis. An overdose of THC is certainly capable of producing a short-lived psychotic break. Whether this adverse event could cause lasting damage is not known.

It is commonly held that THC is psychoactive and CBD is non-psychoactive. But whether THC causes psychosis and schizophrenia remains controversial. There has been endless scientific debate about whether cannabis use is a causal factor in the development of schizophrenia and other psychotic disorders.[150] A tenuous link between cannabis use and the incidence of psychotic disorders appeared to have been established, but confidence is now quite low that the development of mental illness is solely due to cannabis use.[151]

There is increasing evidence that THC tends be pro-psychotic and CBD is antipsychotic. These oppositional effects have been demonstrated by brain imaging. In nearly every region of the brain associated with psychosis, THC tends to elicit a pro-psychotic effect, while CBD produces the opposite.[152] Because of this propensity toward eliciting psychotic symptoms, high-THC cannabis is believed to be linked to increased risk of psychosis, especially in the developing adolescent brain.[153] Higher CBD content of cannabis is linked to a reduction in psychotomimetic effects.[154] All of this does not mean that high-THC cannabis will trigger psychosis—but rather it increases its risk, which remains very small. What is increasingly clear though is that the cannabinoid ratio of today's cannabis is skewed completely toward THC, when for hundreds of years it was 50/50 THC and CBD. The imbalance of today's cannabis is the result of a prohibition that favored psychoactive potency.[155]

In an interesting study by Celia Morgan and Valerie Curran of the Clinical Psychopharmacology Unit of University College London, hair samples were taken from a group of individuals undergoing a longitudinal study for past drug use. The hair samples were tested for their residual cannabinoid content and the results divided by whether the hair contained THC only, THC and CBD, or no cannabinoids. The participants were then given a test that measures proneness toward psychosis. The results show higher levels of unusual experiences—akin to hallucinations and delusions associated with psychosis—in individuals who had only THC in their hair compared with those with THC and CBD, and those with no cannabinoids.[156]

Description

Schizophrenia can interfere with a person's ability to think, relate, make decisions, and manage emotions. The symptoms of schizophrenia are typically classified as "positive symptoms," which include delusions, disordered thought, and hallucinations; and "negative symptoms," which include inability to feel pleasure in daily life, reclusiveness, amotivational syndrome, and flat effect.

EFFECTIVENESS—To date, it would appear that cannabinoids, in particular THC, might be more effective at producing psychotic symptoms than relieving them. However, many schizophrenic patients do self-medicate with high-THC cannabis—typically with the more sedative, relaxing, broad-leafleted varieties. It is interesting to note that a recent study showed a lower incidence of diabetes among recreational cannabis users.[157] Both glutamine and dopamine animal models of psychosis have been successfully treated with CBD. A group of Brazilian researchers led by Antonio Waldo Zuardi conducted a successful study that compared the efficacy of CBD versus amisulpride, an atypical antipsychotic drug used to treat schizophrenia and bipolar disorder. CBD was demonstrated in this study to be as effective as the antipsychotic, but with greatly reduced side effects.[158]

PROPOSED MECHANISM—A very recent paper by Philip Robson, Geoffrey Guy, and Vincenzo Di Marzo look at schizophrenia not as a mental illness, but as a metabolic inflammatory disease. The authors note that a significant percentage of schizophrenics exhibit symptoms associated with metabolic syndromes, including type 2 diabetes, obesity, chronic inflammation, and exaggerated biochemical reaction to stress.[159] They propose the

Historical Uses

Schizophrenia has only recently been characterized as a metabolic disorder, akin to diabetes. However, physicians recognized schizophrenia and its link to other metabolic syndromes in the nineteenth century when these doctors noted that diabetes often occurred in families in which insanity was prevalent.[160] "Reefer madness" is a meme supporting the idea that cannabis causes psychosis. It goes back to a popular scare tactic employed by the tabloid press to support the cannabis prohibition efforts of the 1920s and 1930s. The link to cannabis and madness is much older, having originated in the Western Hemisphere with tales of cannabis-induced insanity and violence in Mexican military barracks in the nineteenth century.[161] It was not until the mid-1990s that Brazilian researchers began to examine the potential for cannabinoids such as CBD to be used as antipsychotic medicines.[162]

development of a THCV/CBD combination therapy that could address many of these metabolic and inflammation issues. The treatment would be an adjunct therapy to augment the efficacy of conventional antipsychotic medication, and likely with a reduced side effects profile.

DOSAGE—THC has been used in several studies to precipitate psychosis, therefore the use of high-THC cannabis in the symptomatic relief of schizophrenia must be approached with considerable caution and professional oversight. CBD has been shown to relieve anxiety and may hold considerable promise as an antipsychotic. Moderate dosage with CBD is more likely safer than THC, but higher doses of CBD can produce mental sedation. However, very small-scale studies with CBD on treatment-resistant schizophrenia have employed massive doses of CBD—up to 1.5 grams per day. The results are promising, but must be considered very preliminary. Very little clinical work has been conducted with CBD as an antipsychotic, though trials have been proposed for 2014. THCV dosage should be carefully monitored since high doses of CB_1 receptor antagonists can produce adverse effects including suicidal thoughts.

Methods of Ingestion

ORAL—It is likely that GW Pharmaceuticals will enter clinical trials of a THCV/CBD oral/mucosal spray for treating metabolic aspects of schizophrenia. Conventional CBD tinctures may address some of these metabolic issues in the interim. THCV oral products are not currently available within the medical cannabis community, although that will change.

VAPORIZATION AND SMOKING—Anecdotal accounts indicate that, for decades, smoking cannabis has been popular among schizophrenic patients as a method of self-medication. Vaporized cannabis as a method of administration is rare among schizophrenics frequenting California medical cannabis dispensaries.

INDICATED CHEMOTYPES—High-CBD varieties should be most effective for their anti-inflammatory and pro-homeostatic properties, since some new models of schizophrenia cast the illness as an inflammatory metabolic disorder. THCV varieties are recommended as they become available for their anti-inflammatory effects.

POPULAR VARIETIES—The 30 to one CBD to THC ratio Cannatonic phenotype and any similar ultra-high CBD varieties, such as Charlotte's Web and AC/DC, are likely to be the best varieties for most patients attempting to use CBD as an antipsychotic for treatment-resistant schizophrenia.

SEIZURE DISORDERS

Since 30 percent of epilepsies do not respond to currently available drug treatments,[163] there is great interest in anecdotal accounts of the successful use of cannabis and its derivatives to treat these disorders. Over 20 million people worldwide have pharmacoresistant epilepsies. There is a pressing need for new, effective antiepilepsy drugs, and the use of cannabis and cannabinoid medicines currently seems promising.

Considerable media attention has focused on the use of cannabis to treat a severe form of childhood epilepsy called Dravet Syndrome.[164] Dravet strikes very young children with catastrophic results and can be life threatening. Conventional anticonvulsant medications only provide limited management of seizures. Small clinical trials with cannabinoids (including CBD, CBDV, and THCV) for the treatment of seizure disorders are expected to begin in late 2013 in the United States.

Description

Epilepsies are chronic, often progressive, neurological conditions characterized by seizures. Epilepsies are the third most common class of neurological disorders after migraines and Parkinson's disease.

EFFECTIVENESS—While successful treatment of intractable seizure disorders with cannabis and cannabinoid medicines attracts great attention across the Internet, randomized and controlled trials of cannabis medicines for epilepsies are still in early stages, even though the antiepilepsy effects of cannabinoids have been studied since the mid-1970s.[165] There is concern that cannabinoids appear to be both pro- and anticonvulsant.[166] A 2012 Cochrane review of studies on the use of cannabis medicines to treat epilepsies was sharply critical of the design and scope of all the human studies conducted to date.[167] Recently, the research focus has shifted away from the cannabinoid delta-9-tetrahydrocannabinolic toward investigating the potential antiepilepsy uses of alternative cannabinoids, including CBD, CBDV, and THCV. CBD reliably delivers a range of anticonvulsant effects with few known adverse results and no psychoactivity.[168] THCV in cell and animal models of epilepsies produces contradictory results.[169] Following promising animal studies, clinical trials of CBDV for treatment of seizure disorders could begin soon.[170] CBG is another cannabinoid that may exhibit antiseizure properties. And synthetic cannabinoids that target the CB_1 receptor have so far demonstrated significant antiseizure activity in animal models of chronic epilepsy.[171]

PROPOSED MECHANISM—The mechanism by which cannabinoids inhibit seizure activity is still not

Historical Uses

The earliest descriptions of cannabis use to treat epilepsies are from medieval Arabic medical texts.[172] As early as the tenth century, the Persian medical writer al-Majusi recommended that the juice of hemp leaves be poured into the nose to prevent seizures.[173] In the fifteenth century, the polymath al-Badri clamed that the epilepsy of a son of the caliph's chamberlain was successfully treated with cannabis resin, although modern scholars question the veracity of this account.[174] J. Russell Reynolds, Queen Victoria's physician, wrote that "In true, chronic epilepsy I have found (cannabis) absolutely useless, and this as the result of extensive experience. There are many cases of so-called epilepsy in adults...in which Indian hemp is the most useful agent with which I am acquainted...and fits may be stopped at once by a full dose of hemp."[175]

completely understood, but likely extends beyond interaction with the cannabinoid receptor CB1 to other receptor systems within the body.[176] Recent studies indicate that the effects of CB1 receptor signaling upon seizure activity depends on how that receptor is being activated, and that this activation varies by how a specific cannabinoid interacts with the receptor, either as an agonist or an antagonist.

DOSAGE—Dosage guidance for the use of cannabinoids for seizure disorders depends upon the type of disorder and the kind of cannabinoid being used. Consultation with a physician is highly recommended to help determine appropriate dosage guidelines because of the risk that the use of specific cannabinoids poses toward increased seizure activity.

Methods of Ingestion

ORAL—Sublingual and buccal administration is preferred to conventional oral use, since swallowed oral metabolism may be less effective.

VAPORIZATION AND SMOKING—In adults, vaporized and smoked cannabis are commonly used by patients with seizure disorders.

INDICATED CHEMOTYPES—Recently, CBD varieties have become more popular among patients with seizure disorders, though the use of THC-dominant varieties with patients goes back to the 1960s. CBDV and THCV varieties are very rare and few patients have access to them.

POPULAR VARIETIES—The best-known medical cannabis variety currently used for epilepsies is Cannatonic, a Spanish high-CBD variety from Resin Seeds. One of the Cannatonic phenotypes produces almost no THC, but can produce nearly 19 percent CBD by dry weight. This phenotype is also known as AC/DC and Charlotte's Web, and is the "highless" cannabis touted by Israeli researchers.[177]

SKIN CONDITIONS

Until relatively recently, little attention has been paid to the potential efficacy of cannabinoids in the treatment of skin conditions. But as the endocannabinoid system is more fully understood, the role it plays in allergic response and inflammation of the skin has become increasingly important. In the near future it is likely that cannabinoid medicines might help treat skin conditions ranging from minor itching and dermatitis to eczema and psoriasis, and even skin tumors including malignant melanoma.[178]

Description

From the tiny nerves attached to hair follicles to the nerves within the epidermis, to nearly every layer of the skin, there is evidence of the presence of the cannabinoid receptors, CB1 and CB2.[179]

EFFECTIVENESS—Topical application of THC has been shown to reduce skin inflammation.[180] There is interest in the potential use of topical cannabis in treating painful skin conditions and itching.[181] There is also research underway to examine whether cannabinoids might be used to treat skin tumors.[182]

PROPOSED MECHANISM—The endocannabinoid system appears to play a protective role in reducing allergic inflammation of the skin.[183] The regulatory role played by the endocannabinoid system within the nervous system and the immune system ultimately may have a significant impact on skin diseases.

DOSAGE—Dosage of topical cannabinoids is not currently well understood. Anecdotal accounts of hash oil being applied with no adverse effects would support the tolerance of relatively high doses, since these oils can exceed 70 percent THC in potency.

Methods of Ingestion

ORAL—Oral cannabis, especially with CBD tinctures, is useful for treatment of inflammation. THC taken orally seems to reduce itching.

VAPORIZATION AND SMOKING—Because of its rapid uptake, smoked and vaporized cannabis is useful for treatment of itching associated with a wide variety of skin conditions, especially intractable itching caused by liver disease.

TOPICAL—Effective in hemp oil and creams.

INDICATED CHEMOTYPES—Both CBD and THC varieties may be infused and used topically.

POPULAR VARIETIES—Harlequin, Cannatonic, and purple, broad-leafleted varieties such as Purple Urkle.

STRESS

Richard Lazarus famously wrote, "Stress occurs when an individual perceives that the demands of an external situation are beyond his or her perceived ability to cope with them."[184] Life is often stressful and it is well understood that elevated stress response can have a profoundly negative impact on health. Stress induces the production of hormones that elevate heart rate and blood pressure, stimulates the gut to speed up digestion, and aggravates many medical conditions. The "fight or flight" response is triggered by stress. Anxiety and depression are often the result of chronic stress. Nearly all cannabis users, medical or recreational, note that cannabis helps counteract the effects of stress. Because chronic cannabis use is associated with higher blood levels of stress hormones, it be might be that heavy cannabis use risks initiating a cycle of stress release, followed by increased stress response.

Historical Uses

The sixteenth-century Portuguese physician Garcia De Orta studied the use of cannabis as a medicine while stationed in India. De Orta went on to write the greatest herbal medicine treatise of his time, *Colloquies on the Simples and Drugs of India*. De Orta noted that the locals, and some of his fellow Portuguese, regularly used cannabis to relieve the stresses of daily life, primarily as an inebriant, but also medicinally. De Orta observed that cannabis seemed to lift users above their anxieties and cares.

Description

Hans Selye coined the word stress in his 1936 study, "A syndrome produced by diverse nocuous agents."[185] Seyle defines stress as the "non-specific response of the body to any demand for change." The rise of cannabis use as an intoxicant and euphoriant in the twentieth century certainly parallels the increase in stress-related disorders in contemporary society. The characterization of human stress and coping response in the 1960s by Professor Richard Lazarus at University of California, Berkeley, came at the time when cannabis became popular in the U.S. as a recreational drug.

EFFECTIVENESS—Cannabis users score lower on measures of hypothalamic-pituitary-adrenal (HPA) axis reactivity than nonusers, which is an excellent measure of acute stress response.[186] But cannabis users often have higher plasma levels of cortisol. It may be that these elevated levels are part of what the cannabis user is seeking—because of lower than normal cortisol levels which have been has been associated with sensation-seeking behaviors such as cannabis use.

PROPOSED MECHANISM—Stress response is mediated by the HPA axis, which consists of the hypothalamus and pituitary gland within the brain, and the adrenal glands on the kidneys. The HPA axis is regulated by the endocannabinoid system.[187] Therefore the endocannabinoid system both reacts to stress and assists with adaptation to stress.[188] The endocannabinoid system also regulates emotional memory associated with stress.[189] The HPA axis effectively regulates stress responses and other bodily processes including immunity, digestion, emotions, sexual response, and energy expenditure. The HPA regulates all this through the release of steroid hormones such as cortisol, commonly described as the "stress hormone." Endocannabinoid signaling has been proven to be essential to enable adaptation to stress.[190] Cannabidiol is quite effective in animal models for reducing stress-related anxiety and lingering anxiety post-stress.[191] The ability of CBD to reduce stress-related anxiety was linked to CBD's ability to encourage nerve production within the hippocampus.[192]

DOSAGE—High doses of cannabis can actually trigger HPA axis reactivity and an increase in cortisol production.[193] This finding lends credence to the observation that chronic overdosage of cannabis can reduce the ability of cannabis to reduce symptoms of stress, which would be the likely outcome of cannabinoid receptor downregulation. Male chronic cannabis users seem to have higher cortisol levels than females, though this could be due to residual THC and THC metabolites that build up in chronic users. There appears to be no correlation between cortisol and the amount of marijuana use, although this may be due to cannabis tolerance among chronic users. Chronic delta-9-tetrahydrocannabinol administration downregulates CB_1 receptors, and chronic cannabis users typically exhibit reduced cortisol reactivity.[194] It may be that the most effective THC dose for stress relief is quite small and perhaps below the threshold of psychoactivity—in some cases, at around 2 milligrams of THC.

Methods of Ingestion

ORAL—Oral or sublingual cannabis is a discreet and effective mode of administration for stress relief.

VAPORIZATION AND SMOKING—Single inhalations of small doses of vaporized or smoked cannabis are effective.

INDICATED CHEMOTYPES—Typically, mildly sedative THC-dominant chemotypes. CBD strains are also effective. Terpenes such as myrcene, linalool, and limonene should increase effectiveness.

POPULAR VARIETIES—Bubba Kush, purple varieties, and high-CBD varieties such as Cannatonic are recommended.

CANNABIS AND ADOLESCENCE

Medical cannabis use presents special challenges and risks for adolescents. The majority of young medical cannabis users are unlikely to suffer any long-term damage over a treatment course at reasonable doses. However, cannabis appears to interact differently with the developing brain than the adult brain. There is concern that a small number of adolescents susceptible to schizophrenia may increase their risk of developing the illness by using cannabis.

Strong evidence exists that heavy use of cannabis among young people leads to increased rates of dependence.[195] A long-term study indicates that the more cannabis consumed in adolescence, the higher the rate of adult schizophrenia, but the connection remains disputed.[196] Miriam Schneider of the German Central Institute of Mental Health made a widely cited risk assessment: "...young people, in particular during the susceptible period around pubertal development, represent a highly vulnerable cannabis consumer group and seem to be at a higher risk of suffering from adverse consequences of cannabinoid exposure than adult consumers."[197] There is little evidence in the literature that moderate medical cannabis use functions as a "gateway" to illicit drugs. Medical use of cannabis by adolescents must be within a defined treatment course with dosage guidelines. Dosage with non-psychoactive THCA and alternative cannabinoids may also reduce some of the risks and adverse effects.

The Risks of Adolescent Cannabis Use

Cannabis use presents challenges to adolescent development, from both developmental and social perspectives. In a 2012 review of the uses and risks of cannabis, medicinally and recreationally, J. M. Bostwick of the Department of Psychiatry and Psychology at the Mayo Clinic emphasized addiction, psychosis, and other risks that cannabis use can pose to adolescents.[198] He noted that effects on the developing brain are more profound because the adolescent organ is undergoing maturation. Uncontrolled doses of cannabis could interfere with the endocannabinoid system's role in brain development. Also, some adolescents using cannabis may be more vulnerable to developing schizophrenia if they carry a specific gene variation.[199] Heavy use of cannabis may result in memory and attention deficits, anxiety, and mood problems. However, many of these "symptoms" also fall within the range of common adolescent behavior. In brain scan studies of adolescent cannabis users, researchers have noted that most of the abnormalities are mild and tend to disappear after three months of abstinence. During the period of adolescent cannabis use, these temporary cognitive deficits can negatively impact schoolwork, sleep quality, and decision-making.[200] Adults in consultation with their physician should carefully monitor any adolescent use of medical cannabis.

CANNABIS AND CHILDREN

Any consideration of cannabis as a medicine for infants or children must be approached with special caution and informed, professional medical oversight. Because cannabis constituents interact with the receptors that regulate physical development and a variety of functions throughout the body—including receptors associated with brain development—great care must be exercised.

With pediatric patients, the principal conditions for which medical cannabis is used are epilepsy and autism spectrum disorders that do not respond to conventional treatments. Because there are so few emerging pharmaceuticals for childhood cancers, increasingly parents are investigating the use of alternative treatments, including cannabis. All of these disorders are devastating to affected children and their families, so the hope that cannabis might bring relief can be very compelling.

Preliminary Findings

Across the Internet, people share stories and videos of children whose serious neurological conditions have been successfully treated with cannabis medicines, especially CBD (cannabidiol). The evidence supporting these accounts is primarily anecdotal, although in 2013, researchers at Stanford University presented a preliminary survey of the use of CBD cannabis with pediatric epilepsy patients in California.[201] However, increasingly researchers and physicians are examining the potential of cannabis-based medicines for pediatric patients. Dr. Elizabeth Anne Thiele, professor of neurology at Harvard Medical School and director of the Pediatric Epilepsy Service at Massachusetts General Hospital, gave testimony at the Massachusetts Department of Public Health hearings on medical marijuana, in which she stated that: "Based on a review of the literature and firsthand experience treating pediatric epilepsy patients, it is my opinion that medical marijuana—and, particularly, the non-psychoactive ingredient in medical marijuana, cannabidiol (CBD)—may have substantial medical benefit for pediatric epilepsy patients, as well as significantly fewer adverse side effects than many of the other antiepileptic therapies available today. Accordingly, I believe the proposed regulation's [Massachusetts's medical marijuana law] proscription of the use of medical marijuana by children under 18 who do not have a 'life-limiting illness'—i.e., an illness for which 'reasonable estimates of prognosis suggest death may occur within six months'—would do a significant disservice to the pediatric epilepsy population in Massachusetts."[202]

While these preliminary findings are encouraging, they do not approach the amount of evidence typically required for a drug to be approved for use by children. The Miami

Children's Brain Institute at Miami Children's Hospital put up a FAQ webpage in response to the numerous inquiries about CBD from parents of children with epilepsy. The institute stated that: "Anyone who takes care of children with epilepsy hopes [that CBD works]. But the bar is the same height for all potential treatments: a statistically measurable improvement in a blinded observer. And that bar has not yet been reached for CBD in epilepsy. There is nothing wrong with people wanting to share their successes with other patients, especially in children with intractable epilepsy who we are so desperate to help. Unfortunately, the experience is not enough for us to say that CBD works."[203]

And there is the crux of the issue: Should unproven cannabis treatments be used with pediatric patients? This is a question that must be answered by parents, researchers, and physicians working together.

It is important to understand that when using cannabis with severely-ill children, the herb is not always effective in delivering symptomatic relief. Suzanne Leigh, a reporter who writes on health and fitness, sought medical marijuana for her 11-year-old daughter, Natasha. Suzanne hoped to stimulate her daughter's appetite during a reoccurrence of the little girl's brain cancer, which eventually would take her life. Medical marijuana did not stimulate Natasha's appetite, despite her mother trying many combinations of oral medical marijuana products containing different ratios of THC and CBD over the course of a year. As Ms. Leigh wrote in the *Huffington Post*, "Marijuana never did save Natasha's life. But neither did the mainstream treatments."[204] In late 2013, the U.S. Food and Drug Administration approved an Investigational New Drug study to be conducted at New York University and University of California, San Francisco, using CBD on intractable pediatric epilepsies. The CBD is furnished by GW Pharmaceuticals in the form of an extract called Epidiolex. This is a very small-scale study enrolling 25 patients at each facility. It is expected that if the preliminary results are encouraging, the study may be expanded to other university research programs at medical schools around the United States. At the same time, news reports from Colorado reported that a number of parents whose children have these epilepsies are moving to Colorado to take advantage of laws legalizing marijuana in the state. A cannabis dispensary in Colorado is cultivating high-CBD cannabis and extracting oil from it for the use of these families.

DOSAGE—The question of dose becomes especially critical with pediatric patients, yet this issue can be very challenging. There are few studies that have determined the effective dose of cannabis medicines for medical conditions among the adult population, and even fewer for children. The key here is to determine the smallest possible dose that might provide symptomatic relief, but which also minimizes the likelihood or impact of potential adverse effects.

CANNABIS AND PREGNANCY

Women using cannabis have a slightly elevated risk of infertility due to ovulatory abnormalities.[205] Some women choose to continue to use cannabis during pregnancy to reduce nausea from morning sickness and depression, despite somewhat contradictory evidence that cannabis use could have negative effects on prenatal, neonatal, and child development.[206] A 2014 Swedish animal study indicated that pure THC interferes with fetal brain development.

A study of 600 British women who smoked cannabis was examined to assess the impact on their pregnancies. Cannabis use during pregnancy was not associated with increased risk of infant mortality. However, frequent use of cannabis throughout pregnancy may be associated with reduced birth weight.[207] There have been two large studies of heavy prenatal use of cannabis: the Ottawa Prenatal Prospective Study (OPPS)[208] and the Maternal Health Practices and Child Development Study (MHPCD).[209] OPPS examined the effects of cannabis and tobacco use on the offspring of primarily white, middle-class Canadian mothers, while the MHPCD studied the effects of prenatal cannabis exposure among the offspring of a group of mothers, half of whom were African American, half Caucasian. Neither of these studies found higher rates of miscarriage, premature birth, or incidence of complications during the pregnancy term or childbirth associated with cannabis use. For three- to four-year-old children, prenatal cannabis exposure negatively affected the verbal and memory domains of children in both the OPPS and MHPCD groups. Cognitive development assessed by IQ (intelligence quotient) testing demonstrated a negative impact on short-term memory and verbal reasoning associated with first- and/or second-trimester marijuana usage. As the cannabis-exposed children grew older, the results of the OPPS and MHPCD diverged. When they reached school age, the OPPS children had no memory deficits, but the MHPCD children appeared to have short-term memory deficits associated with heavy cannabis use by the mother during the second trimester of pregnancy. This deficit in the school-age MHPCD children was countered by the children's increased attention span when compared with nonexposed children. However, one trend that appeared to be confirmed in both the OPPS and MHPCD studies is that cannabis use during pregnancy is associated with impaired cognitive function in the offspring, including attention deficits and executive function. Despite evidence that children of mothers who smoked cannabis for morning sickness, depression, or anxiety did not harm their offspring, recent animal research encourages caution.

CANNABIS AND PREVENTIVE MEDICINE

Could cannabis prevent some diseases and conditions in addition to providing symptomatic relief? The preliminary evidence seems to support this idea. Vincenzo Di Marzo, the noted Italian scientist, has stated that cannabinoids help us relax, eat, rest, forget, and protect ourselves.[210] Judicious application of phytocannabinoids may augment this process. It has been demonstrated that drugs that are antagonistic to cannabinoid receptors can cause numerous adverse effects, so it could be possible that drugs that play nicely with these receptors may support good health.

Historical Uses

The fact that humans have chosen to consume the cannabis plant for over 10,000 years suggests that the plant's balance of cannabinoids and terpenes is generally beneficial. The tonic nature of the plant was first formally recognized in the use of female cannabis plants as yin tonics in traditional Chinese medicine. Cannabis was included in some general tonics marketed in the United States in the nineteenth century, typically in combination with a wide variety of other drugs—some now recognized as safe and others toxic. Chlorodyne, a popular patent medicine, contained a smorgasbord of drugs besides cannabis extract, including morphine, nitroglycerin, and the plant alkaloid, hyoscyamine, found in jimsonweed.

Dr. Donald Tashkin's long-term study of cannabis smokers indicates a small reduction in head, neck, and lung cancers among cannabis smokers that did not also use tobacco. Long-term cannabis users had 3.7 percent lower incidence of lung cancer than nonsmokers.[211] A 2013 study showed that cannabis users had lower resting insulin levels and waist measurements than nonusers.[212] Cell studies and animal models have shown that cannabinoids such as CBD may arrest and even prevent the occurrence of some tumors.[213] Ethan B. Russo's proposed clinical endocannabinoid deficiency might be treated with small doses of phytocannabinoids as prophylaxis.[214] Cannabinoids are also multi-target drugs that may be of interest in preventing complex diseases such as Alzheimer's.[215] Clint Werner, in his book *Marijuana: Gateway to Health*, suggests that the National Football League may someday wish to consider using cannabinoids such as CBD to protect its players from the effects of violent collisions that can cause cumulative brain injury.[216]

EFFECTIVENESS—The protective effects of phytocannabinoids such as CBD are increasingly well understood and demonstrated in preclinical studies. CBD has been shown to be strongly neuroprotective and cardioprotective. These protective abilities may lead to its use with patients at risk from stroke, Alzheimer's disease, and heart attacks. Cannabinoid supplementation may also prevent small tumors from finding the blood supplies needed for their growth and subsequent proliferation.[217]

APPROACHES—Surveying the literature, it appears that there is a defensible argument for the use of small doses of cannabis medicines to support homeostasis and general tone across the range of systems regulated by the endocannabinoid system. Preliminary indications are that caution must be observed in order to avoid effects caused by the use of a single cannabinoid, rather than a combination of cannabinoids that ameliorate each others' adverse effects profile.[218] Dose is important since more and more studies indicate that there is a sweet spot of effective THC dosage, which may be at the threshold of psychoactivity.[219] There is no small irony in the fact that cannabis produced by the U.S. government, which has been criticized as too low in THC content, may be more beneficial for precision dosing than previously understood. A study of heavy, chronic users (with a median use of six joints per day) showed that mild metabolic derangement occurs in young cannabis users (of a median age of 25). These users had more intra-abdominal fat than subcutaneous fat, which is an indicator of metabolic shift in how and where fat is deposited.[220] To avoid this sort of metabolic shift, likely from cannabinoid receptor downregulation, dose control to avoid the buildup of cannabis tolerance becomes more important. And use of cannabis among young adult men living in states with medical marijuana laws may be linked to fewer suicides, as the suicide rate among this population has dropped considerably in these locales.[221]

DOSAGE—Researcher Yannick Marchalant has been quoted as stating, "a puff is enough."[222] While speculative, doses below 2.5 milligrams of THC with an equal amount of non-psychoactive cannabinoids, such as CBD, appear promising. Anecdotal observation in California dispensaries has shown that low-dose prophylaxis with cannabis, vaporized or orally administered, appears to be effective in reducing the frequency of migraine attacks in susceptible patients.

INDICATED CHEMOTYPES—For prophylaxis and preventive health, cannabis varieties with entourages of cannabinoids beyond THC—for example, CBD or CBG—are most interesting. Additionally, if these multi-cannabinoid varieties also produce a broad range of terpenes, this will likely reduce the incidence of adverse effects.

POPULAR VARIETIES—Pincher's Creek, Cannatonic, Harlequin.

CANNABIS AND WOMEN'S HEALTH

According to numerous anecdotal accounts, cannabis has long been considered effective for a range of women's health issues, including dysmenorrhea, excessive menstrual bleeding, and premenstrual syndrome.[223] Sadly, there is a surprising lack of formal research into the potential uses of cannabis medicines to address symptoms and conditions faced by women. Hopefully, this will change over the next decade as our understanding of sex differences found in the endocannabinoid system are elucidated.

Description

In 2011, women made up 27 percent of the patient population utilizing medical cannabis dispensaries in California.[224]

EFFECTIVENESS—There is research underway to examine the potential role of CBD in the treatment of some breast cancer lines.[225] Anecdotal reports from dispensary patients indicate that women are using cannabis to relieve symptoms of menopause, a treatment which helps to regulate hormonal balance.[226]

PROPOSED MECHANISM—Endocannabinoid system receptors and endocannabinoids are found within a range of tissues throughout the uterus and female reproductive system.[227] It is believed that the endocannabinoids, especially anandamide, play a significant role in regulating fertility and early pregnancy.[228] It is known that endocannabinoids regulate aspects of endometriosis.[229] John McPartland has also postulated that dysmenorrhea may be an inflammatory disorder.[230]

DOSAGE—For use with morning sickness, consult your doctor, since high doses of cannabinoids are typically required for nausea.

Methods of Ingestion

ORAL—Low doses of oral cannabis medicines are increasingly popular with patients for their convenience and the length of the effects.

VAPORIZATION AND SMOKING—Vaporization and smoking are by far the preferred method among patients; vaporization is recommended since it reduces exposure to combustion toxins.

INDICATED CHEMOTYPES—Wide-leafleted indicas are reported by patients to be particularly effective for dysmenorrhea.

POPULAR VARIETIES—Women report that narrow-leafleted hybrids such as Blueberry and Blue Dream are effective for the pain of cramping. For premenstrual syndrome, mood-elevating, narrow-leafleted varieties such as Jack Herer and Trainwreck are popular.

CANNABIS DEPENDENCE AND WITHDRAWAL

In 1930s, cannabis was portrayed as an addictive drug capable of producing psychotic cravings in its users. These descriptions were exaggerated, and the reality is that true cannabis dependence appears to be rare except among the heaviest and most frequent users. Withdrawal symptoms appear mild when compared with drugs such as opiates and cocaine, but they have been confirmed experimentally using cannabinoid receptor antagonists, which force withdrawal symptoms when administered to dependent users.[231]

There is more to cannabis dependency than just cannabinoid receptor interaction. The mu-opioid receptor, which is directly responsible for one of the brain's reward mechanisms underlying heroin addiction, is also involved. When a cannabinoid such as THC interacts with a CB1 cannabinoid receptor, it induces the release of opioid peptide molecules, which activate mu-opioid receptors. And the same mu-opioid receptor activation underlies the reward pathways associated with alcohol and nicotine dependency. It appears to be a primary brain receptor causing drug addiction.[232] Additionally, recent studies indicate that there may be genetic, age, and sex differences associated with how cannabis affects brain structures in cannabinoid dependence among chronic users. For example, adolescent, cannabis-dependent males may suffer changes in the morphology of the amygdala, a brain structure that is primary in memory and emotional responses. These changes in the amygdala do not appear in cannabis-dependent adolescent females.[233] Though some of these criteria have been discounted as being more indicative of cannabis prohibition than drug addiction, the appearance of three or more of the following is often considered evidence of cannabis dependency:

- Excessive, often daily, use of cannabis
- Tolerance which requires increased dose to achieve effect
- Compulsion to use cannabis whenever available or offered
- Excessive ritualization and time spent on the acquisition, possession, and intake of cannabis
- Withdrawal symptoms emerging after cessation of cannabis use

How Common Is Dependency?

Statistics are often quoted about the increased incidence of cannabis dependency, based on the number of individuals seeking treatment. However, because drug treatment and rehabilitation is often the court-ordered diversion for individuals arrested for possession of small amounts of cannabis, the numbers of individuals entering cannabis treatment may not accurately reflect the incidence of actual cannabis dependency. In 2007, treatment episode data sets from the federal Substance Abuse and Mental Health Services Administration reported that 288,000 people had undergone treatment for cannabis use.[234] Fifty-seven percent of those individuals were court-ordered into treatment; 28 percent were referred by families, schools, employers, or medical professionals; and 14.8 percent were self-referred. Contrast this with self-referral into treatment for alcohol (29 percent), cocaine (36 percent), or heroin (58 percent). People in treatment for cannabis use were also considerably younger with 40 percent under 19 years old, as compared to 11 percent for alcohol treatment. The most telling fact for how skewed these cannabis treatment figures are is that 37.7 percent of those entering treatment for cannabis had not used cannabis in the last month, and 53 percent had only used cannabis one to three times in the last month—which means that the majority of those entering treatment would likely not meet the standard for a cannabis use disorder. So what are the real risks of cannabis dependence? The risks are likely lower than the widely cited claim that 9 percent of cannabis users become drug dependent. The actual number may be considerably lower. There needs to be more independent research, outside the drug treatment/addiction medicine community, to independently validate the common assertion that cannabis use can lead to dependency as it does with other drugs such as alcohol, opiates, and nicotine. Medical users of cannabis with a recommended course of treatment from their physician are thought to be at less risk.

In studies, cannabis dependence appears to be closely linked to a prolonged period of high doses. Dose control may reduce the risk of dependence. The use of highly concentrated cannabis extracts, if not monitored by the user and physician, could lead to increased risk of dependence; cannabis tolerance that develops from continued exposure to high doses of cannabinoids will require higher doses to achieve the same level of effect.

Cannabis Withdrawal

Cannabis withdrawal symptoms include insomnia, irritability, reduced appetite, anxiety, mild depression, moodiness, and stomach upset or nausea. Cannabis withdrawal can cause some functional impairments that interfere with daily life. Researchers at the University of New South Wales in Australia recommend targeting the withdrawal symptoms that contribute most to functional impairment. Their treatment approach involves, for example, stress management techniques and pharmacological interventions for alleviating loss of appetite and insomnia. Symptoms rarely persist more than 14 days.[235]

Quitting Cannabis Successfully

Successful cessation of cannabis use among dependent users is linked to developing strategies that help the individual cope with exposure to other cannabis smokers—as well as strategies that help the user deal with fear, anger, shame, and other aversive feelings without relapsing into cannabis use. Motivational enhancement techniques do not appear to help in cessation of cannabis use among dependent young adults.[236]

APPENDIX

NOTES

Part 1: Cannabis as a Medicine

[1] Dave Olson, "Hemp Culture in Japan," *Journal of the International Hemp Association* 4, no. 2 (June 1997): 40–50.
[2] Hui-Lin Li, "An Archaeological and Historical Account of Cannabis in China," *Economic Botany* 28, no. 4 (December 1974): 446.
[3] Martin Booth, *Cannabis: A History* (New York: Picador, 2005).
[4] Sula Benet, "Early Diffusion and Folk Uses of Hemp in Cannabis and Culture," in *Cannabis and Culture*, ed. Vera D. Rubin (The Hague: Mouton, 1975): 39–49.
[5] Ernest L. Abel, *Marihuana: The First Twelve Thousand Years* (New York: Plenum Press, 1980).
[6] I. M. Turner, "The Contribution of Sir William Brooke O'Shaughnessy (1809–1889) to Plant Taxonomy," *Phytotaxa* 15 (January 28, 2011): 57–63.
[7] Mel Gorman, "Sir William Brooke O'Shaughnessy: Pioneer Chemist in a Colonial Environment," *Journal of Chemical Education* 46, no. 2 (1969): 99.
[8] *Report of the Indian Hemp Drugs Commission, 1893–94*, 7 vols. (Simla, India: Government Central Printing House, 1894).
[9] William Brooke O'Shaughnessy, "On the preparations of the Indian hemp, or gunjah (*Cannabis indica*); Their effects on the animal system in health, and their utility in the treatment of tetanus and other convulsive diseases," *Transactions of the Medical and Physical Society of Bengal* (1838): 71–102, 421, 461.
[10] J. Russell Reynolds, "On the therapeutical uses and toxic effects of cannabis indica," *Lancet* 135, no. 3473 (1890): 637–38.
[11] Oakley Ray and Charles Ksir, *Drugs, Society, and Human Behavior*, 10th ed. (New York: McGraw-Hill, 2004), 456.
[12] *U.S. Congress, Senate Committee on Finance, Taxation of Marihuana, Hearing on H.R. 6906, 75th Cong., 1st sess., July 12, 1937* (Washington: Government Printing Office, 1937), 33.
[13] David Potter, "Growth and Morphology of Medicinal Cannabis," in *The Medicinal Uses of Cannabis and Cannabinoids*, ed. Geoffrey W. Guy, Brian A. Whittle, and Philip J. Robson (London: Pharmaceutical Press, 2004): 17–54.
[14] J. C. Callaway, "Hempseed as a Nutritional Resource: An Overview," *Euphytica* 140, no. 1 (2004): 65–72.
[15] Charles Ainsworth, "Boys and Girls Come out to Play: The Molecular Biology of Dioecious Plants," *Annals of Botany* 86, no. 2 (2000): 211–21.
[16] Koichi Sakamoto, Tomoko Abe, Tomoki Matsuyama, Shigeo Yoshida, Nobuko Ohmido, Kiichi Fukui, and Shinobu Satoh, "RAPD Markers Encoding Retrotransposable Elements Are Linked to the Male Sex in *Cannabis sativa L.*," *Genome* 48, no. 5 (2005): 931–36.
[17] Robert C. Clarke and David P. Watson, "Cannabis and Natural Cannabis Medicines," *Marijuana and the Cannabinoids* (2007): 1–15.
[18] H. C. Kerr, *Report of the Cultivation of, and Trade in, Ganja in Bengal*, British Parliamentary Papers (1893–94): 66, 94–154.
[19] Mountain Girl, *The Primo Plant: Growing Sinsemilla Marijuana* (Berkeley: Leaves of Grass/Wingbow Press, 1977).
[20] Jim Richardson and Arik Woods, *Sinsemilla: Marijuana Flowers* (Berkeley: And/Or Press, 1976).
[21] Y. Liu and X. Tang, "Green Seedling of Hemp Acquired by Tissue Culture," *China's Fibre Crops* 2 (1984): 19–29. Cited in Clarke and Watson, "Cannabis and Natural Cannabis Medicines," 2007.
[22] Hemant Lata, Suman Chandra, Ikhlas A. Khan, and Mahmoud A. ElSohly, "Propagation through Alginate Encapsulation of Axillary Buds of *Cannabis sativa L.*—An Important Medicinal Plant," *Physiology and Molecular Biology of Plants* 15, no. 11 (2009): 79–86.
[23] Arno Hazecamp, Mark A. Ware, Kirsten R. Muller-Vahl, Donald Abrams, and Franjo Grotenhermen, "The Medicinal Use of Cannabis and Cannabionoids—An International Cross-Sectional Survey on Administration Forms," *Journal of Psychoactive Drugs* 45, no. 3 (2013): 199–210, doi: 10,1080/02791072.2013.805976.
[24] Franjo Grotenhermen, "Pharmacokinetics and Pharmacodynamics of Cannabinoids," *Clinical*

Pharmacokinetics 42, no. 4 (2003): 327–60.
[25] Erin L. Karschner, "Plasma Cannabinoid Pharmacokinetics following Controlled Oral Delta-9-Tetrahydrocannabinol and Oromucosal Cannabis Extract Administration," *Clinical Chemistry* 57, no. 1 (2011): 66–75.
[26] Franjo Grotenhermen, "Pharmacokinetics and Pharmacodynamics of Cannabinoids," *Clinical Pharmacokinetics* 42, no. 4 (2003): 327–60.
[27] J. Hirvonen, R. S. Goodwin, C. T. Li, G. E. Terry, S. S. Zoghbi, C. Morse, V. W. Pike, N. D. Volkow, M. A. Huestis, and R. B. Innis, "Reversible and Regionally Selective Downregulation of Brain Cannabinoid CB1 Receptors in Chronic Daily Cannabis Smokers," *Molecular Psychiatry* 17, no. 6 (2011): 642–49.
[28] Douglas A. Simonetto, Amy S. Oxentenko, Margot L. Herman, and Jason H. Szostek, "Cannabinoid Hyperemesis: A Case Series of 98 Patients," *Mayo Clinic Proceedings* 87, no. 2 (2012).
[29] Valérie Wolff, J. P. Armspach, V. Lauer, O. Rouyer, M. Bataillard, C. Marescaux, B. Geny, "Cannabis-Related Stroke: Myth or Reality?," *Stroke* 44, no. 2 (2013): 558–63; Murray A. Mittleman, Rebecca A. Lewis, Malcolm Maclure, Jane B. Sherwood, and James E. Muller, "Triggering Myocardial Infarction by Marijuana," *Circulation* 103, no. 23 (2001): 2805–9; and Dimitri Renard, Guillaume Taieb, Guillaume Gras-Combe, and Pierre Labauge, "Cannabis-Related Myocardial Infarction and Cardioembolic Stroke," *Journal of Stroke and Cerebrovascular Diseases* 21, no. 1 (2012): 82–83.
[30] Kenneth J. Mukamal, Malcolm Maclure, James E. Muller, and Murray A. Mittleman, "An Exploratory Prospective Study of Marijuana Use and Mortality following Acute Myocardial Infarction," *American Heart Journal* 155, no. 3 (2008): 465–70.
[31] Mahmoud A. ElSohly and Desmond Slade, "Chemical Constituents of Marijuana: The Complex Mixture of Natural Cannabinoids," *Life Sciences* 78, no. 5 (2005): 539–48.
[32] Ethan B. Russo, "Taming THC: Potential Cannabis Synergy and Phytocannabinoid-Terpenoid Entourage Effects," *British Journal of Pharmacology* 163, no. 7 (2011): 1344–64.
[33] A. J. Hampson, M. Grimaldi, J. Axelrod, and D. Wink, "Cannabidiol and Delta-9-Tetrahydrocannabinol Are Neuroprotective Antioxidants," *Proceedings of the National Academy of Sciences of the United States* 95, no. 14 (1998): 8268–73.
[34] Pál Pacher, Sándor Bátkai, and George Kunos, "The Endocannabinoid System as an Emerging Target of Pharmacotherapy," *Pharmacological Reviews* 58, no. 3 (2006): 389–462.
[35] Martin Eichler, L. Spinedi, S. Unfer-Grauwiler, M. Bodmer, C. Surber, M. Luedi, and J. Drewe, "Heat Exposure of Cannabis Sativa Extracts Affects the Pharmacokinetic and Metabolic Profile in Healthy Male Subjects," *Planta Medica* 78, no. 7 (2012): 686.
[36] Ethan B. Russo and Geoffrey W. Guy, "A Tale of Two Cannabinoids: The Therapeutic Rationale for Combining Tetrahydrocannabinol and Cannabidiol," *Medical Hypotheses* 66, no. 2 (2006): 234–46.
[37] Nicholas A. Jones, Andrew J. Hill, Imogen Smith, Sarah A. Bevan, Claire M. Williams, Benjamin J. Whalley, and Gary J. Stephens, "Cannabidiol Displays Antiepileptiform and Antiseizure Properties In Vitro and In Vivo," *Journal of Pharmacology and Experimental Therapeutics* 332, no. 2 (2010): 569–77.
[38] Ethan B. Russo, "Taming THC: Potential Cannabis Synergy and Phytocannabinoid-Terpenoid Entourage Effects," *British Journal of Pharmacology* 163, no. 7 (2011): 1344–64.
[39] Francesca Borrelli, I. Fasolino, B. Romano, R. Capasso, F. Maiello, D. Coppola, P. Orlando, G. Battista, E. Pagano, V. Di Marzo, and A. A. Izzo, "Beneficial Effect of the Non-Psychotropic Plant Cannabinoid Cannabigerol on Experimental Inflammatory Bowel Disease," *Biochemical Pharmacology* 85, no. 9 (May 2013): 1306–16, doi: 10.1016/j.bcp.2013.01.017.
[40] M. G. Cascio, L. A. Gauson, L. A. Stevenson, R. A. Ross, and R. G. Pertwee, "Evidence That the Plant Cannabinoid Cannabigerol Is a Highly Potent a2-Adrenoceptor Agonist and Moderately Potent 5HT1A Receptor Antagonist," *British Journal of Pharmacology* 159, no. 1 (2010): 129–41.
[41] Giovanni Appendinoa et al., "*NPC Natural Product Communications* 2008," NPC Natural Product Communications: 1977.
[42] Sami Sarfaraz, V. M. Adhami, D. N. Syed, F. Afaq, and H. Mukhtar, "Cannabinoids for Cancer Treatment: Progress and Promise," *Cancer Research* 68, no. 2 (2008): 339–42.
[43] David Potter, "The Propagation, Characterisation and Optimisation of Cannabis sativa L. as a Phytopharmaceutical" (diss., King's College London, 2009).
[44] B. K. Colasanti, R. E. Brown, and C. R. Craig, "Ocular Hypotension, Ocular Toxicity, and Neurotoxicity in Response to Marijuana Extract and Cannabidiol," *General Pharmacology* 15, no. 6 (1984): 479.

[45] H. N. ElSohly, C. E. Turner, A. M. Clark, and Mahmoud A. ElSohly, "Synthesis and Antimicrobial Activity of Certain Cannabichromene and Cannabigerol Related Compounds," *Journal of Pharmaceutical Sciences* 71 (1982): 1319–23.
[46] R. Deyo and R. Musty, "A Cannabichromene (CBC) Extract Alters Behavioral Despair on the Mouse Tail Suspension Test of Depression," *Proceedings 2003 Symposium on the Cannabinoids* (Cornwall, ON: International Cannabinoid Research Society, 2003).
[47] N. Qin, M. P. Neeper, Y. Liu, T. L. Hutchinson, M. L. Lubin, C. M. Flores, "TRPV2 Is Activated by Cannabidiol and Mediates CGRP Release in Cultured Rat Dorsal Root Ganglion Neurons," *Journal of Neuroscience* 28 (2008): 6231–38.
[48] E. W. Gill, W. D. M. Paton, and R. G. Pertwee, "Preliminary Experiments on the Chemistry and Pharmacology of Cannabis," *Nature* 228 (1970): 134–36; L. E. Hollister, "Structure Activity Relationship in Man of Cannabis Constituents and Homologues of Delta-9-Tetrahydrocannabinol," *Pharmacology* 11 (1974): 3–11.
[49] R. G. Pertwee, "The Diverse CB1 and CB2 Receptor Pharmacology of Three Plant Cannabinoids: Delta-9-Tetrahydrocannabinol, Cannabidiol and Delta-9-Tetrahydrocannabivarin," *British Journal of Pharmacology* 153, no. 2 (2008): 199–215.
[50] G. Riedel, P. Fadda, S. McKillop-Smith, R. G. Pertwee, B. Platt, and L. Robinson, "Synthetic and Plant-Derived Cannabinoid Receptor Antagonists Show Hypophagic Properties in Fasted and Non-Fasted Mice," *British Journal of Pharmacology* 156, no. 7 (2009): 1154–66.
[51] Nicholas A. Jones, Andrew J. Hill, Imogen Smith, Sarah A. Bevan, Claire M. Williams, Benjamin J. Whalley, and Gary J. Stephens, "Cannabidiol Displays Antiepileptiform and Antiseizure Properties In Vitro and In Vivo," *Journal of Pharmacology and Experimental Therapeutics* 332, no. 2 (2010): 569–77.
[52] Rudolf Brenneisen, "Chemistry and Analysis of Phytocannabinoids and Other Cannabis Constituents," *Marijuana* (2007): 17.
[53] John M. McPartland and Ethan B. Russo, "Cannabis and Cannabis Extracts: Greater than the Sum of Their Parts?," *Journal of Cannabis Therapeutics* 3, no. 4 (2001): 103–32.
[54] Ethan B. Russo, "Taming THC: Potential Cannabis Synergy and Phytocannabinoid-Terpenoid Entourage Effects," *British Journal of Pharmacology* 163, no. 7 (2011): 1344–64.
[55] Xuetong Fan and Robert A. Gates, "Degradation of Monoterpenes in Orange Juice by Gamma Radiation," *Journal of Agricultural and Food Chemistry* 49, no. 5 (2001): 2422–26.
[56] M. Miyazawa and C. Yamafuji, "Inhibition of Acetylcholinesterase Activity by Bicyclic Monoterpenoids," *Journal of Agricultural and Food Chemistry* 53, no. 5 (2005): 1765–68, doi: 10.1021/jf040019b.
[57] T. Komori, R. Fujiwara, M. Tanida, J. Nomura, and M. M. Yokoyama, "Effects of Citrus Fragrance on Immune Function and Depressive States," *Neuroimmunomodulation* 2, no. 3 (1995): 174–80.
[58] T. G. do Vale, E. C. Furtado, J. G. Santos Jr., and G. S. Viana, "Central Effects of Citral, Myrcene and Limonene, Constituents of Essential Oil Chemotypes from Lippia Alba (Mill.) n.e. Brown," *Phytomedicine* 9, no. 8 (2002): 709–14.
[59] Rudolf Brenneisen, "Chemistry and Analysis of Phytocannabinoids and Other Cannabis Constituents," *Marijuana* (2007): 17.
[60] G. W. Guy and C. G. Stott, "The Development of Sativex—A Natural Cannabis-Based Medicine," in *Cannabinoids as Therapeutics*, ed. R. Mechoulam (Basel: Birkhäuser Verlag, 2005), 231–63.
[61] Ethan B. Russo, "Taming THC: Potential Cannabis Synergy and Phytocannabinoid-Terpenoid Entourage Effects," *British Journal of Pharmacology* 163, no. 7 (2011): 1344–64.
[62] Karl William Hillig, "A Systematic Investigation of Cannabis" (PhD diss., Indiana University, 2005).
[63] S. Casano, G. Grassi, V. Martini, and M. Michelozzi, "Variations in Terpene Profiles of Different Strains of *Cannabis sativa L.*," *XXVIII International Horticultural Congress on Science and Horticulture for People (IHC2010): A New Look at Medicinal and Aromatic Plants Seminar*, 2010.

Part 2: Using Medical Cannabis

[1] Robert Connell Clarke, *Hashish!* (Los Angeles: Red Eye Press, 1998).
[2] Ibid., 64
[3] Geoffrey W. Guy, "New Developments in Cannabinoid Research: Making a Modern Medicine from the Cannabis Plant" (lecture, University of California, Los Angeles/Semel Institute, May 8, 2007).
[4] Aurelia Tubaro, A. Giangaspero, S. Sosa, R. Negri, G. Grassi, S. Casano, R. Della Loggia, and G. Appendino, "Comparative Topical Anti-Inflammatory Activity of Cannabinoids and Cannabivarins," *Fitoterapia* 81, no. 7 (2010): 816–19.
[5] Donald Abrams, "Cannabis in Medicine: A Primer for Health Care Professionals" (lecture, University of California, San Francisco, October 24, 2012).
[6] Ethan B. Russo, "Taming THC: Potential Cannabis Synergy and Phytocannabinoid-Terpenoid Entourage Effects," *British Journal of Pharmacology* 163, no. 7

(2011): 1344–64.
[7] A. Ohlsson, J. E. Lindgren, A. Wahlen, S. Agurell, L. E. Hollister, and H. K. Gillespie, "Plasma Delta-9 Levels of Tetrahydrocannabinol after Intravenous, Oral, and Smoke Administration," *Problems of Drug Dependence* (1981): 250.
[8] G. K. Sharma, "Ethnobotany and Its Significance for Cannabis Studies in the Himalayas," *Journal of Psychoactive Drugs* 9, no. 4 (1977): 337–39.
[9] Dolores Hernán Pérez de la Ossa, M. Lorente, M. E. Gil-Alegre, S. Torres, E. García-Taboada, R. Mdel Aberturas, J. Molpeceres, G. Velasco, and A. I. Torres-Suárez, "Local Delivery of Cannabinoid -Loaded Microparticles Inhibits Tumor Growth in a Murine Xenograft Model of Glioblastoma Multiforme," *PLoS ONE* 8, no. 1 (2013): e54795, doi:10.1371/journal.pone.0054795.
[10] Linda B. Hollinshead, "Medical Marijuana and the Workplace," *Employment Relations Today* 40, no. 1 (2013): 71–79.
[11] R. Sewell, R. Andrew, James Poling, and Mehmet Sofuoglu, "The Effect of Cannabis Compared with Alcohol on Driving," The *American Journal on Addictions* 18, no. 3 (2009): 185–93.

Part 4: Medical Uses of Cannabis

[1] V. A. Campbell and A. Gowran, "Alzheimer's Disease; Taking the Edge Off with Cannabinoids?," *British Journal of Pharmacology* 152, no. 5 (November 2007): 655–62, doi:10.1038/sj .bjp.0707446.
[2] J. Russell Reynolds, "On the therapeutical uses and toxic effects of cannabis indica," *Lancet* 135, no. 3473 (1890): 637–38.
[3] José Alexandre Crippa, Antonio Waldo Zuardi, and Jaime E. C. Hallak, "Therapeutical Use of the Cannabinoids in Psychiatry," *Revista Brasileira de Psiquiatria* 32 (2010): 556–66.
[4] José Alexandre Crippa, Antonio Waldo Zuardi, Rocio Martín-Santos, Sagnik Bhattacharyya, Zerrin Atakan, Philip McGuire, Paolo Fusar-Poli, "Cannabis and Anxiety: A Critical Review of the Evidence" *Human Psychopharmacology: Clinical and Experimental* 24, no. 7 (2009): 515–23.
[5] Julia D. Buckner, Russell A. Matthews, and Jose Silgado, "Marijuana-Related Problems and Social Anxiety: The Role of Marijuana Behaviors in Social Situations," *Psychology of Addictive Behaviors* 26, no. 1 (2012): 151.
[6] G. A. Grierson, "The Hemp Plant in Sanskrit and Hindi Literature," *Indian Antiquary* (September 1894): 260–62.
[7] F. Markus Leweke and Dagmar Koethe, "Cannabis and Psychiatric Disorders: It Is Not Only Addiction," *Addiction Biology* 13, no. 2 (2008): 264–75, doi:10.1111/j.1369-1600.2008.00106.x.
[8] Vivian Crawford, "A Homelie Herbe: Medicinal Cannabis in Early England," *Journal of Cannabis Therapeutics* 2 (2002): 71–79.
[9] Robert B. Zurier, "Prospects for Cannabinoids as Anti-Inflammatory Agents," *Journal of Cellular Biochemistry* 88, no. 3 (2003): 462–66.
[10] Fred J. Evans, "Cannabinoids: The Separation of Central from Peripheral Effects on a Structural Basis," *Planta Medica* 57, no. S1 (1991): S60–S67.
[11] Louis Vachon, M. X. Fitzgerald, N. H. Sulliday, I. A. Gould, and E. A. Gaensnier, "Single-Dose Effect of Marihuana Smoke: Bronchial Dynamics and Respiratory-Center Sensitivity in Normal Subjects," *New England Journal of Medicine* 288, no. 19 (1973): 985–89.
[12] Mark Jackson, "'Divine Stramonium': The Rise and Fall of Smoking for Asthma," *Medical History* 54, no. 2 (2010): 171.
[13] James Mills, *Cannabis Britannica: Empire, Trade, and Prohibition 1800–1928* (Oxford: Oxford University Press, 2003).
[14] A. Calignano, I. Kátona, F. Désarnaud, A. Giuffrida, G. La Rana, K. Mackie, T. F. Freund, D. Piomelli, "Bidirectional Control of Airway Responsiveness by Endogenous Cannabinoids," *Nature* 408, no. 6808 (2000): 96–101.
[15] Donald P. Tashkin., G. C. Baldwin, T. Sarafian, S. Dubnett, and M. D. Roth, "Respiratory and Immunologic Consequences of Marijuana Smoking," *Journal of Clinical Pharmacology* 42, no. 11 supplement (2002): 71S–81S.
[16] Jeanette M. Tetrault, K. Crothers, B. A. Moore, R. Mehra, J. Concato, and D. A. Fiellin, "Effects of Marijuana Smoking on Pulmonary Function and Respiratory Complications: A Systematic Review," *Archives of Internal Medicine* 167, no. 3 (2007): 221.
[17] Mark J. Pletcher, Eric Vittinghoff, Ravi Kalhan, Joshua Richman, Monika Safford, Stephen Sidney, Feng Lin, and Stefan Kertesz, "Association between Marijuana Exposure and Pulmonary Function over 20 Years," *Journal of the American Medical Association* 307, no. 2 (2012): 173–81.
[18] Donald P. Tashkin, B. J. Shapiro, Y. E. Lee, and C. E. Harper, "Effects of Smoked Marijuana in Experimentally Induced Asthma," *American Review of Respiratory Disease* 112, no. 3 (1975): 377–86.
[19] S. J. Williams, J. P. Hartley, and J. D. Graham, "Bronchodilator Effect of Delta1-Tetrahydrocannabinol

Administered by Aerosol of Asthmatic Patients," *Thorax* 31, no. 6 (1976): 720–23; and J. P. Hartley, S. G. Nogrady, and A. Seaton, "Bronchodilator Effect of Delta1-Tetrahydrocannabinol," *British Journal of Clinical Pharmacology* 5, no. 6 (1978): 523–25.

[20] Peter Strohbeck-Kuehner, Gisela Skopp, and Rainer Mattern, "Cannabis Improves Symptoms of ADHD," *Cannabinoids* 3(2008): 1–3.

[21] Gisela Uhlig, "Correspondence (Letter to the Editor): ADHD and Consumption of THC," *Deutsches Arzteblatt International* 105, no. 44 (2008): 765.

[22] Maura Castelli, M. Federici, S. Rossi, V. De Chiara, F. Napolitano, V. Studer, C. Motta, L. Sacchetti, R. Romano, A. Musella, G. Bernardi, A. Siracusano, H. H. Gu, N. B. Mercuri, A. Usiello, and D. Centonze, "Loss of Striatal Cannabinoid CB1 Receptor Function in Attention-Deficit/Hyperactivity Disorder Mice with Point-Mutation of the Dopamine Transporter," *European Journal of Neuroscience* 34, no. 9 (2011): 1369–77.

[24] Lester Grinspoon, "A Novel Approach to the Symptomatic Treatment of Autism," *O'Shaughnessy's: The Journal of Cannabis in Clinical Practice*, Spring 2010.

[23] Judith H. Miles, "Autism Spectrum Disorders—A Genetics Review," *Genetics in Medicine* 13, no. 4 (2011): 278–94.

[25] Diane Dufour-Rainfray, P. Vourc'h, S. Tourlet, D. Guilloteau, S. Chalon, and C. R. Andres, "Fetal Exposure to Teratogens: Evidence of Genes Involved in Autism," *Neuroscience and Biobehavioral Reviews* 35, no. 5 (2011): 1254–65.

[26] Tarah Kruger and Ed Christophersen, "An Open Label Study of the Use of Dronabinol (Marinol) in the Management of Treatment-Resistant Self-Injurious Behavior in 10 Retarded Adolescent Patients," *Journal of Developmental and Behavioral Pediatrics* 27, no. 5 (2006): 433.

[27] Sreemanti Basu and Bonnie N. Dittel, "Unraveling the Complexities of Cannabinoid Receptor 2 (CB2) Immune Regulation in Health and Disease," *Immunologic Research* 51, no. 1 (2011): 26–38.

[28] J. Ludovic Croxford and Takashi Yamamura, "Cannabinoids and the Immune System: Potential for the Treatment of Inflammatory Diseases?," *Journal of Neuroimmunology* 166, no. 1 (2005): 3–18.

[29] Florian Strasser, D. Luftner, K. Possinger, G. Ernst, T. Ruhstaller, W. Meissner, Y. D. Ko, M. Schnelle, M. Reif, and T. Cerny, "Comparison of Orally Administered Cannabis Extract and Delta-9-Tetrahydrocannabinol in Treating Patients with Cancer-Related Anorexia-Cachexia Syndrome: A Multicenter, Phase III, Randomized, Double-Blind, Placebo-Controlled Clinical Trial from the Cannabis-In-Cachexia-Study-Group," *Journal of Clinical Oncology* 24, no. 21 (2006): 3394–400.

[30] Chandrama P. Khare, ed., *Indian Herbal Remedies: Rational Western Therapy, Ayurvedic and Other Traditional Usage, Botany* (New York: Springer, 2004).

[31] Kenneth Fearon, F. Strasser, S. D. Anker, I. Bosaeus, E. Bruera, R. L. Fainsinger, A. Jatoi, C. Loprinzi, N. MacDonald, G. Mantovani, M. Davis, M. Muscaritoli, F. Ottery, L. Radbruch, P. Ravasco, D. Walsh, A. Wilcock, S. Kaasa, V. E. Baracos, "Definition and Classification of Cancer Cachexia: An International Consensus," *Lancet Oncology* 12, no. 5 (2011): 489–95.

[32] Gil Bar-Sela, M. Vorobeichik, S. Drawsheh, A. Omer, V. Goldberg, E. Muller, "The Medical Necessity for Medicinal Cannabis: Prospective, Observational Study Evaluating the Treatment in Cancer Patients on Supportive or Palliative Care," *Evidence-Based Complementary and Alternative Medicine* (2013).

[33] Daniel W. Bowles, C. L. O'Bryant, D. R. Camidge, and A. Jimeno, "The Intersection between Cannabis and Cancer in the United States," *Critical Reviews in Oncology/Hematology* 83, no. 1 (2012): 1–10.

[34] Detal Cota, G. Marsicano, B. Lutz, V. Vicennati, G. K. Stalla, R. Pasquali, and U. Pagotto, "Endogenous Cannabinoid System as a Modulator of Food Intake," *International Journal of Obesity* 27, no. 3 (2003): 289–301.

[35] Donald I. Abrams and Manuel Guzman, "Cannabinoids and Cancer," in *Integrative Oncology* (Oxford: Oxford University Press, 2008), 147–70.

[36] Daniel W. Bowles, et al. See note 33.

[37] Amy Alexander, Paul F. Smith, and Rhonda J. Rosengren, "Cannabinoids in the Treatment of Cancer," *Cancer Letters* 285, no. 1 (2009): 6–12.

[38] Caihua Liang, M. D. McClean, C. Marsit, B. Christensen, E. Peters, H. H. Nelson, and K. T. Kelsey, "A Population-Based Case-Control Study of Marijuana Use and Head and Neck Squamous Cell Carcinoma," *Cancer Prevention Research* 2, no. 8 (2009): 759–68; and Donald P. Tashkin, "Effects of Marijuana Smoking on the Lung," *Annals of the American Thoracic Society* 10, no. 3 (2013): 239–47.

[39] Daniel W. Bowles, C. L. O'Bryant, D. R. Camidge, and A. Jimeno, "The Intersection between Cannabis and Cancer in the United States," *Critical Reviews in Oncology/Hematology* 83, no. 1 (2012): 1–10.

[40] M. R. Tramer, D. Carroll, F. A. Campbell, D. J. Reynolds, R. A. Moore, and H. J. McQuay, "Cannabinoids for Control of Chemotherapy-Induced Nausea and Vomiting: Quantitative Systematic Review," *British Medical Journal* 323 (2001): 16–21.

[41] Richard D. Mattes, Karl Engelman, Leslie M. Shaw, and Mahmoud A. ElSohly, "Cannabinoids and Appetite Stimulation," *Pharmacology Biochemistry and Behavior* 49, no. 1 (1994): 187–95.
[42] Marta Duran, Eulalia Perez, Sergio Abanades, Xavier Vidal, Cristina Saura, Margarita Majem, Edurne Arriola et al, "Preliminary efficacy and safety of an oromucosal standardized cannabis extract in chemotherapy-induced nausea and vomiting." *British Journal of Clinical Pharmacology* 70, no. 5 (2010) 656–663.
[43] Russell Noyes Jr., S. Fred Brunk, David A. Baram, and Arthur Canter, "Analgesic Effect of Delta-9-Tetrahydrocannabinol," *Journal of Clinical Pharmacology* 15, nos. 2–3 (1975): 139–43.
[44] Sara Jane Ward, M. D. Ramirez, H. Neelakantan, and E. A. Walker, "Cannabidiol Prevents the Development of Cold and Mechanical Allodynia in Paclitaxel-Treated Female C57Bl6 Mice," *Anesthesia and Analgesia* 113, no. 4 (2011): 947–50.
[45] D. I. Abrams, P. Couey, S. B. Shade, M. E. Kelly, and N. L. Benowitz, "Cannabinoid–Opioid Interaction in Chronic Pain," *Clinical Pharmacology and Therapeutics* 90, no. 6 (2011): 844–51.
[46] Ethan B. Russo, Geoffrey W. Guy, and Philip J. Robson, "Cannabis, Pain, and Sleep: Lessons from Therapeutic Clinical Trials of Sativex®, a Cannabis-Based Medicine," *Chemistry and Biodiversity* 4, no. 8 (2007): 1729–43.
[47] Alejandro Aparisi Rey, M. Purrio, M. P. Viveros, and B. Lutz, "Biphasic Effects of Cannabinoids in Anxiety Responses: CB1 and GABAB Receptors in the Balance of GABAergic and Glutamatergic Neurotransmission," *Neuropsychopharmacology* 37, no. 12 (2012): 2624–34, doi:10.1038/npp.2012.123.
[48] Luciano De Petrocellis, A. Ligresti, A. Schiano Moriello, M. Iappelli, R. Verde, C. G. Stott, L. Cristino, P. Orlando, and V. Di Marzo, "Non-THC Cannabinoids Inhibit Prostate Carcinoma Growth In Vitro and In Vivo: Pro-Apoptotic Effects and Underlying Mechanisms," *British Journal of Pharmacology* 168, no. 1 (2013): 79–102.
[49] Pál Pacher, "Towards the Use of Non-Psychoactive Cannabinoids for Prostate Cancer," *British Journal of Pharmacology* 168, no. 1 (2013): 76–78.
[50] Keiji Fukuda, S. E. Straus, I. Hickie, M. C. Sharpe, J. G. Dobbins, and A. Komaroff, "The Chronic Fatigue Syndrome: A Comprehensive Approach to Its Definition and Study," *Annals of Internal Medicine* 121, no. 12 (1994): 953–59.
[51] John E. Casida, Daniel K. Nomura, Sarah C. Vose, and Kazutoshi Fujioka, "Organophosphate-Sensitive Lipases Modulate Brain Lysophospholipids, Ether Lipids and Endocannabinoids," *Chemico-Biological Interactions* 175, no. 1 (2008): 355–64.
[52] Francesca Comelli, I. Bettoni, M. Colleoni, G. Giagnoni, and B. Costa, "Beneficial Effects of a Cannabis Sativa Extract Treatment on Diabetes-Induced Neuropathy and Oxidative Stress," *Phytotherapy Research* 23, no. 12 (2009): 1678–84.
[53] American Diabetes Association, "Economic Costs of Diabetes in the U.S. in 2012," *Diabetes Care* 36, no. 4 (April 2013): 1033–46.
[54] Joseph S. Alpert, "Marijuana for Diabetic Control," *American Journal of Medicine* 126, no. 7 (2013): 557–58.
[55] A. M. Malfait, R. Gallily, P. F. Sumariwalla, A. S. Malik, E. Andreakos, R. Mechoulam, and M. Feldmann, "The Nonpsychoactive Cannabis Constituent Cannabidiol Is an Oral Anti-Arthritic Therapeutic in Murine Collagen-Induced Arthritis," *Proceedings of the National Academy of Sciences* 97, no. 17 (2000): 9561–66.
[56] L. Weiss, M. Zeira, S. Reich, M. Har-Noy, R. Mechoulam, S. Slavin, and R. Gallily, "Cannabidiol Lowers Incidence of Diabetes in Non-Obese Diabetic Mice," *Autoimmunity* 39, no. 2 (2006): 143–51.
[57] Vincenzo Di Marzo, Fabiana Piscitelli, and Raphael Mechoulam, "Cannabinoids and Endocannabinoids in Metabolic Disorders with Focus on Diabetes," *Handbook of Experimental Pharmacology* 203 (2011): 75–104.
[58] Elizabeth A. Penner, Hannah Buettner, and Murray A. Mittleman, "The Impact of Marijuana Use on Glucose, Insulin, and Insulin Resistance among US Adults," *American Journal of Medicine* 126, no. 7 (July 2013), 583–89, doi:10.1016/j.amjmed.2013.03.002.
[59] Centers for Disease Control and Prevention, "National Diabetes Fact Sheet: National Estimates and General Information on Diabetes and Prediabetes in the United States, 2011," *US Department of Health and Human Services* (2011).
[60] Pál Pacher, Joseph S. Beckman, and Lucas Liaudet, "Nitric Oxide and Peroxynitrite in Health and Disease," *Physiological Reviews* 87, no. 1 (2007): 315–424.
[61] Béla Horváth, P. Mukhopadhyay, G. Haskó, and P. Pacher, "The Endocannabinoid System and Plant-Derived Cannabinoids in Diabetes and Diabetic Complications," *American Journal of Pathology* 180, no. 2 (2012): 432–42.
[62] G. I. Liou, A. El-Remessy, A. Ibrahim, R. Caldwell, Y. Khalifa, A. Gunes, and J. Nussbaum, "Cannabidiol as a Putative Novel Therapy for Diabetic Retinopathy:

A Postulated Mechanism of Action as an Entry Point for Biomarker-Guided Clinical Development," *Current Pharmacogenomics and Personalized Medicine* 7, no. 3 (2009): 215; and A. B. El-Remessy, Y. Khalifa, S. Ola, A. S. Ibrahim, and G. I. Liou, "Cannabidiol Protects Retinal Neurons by Preserving Glutamine Synthetase Activity in Diabetes," *Molecular Vision* 16 (2010): 1487.

[63] Priscilla A. Hollander, A. Amod, L. E. Litwak, U. Chaudhari, and ARPEGGIO Study Group, "Effect of Rimonabant on Glycemic Control in Insulin-Treated Type 2 Diabetes: The ARPEGGIO Trial," *Diabetes Care* 33, no. 3 (2010): 605–7.

[64] Laurence A. Bradley, "Pathophysiology of Fibromyalgia," *American Journal of Medicine* 122, no. 12 (2009): S22–S30.

[65] Aryeh M. Abeles, M. H. Pillinger, B. M. Solitar, and M. Abeles, "Narrative Review: The Pathophysiology of Fibromyalgia," Annals of Internal Medicine 146, no. 10 (2007): 726–34.

[66] Manuel Martinez-Lavin, "Stress, the Stress Response System, and Fibromyalgia," *Arthritis Research and Therapy* 9, no. 4 (2007): 216.

[67] Ethan B. Russo, "Clinical Endocannabinoid Deficiency (CECD): Can This Concept Explain Therapeutic Benefits of Cannabis in Migraine, Fibromyalgia, Irritable Bowel Syndrome and Other Treatment-Resistant Conditions?," *Neuroendocrinology Letters* 25, nos. 1–2 (2004): 31.

[68] Shad B. Smith, D. W. Maixner, R. B. Fillingim, G. Slade, R. H. Gracely, K. Ambrose, D. V. Zaykin, C. Hyde, S. John, K. Tan, W. Maixner, and L. Diatchenko, "Large Candidate Gene Association Study Reveals Genetic Risk Factors and Therapeutic Targets for Fibromyalgia," *Arthritis and Rheumatism* 64, no. 2 (2012): 584–93.

[69] Mark Wallace, G. Schulteis, J. H. Atkinson, T. Wolfson, D. Lazzaretto, H. Bentley, B. Gouaux, and I. Abramson, "Dose-Dependent Effects of Smoked Cannabis on Capsaicin-Induced Pain and Hyperalgesia in Healthy Volunteers," *Anesthesiology* 107, no. 5 (2007): 785–96.

[70] Tim C. Kirkham, C. M. Williams, F. Fezza, and V. Di Marzo, "Endocannabinoid Levels in Rat Limbic Forebrain and Hypothalamus in Relation to Fasting, Feeding and Satiation: Stimulation of Eating by 2-Arachidonoyl Glycerol," *British Journal of Pharmacology* 136, no. 4 (2002): 550–57.

[71] M. R. Tramer, D. Carroll, F. A. Campbell, D. J. Reynolds, R. A. Moore, and H. J. McQuay, "Cannabinoids for Control of Chemotherapy-Induced Nausea and Vomiting: Quantitative Systematic Review," *British Medical Journal* 323 (2001): 16–21.

[72] Hélène Peters and Gabriel G. Nahas, "A Brief History of Four Millennia (BC 2000–AD 1974)," in *Marihuana and Medicine*, ed. Gabriel G. Nahas, Kenneth M. Sutin, David Harvey, Stig Agurell, Nicholas Pace, and Robert Cancro (New York: Humana Press, 1999), 3–7.

[73] Manfred Fankhauser, "History of Cannabis in Western Medicine," in *Cannabis and Cannabinoids: Pharmacology, Toxicology, and Therapeutic Potential*, ed. Franjo Grotenhermen and Ethan Russo (New York: The Haworth Integrative Healing Press, 2002), 37–51.

[74] Paul M. Gahlinger, "Gastrointestinal Illness and Cannabis Use in a Rural Canadian Community," *Journal of Psychoactive Drugs* 16, no. 3 (1984): 263–66.

[75] Alessia Ligresti, T. Bisogno, I. Matias, L. De Petrocellis, M. G. Cascio, V. Cosenza, G. D'argenio, G. Scaglione, M. Bifulco, I. Sorrentini, and V. Di Marzo, "Possible Endocannabinoid Control of Colorectal Cancer Growth," *Gastroenterology* 125, no. 3 (2003): 677–87.

[76] Christel Rousseaux, X. Thuru, A. Gelot, N. Barnich, C. Neut, L. Dubuquoy, C. Dubuquoy, E. Merour, K. Geboes, M. Chamaillard, A. Ouwehand, G. Leyer, D. Carcano, J. F. Colombel, D. Ardid, and P. Desreumaux, "Lactobacillus Acidophilus Modulates Intestinal Pain and Induces Opioid and Cannabinoid Receptors," *Nature Medicine* 13, no. 1 (2006): 35–37.

[77] Ethan B. Russo, "Taming THC: Potential Cannabis Synergy and Phytocannabinoid-Terpenoid Entourage Effects," *British Journal of Pharmacology* 163, no. 7 (2011): 1344–64.

[78] Jean Kalata, "Medical Uses of Marijuana: Opinions of US Residents 45+," report conducted for *AARP the Magazine*, December 2004, www.csdp.org/research/aarp_medical_marijuana.pdf.

[79] "TEDS Report: Marijuana Admissions Reporting Daily Use at Treatment Entry," Substance Abuse and Mental Health Services Administration, Center for Behavioral Health Statistics and Quality, February 2, 2012, www.samhsa.gov/data/2k12/TEDS_SR_029_Marijuana_2012/TEDS_Short_Report_029_Marijuana_2012.pdf.

[80] J. Russell Reynolds, "On the therapeutical uses and toxic effects of cannabis indica," *Lancet* 135, no. 3473 (1890): 637–38.

[81] Robert S. Hepler and Ira R. Frank, "Marihuana Smoking and Intraocular Pressure," *JAMA: The Journal of the American Medical Association* 217, no. 10 (1971): 1392.

[82] Allan J. Flach, "Delta-9-Tetrahydrocannabinol (THC) in the Treatment of End-Stage Open-Angle

Glaucoma," *Transactions of the American Ophthalmological Society* 100 (2002): 215.
[83] Henry Jampel, "American Glaucoma Society Position Statement: Marijuana and the Treatment of Glaucoma," *Journal of Glaucoma* 19, no. 2 (2010): 75–76; and Yvonne M. Buys and Paul E. Rafuse, "Canadian Ophthalmological Society Policy Statement on the Medical Use of Marijuana for Glaucoma," *Canadian Journal of Ophthalmology/Journal Canadien d'Ophtalmologie* 45, no. 4 (2010): 324–26.
[84] Ileana Tomida, A. Azuara-Blanco, H. House, M. Flint, R. G. Pertwee, and P. J. Robson, "Effect of Sublingual Application of Cannabinoids on Intraocular Pressure: A Pilot Study," *Journal of Glaucoma* 15, no. 5 (2006): 349–53.
[85] Laurence Brunet, E. E. Moodie, K. Rollet, C. Cooper, S. Walmsley, M. Potter, and M. B. Klein, "Marijuana Smoking Does Not Accelerate Progression of Liver Disease in HIV–Hepatitis C Coinfection: A Longitudinal Cohort Analysis," *Clinical Infectious Diseases* 57, no. 5 (2013): 663–70, doi:10.1093/cid/cit378.
[86] Christophe Hézode, F. Roudot-Thoraval, S. Nguyen, P. Grenard, B. Julien, E. S. Zafrani, J. M. Pawlotsky, D. Dhumeaux, S. Lotersztajn, and A. Mallat, "Daily Cannabis Smoking as a Risk Factor for Progression of Fibrosis in Chronic Hepatitis C," *Hepatology* 42, no. 1 (2005): 63–71; Christophe Hézode, E. S. Zafrani, F. Roudot-Thoraval, C. Costentin, A. Hessami, M. Bouvier-Alias, F. Medkour, J. M. Pawlostky, S. Lotersztajn, and A. Mallat, "Daily Cannabis Use: A Novel Risk Factor of Steatosis Severity in Patients with Chronic Hepatitis C," *Gastroenterology* 134, no. 2 (2008): 432–39; and Julie H. Ishida, M. G. Peters, C. Jin, K. Louie, V. Tan, P. Bacchetti, and N. A. Terrault, "Influence of Cannabis Use on Severity of Hepatitis C Disease," *Clinical Gastroenterology and Hepatology* 6, no. 1 (2008): 69–75.
[87] Joseph Tam, J. Liu, B. Mukhopadhyay, R. Cinar, G. Godlewski, and G. Kunos, "Endocannabinoids in Liver Disease," *Hepatology* 53, no. 1 (2011): 346–55.
[88] Margaret Haney, E. W. Gunderson, J. Rabkin, C. L. Hart, S. K. Vosburg, S. D. Comer, and R. W. Foltin, "Dronabinol and Marijuana in HIV-Positive Marijuana Smokers: Caloric Intake, Mood, and Sleep," *Journal of Acquired Immune Deficiency Syndromes* 45, no. 5 (2007): 545–54.
[89] D. I. Abrams, C. A. Jay, S. B. Shade, H. Vizoso, H. Reda, S. Press, M. E. Kelly, M. C. Rowbotham, and K. L. Petersen, "Cannabis in Painful HIV-Associated Sensory Neuropathy: A Randomized Placebo-Controlled Trial," *Neurology* 68, no. 7 (2007): 515–21.
[90] Alicja Szulakowska and Halina Milnerowicz, "Cannabinoids—Influence on the Immune System and Their Potential Use in Supplementary Therapy of HIV/AIDS," in *HIV and AIDS—Updates on Biology, Immunology, Epidemiology and Treatment Strategies*, ed. Nancy Dumais (Rijeka, Croatia: InTech, 2011), 665–81.
[91] Patricia E. Molina, P. Winsauer, P. Zhang, E. Walker, L. Birke, A. Amedee, C. V. Stouwe, D. Troxclair, R. McGoey, K. Varner, L. Byerley, and L. LaMotte, "Cannabinoid Administration Attenuates the Progression of Simian Immunodeficiency Virus," *AIDS Research and Human Retroviruses* 27, no. 6 (2011): 585–92.
[92] Neal E. Slatkin, "Cannabinoids in the Treatment of Chemotherapy-Induced Nausea and Vomiting: Beyond Prevention of Acute Emesis," *Journal of Supportive Oncolology* 5, no. 5, supplement 3 (2007): 1–9.
[93] Clinton A. Werner, "Medical Marijuana and the AIDS Crisis," *Journal of Cannabis Therapeutics* 1, nos. 3–4 (2001): 17–33.
[94] Harvey W. Feldman and Jerry Mandel, "Providing Medical Marijuana: The Importance of Cannabis Clubs," *Journal of Psychoactive Drugs* 30, no. 2 (1998): 179–86; and "San Francisco," San Francisco AIDS Foundation, accessed October 4, 2013, www.sfaf.org/hiv-info/statistics.
[95] Cristina Maria Costantino, Achla Gupta, Alice W. Yewdall, Benjamin M. Dale, Lakshmi A. Devi, and Benjamin K. Chen, "Cannabinoid Receptor 2-Mediated Attenuation of CXCR4-Tropic HIV Infection in Primary CD4+ T Cells," *PloS ONE* 7, no. 3 (2012): e33961, doi:10.1371/journal.pone.0033961.
[96] Celia J. A. Morgan, Tom P. Freeman, Gráinne L. Schafer, and H. Valerie Curran, "Cannabidiol Attenuates the Appetitive Effects of Delta 9-Tetrahydrocannabinol in Humans Smoking Their Chosen Cannabis," *Neuropsychopharmacology* 35, no. 9 (2010): 1879–85.
[97] Nicholas Pace, Henry Clay Frick, Kenneth Sutin, William Manger, George Hyman, and Gabriel Nahas, "The Medical Use of Marihuana and THC in Perspective," in *Marihuana and Medicine* (New York: Humana Press, 1999), 767–80.
[98] Ethan Russo, "Hemp for Headache: An In-Depth Historical and Scientific Review of Cannabis in Migraine Treatment," *Journal of Cannabis Therapeutics* 1, no. 2 (2001): 21–92.
[99] William Dymock, *The Vegetable Materia Medica of Western India* (Education Society's Press, 1885), 605.
[100] Manfred Fankhauser, "History of Cannabis in Western Medicine," in *Cannabis and Cannabinoids: Pharmacology, Toxicology, and Therapeutic Potential*, ed. Franjo Grotenhermen and Ethan Russo (Binghamton,

NY: Haworth Integrative Healing Press, 2002), 37–51.
101 M. Fishbein, "Migraine Associated with Menstruation," *Journal of the American Medical Association* 237, no. 326 (1942).
102 Ethan B. Russo, "Clinical Endocannabinoid Deficiency (CECD): Can This Concept Explain Therapeutic Benefits of Cannabis in Migraine, Fibromyalgia, Irritable Bowel Syndrome and Other Treatment-Resistant Conditions?," *Neuroendocrinology Letters* 25, nos. 1–2 (2004): 31–39.
103 P. Brown, "Pathophysiology of Spasticity," *Journal of Neurology, Neurosurgery and Psychiatry* 57 (1994): 773–77; and E. Shohami, A. Cohen-Yeshurun, L. Magid, M. Algali, and R. Mechoulam, "Endocannabinoids and Traumatic Brain Injury," *British Journal of Pharmacology* 163 (2011): 1402–10.
104 J. B. Nielsen, C. Crone, and H. Hultborn, "The Spinal Pathophysiology of Spasticity—from a Basic Science Point of View," *Acta Physiologica* 189 (2007): 171–80.
105 J. Corey-Bloom, T. Wolfson, A. Gamst, S. Jin, T. D. Marcotte, H. Bentley, and B. Gouaux, "Smoked Cannabis for Spasticity in Multiple Sclerosis: A Randomized, Placebo-Controlled Trial," *Canadian Medical Association Journal* 184, no. 10 (2012): 1143–50.
106 J. Zajicek, P. Fox, H. Sanders, D. Wright, J. Vickery, A. Nunn, and A. Thompson, "Cannabinoids for Treatment of Spasticity and Other Symptoms Related to Multiple Sclerosis (CAMS Study): Multicentre Randomised Placebo-Controlled Trial," *Lancet* 362 (2003): 1517–26; and D. T. Wade, P. Makela, P. Robson, H. House, and C. Bateman, "Do Cannabis-Based Medicinal Extracts Have General or Specific Effects on Symptoms in Multiple Sclerosis? A Double-Blind, Randomized, Placebo-Controlled Study on 160 Patients," *Multiple Sclerosis Journal* 10 (2004): 434–41.
107 D. Centonze, F. Mori, G. Koch, F. Buttari, C. Codecà, S. Rossi, M. T. Cencioni, M. Bari, S. Fiore, G. Bernardi, L. Battistini, and M. Maccarrone, "Lack of Effect of Cannabis-Based Treatment on Clinical and Laboratory Measures in Multiple Sclerosis," *Neurological Sciences* 30 (2009): 531–44; and David J. Rog, Turo J. Nurmikko, Tim Friede, and Carolyn A. Young, "Randomized, Controlled Trial of Cannabis-Based Medicine in Central Pain in Multiple Sclerosis," *Neurology* 65 (2005): 812–19.
108 David Baker, Gareth Pryce, Samuel J. Jackson, Chris Bolton, and Gavin Giovannoni, "The Biology That Underpins the Therapeutic Potential of Cannabis-Based Medicines for the Control of Spasticity in Multiple Sclerosis," *Multiple Sclerosis and Related Disorders* 1 (2012): 64–75.
109 Barbara Todaro, "Cannabinoids in the Treatment of Chemotherapy-Induced Nausea and Vomiting," *Journal of the National Comprehensive Cancer Network* 10, no. 4 (2012): 487–92.
110 Stephen E. Sallan, Norman E. Zinberg, and Emil Frei III, "Antiemetic Effect of Delta-9-Tetrahydrocannabinol in Patients Receiving Cancer Chemotherapy," *New England Journal of Medicine* 293, no. 16 (1975): 795–97.
111 Richard E. Doblin and M. A. Kleiman, "Marijuana as Antiemetic Medicine: A Survey of Oncologists' Experiences and Attitudes," *Journal of Clinical Oncology* 9, no. 7 (1991): 1314–19.
112 Francisco C. Machado Rocha, S. C. Stéfano, R. De Cássia Haiek, L. M. Rosa Oliveira, and D. X. Da Silveira, "Therapeutic Use of *Cannabis sativa* on Chemotherapy-Induced Nausea and Vomiting among Cancer Patients: Systematic Review and Meta-Analysis," *European Journal of Cancer Care* 17, no. 5 (2008): 431–43.
113 E. M. Rock, D. Bolognini, C. L. Limebeer, M. G. Cascio, S. Anavi-Goffer, P. J. Fletcher, R. Mechoulam, R. G. Pertwee, and L. A. Parker, "Cannabidiol, a Non-Psychotropic Component of Cannabis, Attenuates Vomiting and Nausea-Like Behaviour via Indirect Agonism of 5-HT1A Somatodendritic Autoreceptors in the Dorsal Raphe Nucleus," *British Journal of Pharmacology* 165, no. 8 (2012): 2620–34.
114 E. M. Rock, R. L. Kopstick, C. L. Limebeer, and L. A. Parker, "Tetrahydrocannabinolic Acid Reduces Nausea-Induced Conditioned Gaping in Rats and Vomiting in *Suncus murinus*," *British Journal of Pharmacology* 170, no. 3 (2013): 641–48, doi:10.1111/bph.12316.
115 Linda A. Parker, Erin M. Rock, and Cheryl L. Limebeer, "Regulation of Nausea and Vomiting by Cannabinoids," *British Journal of Pharmacology* 163, no. 7 (2011): 1411–22.
116 Stephanie Price, C. Fisher, R. Kumar, and A. Hilgerson, "Cannabinoid Hyperemesis Syndrome as the Underlying Cause of Intractable Nausea and Vomiting," *Journal of the American Osteopathic Association* 111, no. 3 (2011): 166–69.
117 Douglas A. Simonetto, Amy S. Oxentenko, Margot L. Herman, and Jason H. Szostek, "Cannabinoid Hyperemesis: A Case Series of 98 Patients," *Mayo Clinic Proceedings* 87, no. 2 (2012).
118 Martin H. Lynch, "Treatment of Neuralgia by Indian Hemp: Physiology of the Nerves," *Provincial Medical Journal and Retrospect of the Medical Sciences* 6, no. 131 (April 1, 1843): 9–11.
119 Igor A. Grant, "Medicinal Cannabis and Painful

Sensory Neuropathy," *American Medical Association Journal of Ethics* 15, no. 5 (May 2013): 466–69.
[120] D. I. Abrams, C. A. Jay, S. B. Shade, H. Vizoso, H. Reda, S. Press, M. E. Kelly, M. C. Rowbotham, and K. L. Petersen, "Cannabis in Painful HIV-Associated Sensory Neuropathy: A Randomized Placebo-Controlled Trial," *Neurology* 68, no. 7 (2007): 515–21.
[121] David J. Rog, Turo J. Nurmikko, and Carolyn A. Young, "Oromucosal Delta-9-Tetrahydrocannabinol /Cannabidiol for Neuropathic Pain Associated with Multiple Sclerosis: An Uncontrolled, Open-Label, 2-Year Extension Trial," *Clinical Therapeutics* 29, no. 9 (2007): 2068–79.
[122] Tannia Gutierrez and Andrea G. Hohmann, "Cannabinoids for the Treatment of Neuropathic Pain: Are They Safe and Effective?," *Future Neurology* 6, no. 2 (2011): 129–33.
[123] Mark A. Ware, T. Wang, S. Shapiro, A. Robinson, T. Ducruet, T. Huynh, A. Gamsa, G. J. Bennett, and J. P. Collet, "Smoked Cannabis for Chronic Neuropathic Pain: A Randomized Controlled Trial," *Canadian Medical Association Journal* 182, no. 14 (2010): E694–E701.
[124] Ethan B. Russo, "Clinical Endocannabinoid Deficiency (CECD): Can This Concept Explain Therapeutic Benefits of Cannabis in Migraine, Fibromyalgia, Irritable Bowel Syndrome and Other Treatment-Resistant Conditions?," *Neuroendocrinology Letters* 25, nos. 1–2 (2004): 31–39.
[125] Sunil K. Aggarwal, "Cannabinergic Pain Medicine: A Concise Clinical Primer and Survey of Randomized-Controlled Trial Results," *Clinical Journal of Pain* 29, no. 2 (2013): 162–71.
[126] Ethan B. Russo and Andrea G. Hohmann, "Role of Cannabinoids in Pain Management," in *Comprehensive Treatment of Chronic Pain by Medical, Interventional, and Integrative Approaches*, ed. Timothy R. Deer, Michael S. Leong, Asokumar Buvanendran, Vitaly Gordin, Philip S. Kim, Sunil J. Panchal, and Albert L. Ray (New York: Springer, 2013), 181–97.
[127] Ibid.
[128] Hobart Amory Hare, "Clinical and Physiological Notes on the Action of *Cannabis indica*," *Therapeutic Gazette* 11 (1887): 225–28.
[129] Daniele Bolognini, Barbara Costa, Sabatino Maione, Francesca Comelli, Pietro Marini, Vincenzo Di Marzo, Daniela Parolaro, Ruth A. Ross, Lisa A. Gauson, Maria G. Cascio, and Roger G. Pertwee, "The Plant Cannabinoid Delta 9-Tetrahydrocannabivarin Can Decrease Signs of Inflammation and Inflammatory Pain in Mice," *British Journal of Pharmacology* 160, no. 3 (2010): 677–87.
[130] Steven G. Kinsey and Erica C. Cole, "Acute Delta-9-Tetrahydrocannabinol Blocks Gastric Hemorrhages Induced by the Nonsteroidal Anti-Inflammatory Drug Diclofenac Sodium in Mice," *European Journal of Pharmacology* (June 11, 2013), doi:10.1016/j.ejphar.2013.06.001.
[131] Mark Wallace, G. Schulteis, J. H. Atkinson, T. Wolfson, D. Lazzaretto, H. Bentley, B. Gouaux, and I. Abramson, "Dose-Dependent Effects of Smoked Cannabis on Capsaicin-Induced Pain and Hyperalgesia in Healthy Volunteers," *Anesthesiology* 107, no. 5 (2007): 785–96.
[132] Russell K. Portenoy, E. D. Ganae-Motan, S. Allende, R. Yanagihara, L. Shaiova, S. Weinstein, R. McQuade, S. Wright, and M. T. Fallon, "Nabiximols for Opioid-Treated Cancer Patients with Poorly-Controlled Chronic Pain: A Randomized, Placebo-Controlled, Graded-Dose Trial," *Journal of Pain* 13, no. 5 (2012): 438–49.
[133] Yukihiro Tambe, H. Tsujiuchi, G. Honda, Y. Ikeshiro, and S. Tanaka, "Gastric Cytoprotection of the Non-Steroidal Anti-Inflammatory Sesquiterpene, Beta-Caryophyllene," *Planta Medica* 62, no. 5 (1996): 469–70.
[134] J. L. Eriksen, Z. Wszolek, and L. Petrucelli, "Molecular Pathogenesis of Parkinson Disease," *Archives of Neurology* 62 (2005): 353–57.
[135] Christophe G. Goetz, "The History of Parkinson's Disease: Early Clinical Descriptions and Neurological Therapies," *Cold Spring Harbor Perspectives in Medicine* 1, no. 1 (2011), doi:10.1101/cshperspect.a008862.
[136] W. R. Gowers, "Paralysis Agitans," in *A System of Medicine*, ed. A. Allbutt and T. Rolleston (London: Macmillan, 1899): 156–78.
[137] Kateñina Venderová, Evžen Růžicka, Viktor Voñíšek, and Peter Višňovský, "Survey on Cannabis Use in Parkinson's Disease: Subjective Improvement of Motor Symptoms," *Movement Disorders* 19, no. 9 (2004): 1102–6.
[138] I. Lotan, T. Treves, Y. Roditi, and R. Djaldetti, "Medical Marijuana (Cannabis) Treatment for Motor and Non-Motor Symptoms in Parkinson's Disease: An Open-Label Observational Study," *Movement Disorders* 28, supplement 1 (2013): 448.
[139] C. García, C. Palomo-Garo, M. García-Arencibia, J. Ramos, R. Pertwee, and J. Fernández-Ruiz, "Symptom-Relieving and Neuroprotective Effects of the Phytocannabinoid Delta 9-THCV in Animal Models of Parkinson's Disease," *British Journal of Pharmacology* 163, no. 7 (2011): 1495–506.
[140] Javier Fernández-Ruiz, O. Sagredo, M. R. Pazos, C. García, R. Pertwee, R. Mechoulam, and

J. Martínez-Orgado, "Cannabidiol for Neurodegenerative Disorders: Important New Clinical Applications for This Phytocannabinoid?," *British Journal of Clinical Pharmacology* 75, no. 2 (2013): 323–33.
141 Vincenzo Di Marzo, "Targeting the Endocannabinoid System: To Enhance or Reduce?," *Nature Reviews Drug Discovery* 7, no. 5 (2008): 438–55.
142 J. Douglas Bremner, S. M. Southwick, A. Darnell, and D. S. Charney, "Chronic PTSD in Vietnam Combat Veterans: Course of Illness and Substance Abuse," *American Journal of Psychiatry* 153, no. 3 (1996): 369–75.
143 Ronald C. Kessler, A. Sonnega, E. Bromet, M. Hughes, C. B. Nelson, "Posttraumatic Stress Disorder in the National Comorbidity Survey," *Archives of General Psychiatry* 52, no. 12 (1995): 1048.
144 Ernest L. Abel, "New Uses for the Old Hemp Plant," *Marihuana* (1980), 105–21; and Cristóbal Acosta, *Tratado de las drogas y medicinas de las Indias Orientales...* (Editorial MAXTOR, 2005).
145 Robert H. Pietrzak, R. B. Goldstein, S. M. Southwick, and B. F. Grant, "Prevalence and Axis I Comorbidity of Full and Partial Posttraumatic Stress Disorder in the United States: Results from Wave 2 of the National Epidemiologic Survey on Alcohol and Related Conditions," *Journal of Anxiety Disorders* 25, no. 3 (2011): 456–65.
146 Torsten Passie, H. M. Emrich, M. Karst, S. D. Brandt, and J. H. Halpern, "Mitigation of Post-Traumatic Stress Symptoms by Cannabis Resin: A Review of the Clinical and Neurobiological Evidence," *Drug Testing and Analysis* 4, nos. 7–8 (2012): 649–59.
147 Roger K. Pitman, Lisa M. Shin, and Scott L. Rauch, "Investigating the Pathogenesis of Posttraumatic Stress Disorder with Neuroimaging," *Journal of Clinical Psychiatry* 62, supplement 17 (2001): 47–54.
148 Giovanni Marsicano, Carsten T. Wotjak, Shahnaz C. Azad, Tiziana Bisogno, Gerhard Rammes, Maria Grazia Cascio, Heike Hermann, Jianrong Tang, Clementine Hofmann, Walter Zieglgänsberger, Vincenzo Di Marzo, and Beat Lutz, "The Endogenous Cannabinoid System Controls Extinction of Aversive Memories," *Nature* 418, no. 6897 (2002): 530–34.
149 A. Neumeister, M. D. Normandin, R. H. Pietrzak, D. Piomelli, M. Q. Zheng, A. Gujarro-Anton, M. N. Potenza, C. R. Bailey, S. F. Lin, S. Najafzadeh, J. Ropchan, S. Henry, S. Corsi-Travali, R. E. Carson and Y. Huang, "Elevated Brain Cannabinoid CB1 Receptor Availability in Post-Traumatic Stress Disorder: A Positron Emission Tomography Study," *Molecular Psychiatry* 18 (September 2013): 1034–40, doi:10.1038/mp.2013.61.
150 Theresa H. M. Moore, S. Zammit, A. Lingford -Hughes, T. R. Barnes, P. B. Jones, M. Burke, and G. Lewis, "Cannabis Use and Risk of Psychotic or Affective Mental Health Outcomes: A Systematic Review," *Lancet* 370, no. 9584 (2007): 319–28.
151 Stanley Zammit, T. H. Moore, A. Lingford-Hughes, T. R. Barnes, P. B. Jones, M. Burke, and G. Lewis, "Effects of Cannabis Use on Outcomes of Psychotic Disorders: Systematic Review," *British Journal of Psychiatry* 193, no. 5 (2008): 357–63.
152 S. Bhattacharyya, P. D. Morrison, P. Fusar-Poli, R. Martin-Santos, S. Borgwardt, T. Winton-Brown, C. Nosarti, C. M. O'Carroll, M. Seal, P. Allen, M. A. Mehta, J. M. Stone, N. Tunstall, V. Giampietro, S. Kapur, R. M. Murray, A. W. Zuardi, J. A. Crippa, Z. Atakan, and P. K. McGuire, "Opposite Effects of Delta-9-Tetrahydrocannabinol and Cannabidiol on Human Brain Function and Psychopathology," *Neuropsychopharmacology* 35, no. 3 (2010): 764–74.
153 Marta Di Forti, C. Morgan, P. Dazzan, C. Pariante, V. Mondelli, T. R. Marques, R. Handley, S. Luzi, M. Russo, A. Paparelli, A. Butt, S. A. Stilo, B. Wiffen, J. Powell, R. M. Murray, "High-Potency Cannabis and the Risk of Psychosis," *British Journal of Psychiatry* 195, no. 6 (2009): 488–91.
154 Celia J. A. Morgan, G. Schafer, T. P. Freeman, and H. V. Curran, "Impact of Cannabidiol on the Acute Memory and Psychotomimetic Effects of Smoked Cannabis: Naturalistic Study," *British Journal of Psychiatry* 197, no. 4 (2010): 285–90.
155 Robert Clarke and Mark Merlin, *Cannabis: Evolution and Ethnobotany* (Berkeley: University of California Press, 2013), 235.
156 Celia J. A. Morgan, G. Schafer, T. P. Freeman, and H. V. Curran, "Impact of Cannabidiol on the Acute Memory and Psychotomimetic Effects of Smoked Cannabis: Naturalistic Study," *British Journal of Psychiatry* 197, no. 4 (2010): 285–90.
157 Ranganath Muniyappa, Sara Sable, Ronald Ouwerkerk, Andrea Mari, Ahmed M. Gharib, Mary Walter, Amber Courville, Gail Hall, Kong Y. Chen, Nora D. Volkow, George Kunos, Marilyn A. Huestis, and Monica C. Skarulis, "Metabolic Effects of Chronic Cannabis Smoking," *Diabetes Care* (2013), doi:10.2337/dc12-2303.
158 Antonio Waldo Zuardi, J. E. Hallak, S. M. Dursun, S. L. Morais, R. F. Sanches, R. E. Musty, and J. A. Crippa, "Cannabidiol Monotherapy for Treatment-Resistant Schizophrenia," *Journal of Psychopharmacology* 20, no. 5 (2006): 683–86.
159 P. J. Robson, G. W. Guy, and V. Di Marzo, "Cannabinoids and Schizophrenia: Therapeutic

Prospects," *Current Pharmaceutical Design* (2013).
[160] Dora Kohen, "Diabetes Mellitus and Schizophrenia: Historical Perspective," *British Journal of Psychiatry* 184, no. 47 (2004): s64–s66.
[161] Isaac Campos, *Home Grown: Marijuana and the Origins of Mexico's War on Drugs* (Chapel Hill: University of North Carolina Press, 2012).
[162] A. W. Zuardi, S. L. Morais, F. S. Guimarães, and R. Mechoulam, "Antipsychotic Effect of Cannabidiol," *Journal of Clinical Psychiatry* 56, no. 10 (1995): 485–86.
[163] P. Kwan and M. J. Brodie, "Emerging Drugs for Epilepsy," *Expert Opinion on Emerging Drugs* 12 (2007): 407–22.
[164] Saundra Young, "Marijuana Stops Child's Severe Seizures," CNN, August 7, 2013, edition.cnn.com/2013/08/07/health/charlotte-child-medical-marijuana/index.html.
[165] P. A. Fried and D. C. McIntyre, "Electrical and Behavioral Attenuation of the Anti-Convulsant Properties of Delta 9-THC following Chronic Administrations," *Psychopharmacologia* 31, no. 3 (1973): 215–27.
[166] Shyamshree S. Manna and Sudhir N. Umathe, "Involvement of Transient Receptor Potential Vanilloid Type 1 Channels in the Pro-Convulsant Effect of Anandamide in Pentylenetetrazole-Induced Seizures," *Epilepsy Research* 100, no. 1 (2012): 113–24.
[167] D. Gloss and B. Vickrey, "Cannabinoids for Epilepsy," *Cochrane Database of Systematic Reviews* 6 (2012), doi:10.1002/14651858.CD009270.pub2.
[168] Andrew J. Hill, C. M. Williams, B. J. Whalley, and G. J. Stephens, "Phytocannabinoids as Novel Therapeutic Agents in CNS Disorders," *Pharmacology and Therapeutics* 133, no. 1 (2012): 79–97.
[169] Samantha Elizabeth Weston, "The Effects of [Delta]-Tetrahydrocannabivarin in an In Vitro Model of Epileptiform Activity and In Vivo Models of Seizure," (PhD diss., University of Reading, 2011).
[170] A. J. Hill, M. S. Mercier, T. D. Hill, S. E. Glyn, N. A. Jones, Y. Yamasaki, T. Futamura, M. Duncan, C. G. Stott, G. J. Stephens, C. M. Williams, and B. J. Whalley, "Cannabidivarin Is Anticonvulsant in Mouse and Rat," *British Journal of Pharmacology* 167, no. 8 (2012): 1629–42; and T. D. M. Hill, M. G. Cascio, B. Romano, M. Duncan, R. G. Pertwee, C. M. Williams, B. J. Whalley, and A. J. Hill, "Cannabidivarin-Rich Cannabis Extracts Are Anticonvulsant in Mouse and Rat via a CB1 Receptor-Independent Mechanism," *British Journal of Pharmacology* 170, no. 3 (2013): 679–92, doi:10.1111/bph.12321.
[171] Roberto Di Maio, "Cannabinoid 1 Receptor as Therapeutic Target in Preventing Chronic Epilepsy," *Faseb Journal* 27 (2013).
[172] B. Whalley, "Cannabis and Epilepsy: From Recreational Abuse to Therapeutic Use," University of Reading, 2007, www.societyofbiology.org/images/ben-whalley.pdf.
[173] Indalecio Lozano, "The Therapeutic Use of *Cannabis sativa* (L.) in Arabic Medicine," *Journal of Cannabis Therapeutics* 1, no. 1 (2001): 63–70.
[174] Franz Rosenthal, *The Herb: Hashish versus Medieval Muslim Society* (Leiden: Brill, 1971).
[175] J. Russell Reynolds, "On the therapeutical uses and toxic effects of cannabis indica," *Lancet* 135, no. 3473 (1890): 637–38.
[176] Ethan B. Russo, A. Burnett, B. Hall, and K. K. Parker, "Agonistic Properties of Cannabidiol at 5-HT1a Receptors," *Neurochemical Research* 30, no. 8 (2005): 1037–43.
[177] Maayan Lubell, "What a Drag, Israeli Firm Grows 'Highless' Marijuana," *Reuters*, July 3, 2012, www.reuters.com/article/2012/07/03/us-israel-marijuana-idUSBRE8620FU20120703.
[178] M. Llanos Casanova, C. Blázquez, J. Martínez-Palacio, C. Villanueva, M. J. Fernández-Aceñero, J. W. Huffman, J. L. Jorcano, and M. Guzmán, "Inhibition of Skin Tumor Growth and Angiogenesis In Vivo by Activation of Cannabinoid Receptors," *Journal of Clinical Investigation* 111, no. 1 (2003): 43–50.
[179] Sonja Ständer, M. Schmelz, D. Metze, T. Luger, and R. Rukwied, "Distribution of Cannabinoid Receptor 1 (CB1) and 2 (CB2) on Sensory Nerve Fibers and Adnexal Structures in Human Skin," *Journal of Dermatological Science* 38, no. 3 (2005): 177–88.
[180] Thomas W. Klein, "Cannabinoid-Based Drugs as Anti-Inflammatory Therapeutics," *Nature Reviews Immunology* 5, no. 5 (2005): 400–11.
[181] F. Scarampella, F. Abramo, and C. Noli, "Clinical and Histological Evaluation of an Analogue of Palmitoylethanolamide, PLR 120 (Comicronized Palmidrol INN) in Cats with Eosinophilic Granuloma and Eosinophilic Plaque: A Pilot Study," *Veterinary Dermatology* 12, no. 1 (2001): 29–39.
[182] E. Perez-Gomez, C. Andradas, J. M. Flores, M. Quintanilla, J. M. Paramio, M. Guzmán, and C. Sánchez, "The Orphan Receptor GPR55 Drives Skin Carcinogenesis and Is Upregulated in Human Squamous Cell Carcinomas," *Oncogene* 32, no. 20 (2012): 2534–42.
[183] Meliha Karsak, Evelyn Gaffal, Rahul Date, Lihua Wang-Eckhardt, Jennifer Rehnelt, Stefania Petrosino, Katarzyna Starowicz, Regina Steuder, Eberhard Schlicker, Benjamin Cravatt, Raphael Mechoulam,

Reinhard Buettner, Sabine Werner, Vincenzo Di Marzo, Thomas Tüting, and Andreas Zimmer, "Attenuation of Allergic Contact Dermatitis through the Endocannabinoid System," *Science* 316, no. 5830 (2007): 1494–97.

[184] Richard S. Lazarus, *Psychological Stress and the Coping Process* (McGraw-Hill, 1966), 31.

[185] Hans Selye, "A Syndrome Produced by Diverse Nocuous Agents," *Nature* 138 (July 4, 1936): 32, doi:10.1038/138032a0.

[186] Andrea Prince van Leeuwen, H. E. Creemers, K. Greaves-Lord, F. C. Verhulst, J. Ormel, and A. C. Huizink, "Hypothalamic-Pituitary-Adrenal Axis Reactivity to Social Stress and Adolescent Cannabis Use: The TRAILS Study," *Addiction* 106, no. 8 (2011): 1484–92.

[187] P. J. Robson, G. W. Guy, and V. Di Marzo, "Cannabinoids and Schizophrenia: Therapeutic Prospects," *Current Pharmaceutical Design* (2013).

[188] Cecilia J. Hillard, "Endocannabinoids, Monoamines and Stress," in *Endocannabinoid Regulation of Monoamines in Psychiatric and Neurological Disorders* (New York: Springer, 2013), 173–212.

[189] Irit Akirav, "Cannabinoids and Glucocorticoids Modulate Emotional Memory after Stress," *Neuroscience and Biobehavioral Reviews* (2013), doi:10.1016/j.neubiorev.2013.08.002.

[190] Matthew N. Hill, R. J. McLaughlin, B. Bingham, L. Shrestha, T. T. Lee, J. M. Gray, C. J. Hillard, B. B. Gorzalka, V. Viau, "Endogenous Cannabinoid Signaling Is Essential for Stress Adaptation," *Proceedings of the National Academy of Sciences* 107, no. 20 (2010): 9406–11.

[191] Leonardo B. M. Resstel, Rodrigo F. Tavares, Sabrina F. S. Lisboa, Sâmia R. L. Joca, Fernando M. A. Corrêa, and Francisco S. Guimarães, "5-HT1A Receptors Are Involved in the Cannabidiol-Induced Attenuation of Behavioural and Cardiovascular Responses to Acute Restraint Stress in Rats," *British Journal of Pharmacology* 156, no. 1 (2009): 181–88.

[192] Alline C. Campos, Z. Ortega, J. Palazuelos, M. V. Fogaça, D. C. Aguiar, J. Díaz-Alonso, S. Ortega-Gutiérrez, H. Vázquez-Villa, F. A. Moreira, M. Guzmán, I. Galve-Roperh, F. S. Guimarães, "The Anxiolytic Effect of Cannabidiol on Chronically Stressed Mice Depends on Hippocampal Neurogenesis: Involvement of the Endocannabinoid System," *International Journal of Neuropsychopharmacology* (2013): 1–13.

[193] M. Ranganathan, G. Braley, B. Pittman, T. Cooper, E. Perry, J. Krystal, and D. C. D'Souza, "The Effects of Cannabinoids on Serum Cortisol and Prolactin in Humans," *Psychopharmacology* 203 (2009): 737–44.

[194] Lorenzo Somaini, M. Manfredini, M. Amore, A. Zaimovic, M. A. Raggi, C. Leonardi, M. L. Gerra, C. Donnini, and G. Gerra, "Psychobiological Responses to Unpleasant Emotions in Cannabis Users," *European Archives of Psychiatry and Clinical Neuroscience* 262, no. 1 (2012): 47–57; and G. R. King, T. Ernst, W. Deng, A. Stenger, R. M. K. Gonzales, H. Nakama, and L. Chang, "Effects of Chronic Active Cannabis Use on Visuomotor Integration, in Relation to Brain Activation and Cortisol Levels," *Journal of Neuroscience* 31, no. 49 (2011): 17923.

[195] George C. Patton, Carolyn Coffey, John B. Carlin, Louisa Degenhardt, Michael Lynskey, and Wayne Hall, "Cannabis Use and Mental Health in Young People: Cohort Study," *British Medical Journal* 325, no. 7374 (2002): 1195–98, doi:http://dx.doi.org/10.1136/bmj.325.7374.1195.

[196] Stanley Zammit, Peter Allebeck, Sven Andreasson, Ingvar Lundberg, and Glyn Lewis, "Self Reported Cannabis Use as a Risk Factor for Schizophrenia in Swedish Conscripts of 1969: Historical Cohort Study," *British Medical Journal* 325, no. 7374 (2002): 1199; and L. J. Phillips, C. Curry, A. R. Yung, H. P. Yuen, S. Adlard, and P. D. McGorry, "Cannabis Use Is Not Associated with the Development of Psychosis in an 'Ultra' High-Risk Group," *Australian and New Zealand Journal of Psychiatry* 36, no. 6 (2002): 800–6.

[197] M. Schneider, "Puberty as a Highly Vulnerable Developmental Period for the Consequences of Cannabis Exposure," *Addiction Biology* 13, no. 2 (2008): 253–63, doi:10.1111/j.1369-1600.2008.00110.x.

[198] J. M. Bostwick, "Blurred Boundaries: The Therapeutics and Politics of Medical Marijuana," *Mayo Clinic Proceedings* 87, no. 2 (2012): 172–86.

[199] Avshalom Caspia, Terrie E. Moffitt, Mary Cannon, Joseph McClay, Robin Murray, HonaLee Harrington, Alan Taylor, Louise Arseneault, Ben Williams, Antony Braithwaite, Richie Poulton, Ian W. Craig, "Moderation of the Effect of Adolescent-Onset Cannabis Use on Adult Psychosis by a Functional Polymorphism in the Catechol-O-Methyltransferase Gene: Longitudinal Evidence of a Gene X Environment Interaction," *Biological Psychiatry* 57, no. 10 (2005): 1117–27, dx.doi.org/10.1016/j.biopsych.2005.01.026.

[200] J. Jacobus, S. Bava, M. Cohen-Zion, O. Mahmood, and S. F. Tapert, "Functional Consequences of Marijuana Use in Adolescents," *Pharmacology Biochemistry and Behavior* 92, no. 4 (2009): 559–65, doi:10.1016/j.pbb.2009.04.001.

[201] An abstract of the Stanford survey that was supervised by Dr. Brenda Porter was presented at the

"Curing the Epilepsies" meeting of the National Institute of Neurological Disorders and Stroke, held from April 17–19, 2013.

[202] Massachusetts Department of Public Health: Public Hearings on Proposed Regulations at 105 CMR 725.000 (April 18, 2013) (testimony of Elizabeth Anne Thiele, MD, PhD, Director, Pediatric Epilepsy Program, Massachusetts General Hospital).

[203] "Cannabidiol for Epilepsy," Miami Children's Brain Institute, www.hemr.org/wiki/Cannabidiol_for_epilepsy.

[204] Suzanne Leigh, "Buying Pot for My 11-Year-Old," *Huffington* Post, July 11, 2013, www.huffingtonpost.com/suzanne-leigh/buying-pot-for-my-11-year-old_b_3538543.html.

[205] Beth A. Mueller, Janet R. Daling, Noel S. Weiss, and Donald E. Moore, "Recreational Drug Use and the Risk of Primary Infertility," *Epidemiology* 1, no. 3 (1990): 195–200.

[206] Derek G. Moore, J. D. Turner, A. C. Parrott, J. E. Goodwin, S. E. Fulton, M. O. Min, H. C. Fox, F. M. Braddick, E. L. Axelsson, S. Lynch, H. Ribeiro, C. J. Frostick, and L. T. Singer, "During Pregnancy, Recreational Drug-Using Women Stop Taking Ecstasy (3, 4-Methylenedioxy-N-Methylamphetamine) and Reduce Alcohol Consumption, but Continue to Smoke Tobacco and Cannabis: Initial Findings from the Development and Infancy Study," *Journal of Psychopharmacology* 24, no. 9 (2010): 1403–10.

[207] David M. Fergusson, L. John Horwood, and Kate Northstone, "Maternal Use of Cannabis and Pregnancy Outcome," *BJOG: An International Journal of Obstetrics & Gynaecology* 109, no. 1 (2002): 21–27.

[208] Peter A. Fried and J. E. Makin, "Neonatal Behavioural Correlates of Prenatal Exposure to Marihuana, Cigarettes and Alcohol in a Low Risk Population," *Neurotoxicology and Teratology* 9, no. 1 (1987): 1–7.

[209] Gale A. Richardson, C. Ryan, J. Willford, N. L. Day, and L. Goldschmidt, "Prenatal Alcohol and Marijuana Exposure: Effects on Neuropsychological Outcomes at 10 Years," *Neurotoxicology and Teratology* 24, no. 3 (2002): 309–20.

[210] V. Di Marzo, D. Melck, T. Bisogno, and L. De Petrocellis, "Endocannabinoids: Endogenous Cannabinoid Receptor Ligands with Neuromodulatory Action," *Trends in Neurosciences* 21, no. 12 (1998): 521–28.

[211] Mia Hashibe, H. Morgenstern, Y. Cui, D. P. Tashkin, Z. F. Zhang, W. Cozen, T. M. Mack, and S. Greenland, "Marijuana Use and the Risk of Lung and Upper Aerodigestive Tract Cancers: Results of a Population-Based Case-Control Study," *Cancer Epidemiology Biomarkers and Prevention* 15, no. 10 (2006): 1829–34; and Zuo-Feng Zhang, H. Morgenstern, M. R. Spitz, D. P. Tashkin, G. P. Yu, J. R. Marshall, T. C. Hsu, S. P. Schantz, "Marijuana Use and Increased Risk of Squamous Cell Carcinoma of the Head and Neck," *Cancer Epidemiology Biomarkers and Prevention* 8, no. 12 (1999): 1071–78.

[212] Elizabeth A. Penner, Hannah Buettner, and Murray A. Mittleman, "The Impact of Marijuana Use on Glucose, Insulin, and Insulin Resistance among US Adults," *American Journal of Medicine* 126, no. 7 (July 2013): 583-89, doi:10.1016/j.amjmed.2013.03.002.

[213] Paola Massi, M. Solinas, V. Cinquina, and D. Parolaro, "Cannabidiol as Potential Anticancer Drug," *British Journal of Clinical Pharmacology* 75, no. 2 (2013): 303–12; and Alessia Ligresti, A. S. Moriello, K. Starowicz, I. Matias, S. Pisanti, L. De Petrocellis, C. Laezza, G. Portella, M. Bifulco, and V. Di Marzo, "Antitumor Activity of Plant Cannabinoids with Emphasis on the Effect of Cannabidiol on Human Breast Carcinoma," *Journal of Pharmacology and Experimental Therapeutics* 318, no. 3 (2006): 1375–87.

[214] Ethan B. Russo, "Clinical Endocannabinoid Deficiency (CECD)," *Neuroendocrinology Letters* 29, no. 2 (2008): 192–200.

[215] Pedro Gonzalez-Naranjo, N. E. Campillo, C. Pérez, and J. A. Páez, "Multitarget Cannabinoids as Novel Strategy for Alzheimer Disease," *Current Alzheimer Research* 10, no. 3 (2013): 229–39.

[216] Clint Werner, *Marijuana: Gateway to Health: How Cannabis Protects Us from Cancer and Alzheimer's Disease* (San Francisco: Dachstar Press, 2011).

[217] Susan Weiss Behrend, "Cannabinoids May Be Therapeutic in Breast Cancer," *Oncology Nursing Forum* 40, no. 2 (2013): 191–92.

[218] Raphael Mechoulam and Linda Parker, "Towards a Better Cannabis Drug," *British Journal of Pharmacology* (2013), doi:10.1111/bph.12400.

[219] Mark A. Ware, T. Wang, S. Shapiro, A. Robinson, T. Ducruet, T. Huynh, A. Gamsa, G. J. Bennett, and J. P. Collet, "Smoked Cannabis for Chronic Neuropathic Pain: A Randomized Controlled Trial," *Canadian Medical Association Journa*l 182, no. 14 (2010): E694–E701.

[220] Ranganath Muniyappa, Sara Sable, Ronald Ouwerkerk, Andrea Mari, Ahmed M. Gharib, Mary Walter, Amber Courville, Gail Hall, Kong Y. Chen, Nora D. Volkow, George Kunos, Marilyn A. Huestis, and Monica C. Skarulis, "Metabolic Effects of Chronic Cannabis Smoking," *Diabetes Care* (2013), doi:10.2337/dc12-2303.

[221] D. Mark Anderson, Daniel I. Rees, and Joseph J. Sabia, "High on Life? Medical Marijuana Laws and Suicide" (January 2012), ftp.iza.org/dp6280.pdf.
[222] Clint Werner, *Marijuana: Gateway to Health: How Cannabis Protects Us from Cancer and Alzheimer's Disease* (San Francisco: Dachstar Press, 2011), 69.
[223] Lester Grinspoon and James B. Bakalar, *Marihuana, the Forbidden Medicine* (New Haven: Yale University Press, 1997).
[224] Craig Reinarman, H. Nunberg, F. Lanthier, and T. Heddleston, "Who Are Medical Marijuana Patients? Population Characteristics from Nine California Assessment Clinics," *Journal of Psychoactive Drugs* 43, no. 2 (2011): 128–35.
[225] Sean D. McAllister, R. Murase, R. T. Christian, D. Lau, A. J. Zielinski, J. Allison, C. Almanza, A. Pakdel, J. Lee, C. Limbad, Y. Liu, R. J. Debs, D. H. Moore, P. Y. Desprez, "Pathways Mediating the Effects of Cannabidiol on the Reduction of Breast Cancer Cell Proliferation, Invasion, and Metastasis," *Breast Cancer Research and Treatment* 129, no. 1 (2011): 37–47.
[226] C. Michael Gammon, G. Mark Freeman Jr., Wihua Xie, Sandra L. Petersen, and William C. Wetsel, "Regulation of Gonadotropin-Releasing Hormone Secretion by Cannabinoids," *Endocrinology* 146, no. 10 (2005): 4491–99.
[227] Anthony H. Taylor, M. S. Abbas, M. A. Habiba, and J. C. Konje, "Histomorphometric Evaluation of Cannabinoid Receptor and Anandamide Modulating Enzyme Expression in the Human Endometrium through the Menstrual Cycle," *Histochemistry and Cell Biology* 133, no. 5 (2010): 557–65.
[228] Mona R. El-Talatini, Anthony H. Taylor, and Justin C. Konje, "The Relationship between Plasma Levels of the Endocannabinoid, Anandamide, Sex Steroids, and Gonadotrophins during the Menstrual Cycle," *Fertility and Sterility* 93, no. 6 (2010): 1989–96.
[229] Natalia Dmitrieva, H. Nagabukuro, D. Resuehr, G. Zhang, S. L. McAllister, K. A. McGinty, K. Mackie, K. J. Berkley, "Endocannabinoid Involvement in Endometriosis," *Pain* 151, no. 3 (2010): 703–10.
[230] John M. McPartland, "Cannabis and Eicosanoids: A Review of Molecular Pharmacology," *Journal of Cannabis Therapeutics* 1, no. 1 (2001): 71–83.
[231] lan J. Budney and John R. Hughes, "The Cannabis Withdrawal Syndrome," *Current Opinion in Psychiatry* 19, no. 3 (2006): 233–38.
[232] Candice Contet, Brigitte L. Kieffer, and Katia Befort, "Mu Opioid Receptor: A Gateway to Drug Addiction," *Current Opinion in Neurobiology* 14, no. 3 (2004): 370–78.
[233] Walter Fratta and Liana Fattore, "Molecular Mechanisms of Cannabinoid Addiction," *Current Opinion in Neurobiology* 23, no. 4 (August 2013): 487–92.
[234] "Mental Health Services Administration: Treatment Episode Data Set (TEDS) — Highlights 2007. National Admissions to Substance Abuse Treatment Services," Substance Abuse and Mental Health Services Administration, Office of Applied Studies, US Government, 2009.
[235] David J. Allsop, Jan Copeland, Melissa M. Norberg, Shanlin Fu, Anna Molnar, John Lewis, and Alan J. Budney, "Quantifying the Clinical Significance of Cannabis Withdrawal," *PLoS ONE* 7, no. 9 (2012): e44864, doi:10.1371/journal.pone.0044864.
[236] Melissa M. Norberg, R. A. Battisti, J. Copeland, D. F. Hermens, and I. B. Hickie, "Two Sides of the Same Coin: Cannabis Dependence and Mental Health Problems in Help-Seeking Adolescent and Young Adult Outpatients," *International Journal of Mental Health and Addiction* 10, no. 6 (2012): 818–28.

SELECTED BIBLIOGRAPHY

Abel, Ernest L. *Marihuana: The First Twelve Thousand Years*. New York: Plenum Press, 1980.

Abrams, Donald I. and Manuel Guzman. "Cannabinoids and Cancer." *Integrative Oncology*. Oxford: Oxford University Press 2008.

Abrams, Donald I., C. A. Jay, S. B. Shade, H. Vizoso, H. Reda, S. Press, M. E. Kelly, M. C. Rowbotham, and K. L. Petersen. "Cannabis in Painful HIV-Associated Sensory Neuropathy: A Randomized Placebo-Controlled Trial." *Neurology* 68, no. 7 (2007): 515–21.

Aggarwal, Sunil K. "Cannabinergic Pain Medicine: A Concise Clinical Primer and Survey of Randomized-Controlled Trial Results." *Clinical Journal of Pain* 29, no. 2 (2013): 162–71.

Alpert, Joseph S. "Marijuana for Diabetic Control." *American Journal of Medicine* 126, no. 7 (2013): 557–58.

Batho, Robert. "Cannabis Indica," *British Medical Journal* 1, no. 1169 (1883): 1002.

Benet, Sula. "Early Diffusion and Folk Uses of Hemp in Cannabis and Culture." In *Cannabis and Culture*, edited by Vera D. Rubin, 39–49. The Hague: Mouton, 1975.

Bostwick, J. M. "Blurred Boundaries: The Therapeutics and Politics of Medical Marijuana." *Mayo Clinic Proceedings* 87, no. 2 (2012): 172–86.

Brenneisen, Rudolf. "Chemistry and Analysis of Phytocannabinoids and Other Cannabis Constituents." *Marijuana* (2007): 17.

Buckner, Julia D., Russell A. Matthews, and Jose Silgado. "Marijuana-Related Problems and Social Anxiety: The Role of Marijuana Behaviors in Social Situations." *Psychology of Addictive Behaviors* 26, no. 1 (2012): 151.

Campos, Alline C., Z. Ortega, J. Palazuelos, M. V. Fogaça, D. C. Aguiar, J. Díaz-Alonso, S. Ortega-Gutiérrez, H. Vázquez-Villa, F. A. Moreira, M. Guzmán, I. Galve-Roperh, F. S. Guimarães. "The Anxiolytic Effect of Cannabidiol on Chronically Stressed Mice Depends on Hippocampal Neurogenesis: Involvement of the Endocannabinoid System." *International Journal of Neuropsychopharmacology* (2013): 1–13.

Campos, Isaac. *Home Grown: Marijuana and the Origins of Mexico's War on Drugs*. Chapel Hill: University of North Carolina Press, 2012.

Clarke, Robert C. *Marijuana Botany, an Advanced Study: The Propagation and Breeding of Distinctive Cannabis*. Ronin Pub, 1981.

———. *Hashish!* Los Angeles: Red Eye Press, 1998.

Clarke, Robert C., and Mark Merlin. *Cannabis: Evolution and Ethnobotany*. Berkeley: University of California Press, 2013.

Clarke, Robert C., and David P. Watson. "Cannabis and Natural Cannabis Medicines." *Marijuana and the Cannabinoids* (2007): 1–15.

Crawford, Vivian. "A Homelie Herbe: Medicinal Cannabis in Early England." *Journal of Cannabis Therapeutics* 2 (2002): 71–79.

Crippa, José Alexandre, Antonio Waldo Zuardi, Rocio Martín-Santos, Sagnik Bhattacharyya, Zerrin Atakan, Philip McGuire, and Paolo Fusar-Poli. "Cannabis and Anxiety: a Critical Review of the Evidence." *Human Psychopharmacology: Clinical and Experimental* 24, no. 7 (2009): 515–23.

De Petrocellis, Luciano, A. Ligresti, A. Schiano Moriello, M. Iappelli, R. Verde, C. G. Stott, L. Cristino, P. Orlando, and V. Di Marzo. "Non-THC Cannabinoids Inhibit Prostate Carcinoma Growth In Vitro and In Vivo: Pro-Apoptotic Effects and Underlying Mechanisms." *British Journal of Pharmacology* 168, no. 1 (2013): 79–102.

Di Marzo, Vincenzo. "Targeting the Endocannabinoid System: To Enhance or Reduce?" *Nature Reviews Drug Discovery* 7, no. 5 (2008): 438–55.

Di Marzo, Vincenzo, Fabiana Piscitelli, and Raphael Mechoulam. "Cannabinoids and Endocannabinoids in Metabolic Disorders with Focus on Diabetes." *Handbook of Experimental Pharmacology*, 203 (2011): 75–104.

Doblin, Richard E., and M. A. Kleiman. "Marijuana as Antiemetic Medicine: A Survey of Oncologists' Experiences and Attitudes." *Journal of Clinical Oncology* 9, no. 7 (1991): 1314–19.

Eichler, Martin, L. Spinedi, S. Unfer-Grauwiler, M. Bodmer, C. Surber, M. Luedi, and J. Drewe. "Heat Exposure of Cannabis Sativa Extracts Affects the Pharmacokinetic and Metabolic Profile in Healthy Male Subjects." *Planta Medica* 78, no. 7 (2012): 686.

ElSohly, H. N., C. E. Turner, A. M. Clark, and Mahmoud A. ElSohly. "Synthesis and Antimicrobial Activity of Certain Cannabichromene and Cannabigerol Related Compounds." *Journal of Pharmaceutical Sciences* 71 (1982): 1319–23.

Fankhauser, Manfred. "History of Cannabis in Western Medicine." In *Cannabis and Cannabinoids: Pharmacology, Toxicology, and Therapeutic Potential*, edited by Franjo Grotenhermen and Ethan Russo, 37–51. New York: The Haworth Integrative Healing Press, 2002.

Fernández-Ruiz, Javier, O. Sagredo, M. R. Pazos, C. García, R. Pertwee, R. Mechoulam, and J. Martínez-Orgado. "Cannabidiol for Neurodegenerative

Disorders: Important New Clinical Applications for This Phytocannabinoid?" *British Journal of Clinical Pharmacology* 75, no. 2 (2013): 323–33.
Fratta, Walter, and Liana Fattore. "Molecular Mechanisms of Cannabinoid Addiction." *Current Opinion in Neurobiology* 23, no. 4 (August 2013): 487–92.
García, C., C. Palomo-Garo, M. García-Arencibia, J. Ramos, R. Pertwee, and J. Fernández-Ruiz. "Symptom-Relieving and Neuroprotective Effects of the Phytocannabinoid Delta-9-THCV in Animal Models of Parkinson's Disease." *British Journal of Pharmacology* 163, no. 7 (2011): 1495–506.
Gieringer, Dale H. "Forgotten Origins of Cannabis Prohibition in California, The." Contemp. Drug Probs. 26 (1999): 237.
Gieringer, Dale, Joseph St. Laurent, and Scott Goodrich. "Cannabis vaporizer combines efficient delivery of THC with effective suppression of pyrolytic compounds." *Journal of Cannabis Therapeutics* 4.1 (2004): 7-27.
Gill, E. W., W. D. M. Paton, and R. G. Pertwee. "Preliminary Experiments on the Chemistry and Pharmacology of Cannabis." *Nature* 228 (1970): 134–36.
Gorman, Mel. "Sir William Brooke O'Shaughnessy: Pioneer Chemist in a Colonial Environment." *Journal of Chemical Education* 46, no. 2 (1969): 99.
Grant, Igor A. "Medicinal Cannabis and Painful Sensory Neuropathy." *American Medical Association Journal of Ethics* 15, no. 5 (May 2013): 466–69.
Grinspoon, Lester. "A Novel Approach to the Symptomatic Treatment of Autism." *O'Shaughnessy's: The Journal of Cannabis in Clinical Practice*, Spring 2010.
Grinspoon, Lester, and James B. Bakalar. *Marihuana, the Forbidden Medicine*. New Haven: Yale University Press, 1997.
Grotenhermen, Franjo. "Pharmacokinetics and Pharmacodynamics of Cannabinoids." *Clinical Pharmacokinetics* 42, no. 4 (2003): 327–60.
Guy, G. W., and C. G. Stott. "The Development of Sativex—A Natural Cannabis-Based Medicine." In *Cannabinoids as Therapeutics*, edited by R. Mechoulam, 23–63. Basel: Birkhäuser Verlag, 2005.
Hampson, A. J., M. Grimaldi, J. Axelrod, and D. Wink. "Cannabidiol and Delta-9-Tetrahydrocannabinol Are Neuroprotective Antioxidants." *Proceedings of the National Academy of Sciences of the United States* 95, no. 14 (1998): 8268–73.
Hazekamp, Arno, Mark A. Ware, Kirsten R. Muller-Vahl, Donald Abrams, and Franjo Grotenhermen. "The Medicinal Use of Cannabis and Cannabionoids—An International Cross-Sectional Survey on Administration Forms." *Journal of Psychoactive Drugs* 45, no. 3 (2013): 199–210. doi: 10,1080/02791072.2013.805976.
Hill, A. J., M. S. Mercier, T. D. Hill, S. E. Glyn, N. A. Jones, Y. Yamasaki, T. Futamura, M. Duncan, C. G. Stott, G. J. Stephens, C. M. Williams, and B. J. Whalley. "Cannabidivarin Is Anticonvulsant in Mouse and Rat." *British Journal of Pharmacology* 167, no. 8 (2012): 1629–42.
Hill, Andrew J., C. M. Williams, B. J. Whalley, and G. J. Stephens. "Phytocannabinoids as Novel Therapeutic Agents in CNS Disorders." *Pharmacology and Therapeutics* 133, no. 1 (2012): 79–97.
Hillig, Karl William. "A Systematic Investigation of Cannabis." PhD diss., Indiana University, 2005.
Hirvonen, J., R. S. Goodwin, C. T. Li, G. E. Terry, S. S. Zoghbi, C. Morse, V. W. Pike, N. D. Volkow, M. A. Huestis, and R. B. Innis. "Reversible and Regionally Selective Downregulation of Brain Cannabinoid CB_1 Receptors in Chronic Daily Cannabis Smokers." *Molecular Psychiatry* 17, no. 6 (2011): 642–49.
Horváth, Béla, P. Mukhopadhyay, G. Haskó, and P. Pacher. "The Endocannabinoid System and Plant-Derived Cannabinoids in Diabetes and Diabetic Complications." *American Journal of Pathology* 180, no. 2 (2012): 432–42.
Iversen, Leslie L. *The Science of Marijuana*. Oxford: Oxford University Press, 2000.
Jones, Nicholas A., Andrew J. Hill, Imogen Smith, Sarah A. Bevan, Claire M. Williams, Benjamin J. Whalley, and Gary J. Stephens. "Cannabidiol Displays Antiepileptiform and Antiseizure Properties In Vitro and In Vivo." *Journal of Pharmacology and Experimental Therapeutics* 332, no. 2 (2010): 569–77.
Kerr, H. C. *Report of the Cultivation of, and Trade in, Ganja in Bengal*. British Parliamentary Papers (1893–94): 66, 94–154.
King, G. R., T. Ernst, W. Deng, A. Stenger, R. M. K. Gonzales, H. Nakama, and L. Chang. "Effects of Chronic Active Cannabis Use on Visuomotor Integration, in Relation to Brain Activation and Cortisol Levels." *Journal of Neuroscience* 31, no. 49 (2011): 17923.
Klein, Thomas W. "Cannabinoid-Based Drugs as Anti-Inflammatory Therapeutics." *Nature Reviews Immunology* 5, no. 5 (2005): 400–11.
Lata, Hemant, Suman Chandra, Ikhlas A. Khan, and Mahmoud A. ElSohly. "Propagation through Alginate Encapsulation of Axillary Buds of *Cannabis sativa L.*—An Important Medicinal Plant." *Physiology and Molecular Biology of Plants* 15, no. 11 (2009): 79–86.
Ligresti, Alessia, T. Bisogno, I. Matias, L. De Petrocellis, M. G. Cascio, V. Cosenza, G. D'argenio, G. Scaglione, M. Bifulco, I. Sorrentini, and V.

Di Marzo. "Possible Endocannabinoid Control of Colorectal Cancer Growth." *Gastroenterology* 125, no. 3 (2003): 677–87.

Ligresti, Alessia, A. S. Moriello, K. Starowicz, I. Matias, S. Pisanti, L. De Petrocellis, C. Laezza, G. Portella, M. Bifulco, and V. Di Marzo. "Antitumor Activity of Plant Cannabinoids with Emphasis on the Effect of Cannabidiol on Human Breast Carcinoma." *Journal of Pharmacology and Experimental Therapeutics* 318, no. 3 (2006): 1375–87.

Liou, G. I., A. El-Remessy, A. Ibrahim, R. Caldwell, Y. Khalifa, A. Gunes, and J. Nussbaum. "Cannabidiol as a Putative Novel Therapy for Diabetic Retinopathy: A Postulated Mechanism of Action as an Entry Point for Biomarker-Guided Clinical Development." *Current Pharmacogenomics and Personalized Medicine* 7, no. 3 (2009): 215.

Lotan, I., T. Treves, Y. Roditi, and R. Djaldetti, "Medical Marijuana (Cannabis) Treatment for Motor and Non-Motor Symptoms in Parkinson's Disease: An Open-Label Observational Study." *Movement Disorders* 28, supplement 1 (2013): 448.

Massi, Paola, M. Solinas, V. Cinquina, and D. Parolaro. "Cannabidiol as Potential Anticancer Drug." *British Journal of Clinical Pharmacology* 75, no. 2 (2013): 303–12.

McPartland, John M. "Cannabis and Eicosanoids: A Review of Molecular Pharmacology." *Journal of Cannabis Therapeutics* 1, no. 1 (2001): 71–83.

McPartland, John M., and Ethan B. Russo. "Cannabis and Cannabis Extracts: Greater than the Sum of Their Parts?" *Journal of Cannabis Therapeutics* 3, no. 4 (2001): 103–32.

Mechoulam, Raphael. "The Pharmacohistory of *Cannabis sativa*." In *Cannabis as Therapeutic Agent.* Boca Raton, FL: CRC Press, 1986: 1–19.

Mechoulam, Raphael, and L. Hanus. "A Historical Overview of Chemical Research on Cannabinoids." *Chemistry and Physics of Lipids* 108 (2000): 1–13.

Mechoulam, Raphael and Linda Parker. "Towards a Better Cannabis Drug." *British Journal of Pharmacology* (2013). doi:10.1111/bph.12400.

Mills, James. *Cannabis Britannica: Empire, Trade, and Prohibition 1800–1928*. Oxford: Oxford University Press, 2003.

Mittleman, Murray A., Rebecca A. Lewis, Malcolm Maclure, Jane B. Sherwood, and James E. Muller "Triggering Myocardial Infarction by Marijuana." *Circulation* 103, no. 23 (2001): 2805–9.

Molina, Patricia E., P. Winsauer, P. Zhang, E. Walker, L. Birke, A. Amedee, C. V. Stouwe, D. Troxclair, R. McGoey, K. Varner, L. Byerley, and L. LaMotte. "Cannabinoid Administration Attenuates the Progression of Simian Immunodeficiency Virus." *AIDS Research and Human Retroviruses* 27, no. 6 (2011): 585–92.

Morgan, Celia J. A., Tom P. Freeman, Gráinne L. Schafer, and H. Valerie Curran. "Cannabidiol Attenuates the Appetitive Effects of Delta 9-Tetrahydrocannabinol in Humans Smoking Their Chosen Cannabis." *Neuropsychopharmacology* 35, no. 9 (2010): 1879–85.

Morgan, Celia J. A., G. Schafer, T. P. Freeman, and H. V. Curran. "Impact of Cannabidiol on the Acute Memory and Psychotomimetic Effects of Smoked Cannabis: Naturalistic Study." *British Journal of Psychiatry* 197, no. 4 (2010): 285–90.

Mountain Girl. *The Primo Plant: Growing Sinsemilla Marijuana*. Berkeley: Leaves of Grass/Wingbow Press, 1977.

Muniyappa, Ranganath, Sara Sable, Ronald Ouwerkerk, Andrea Mari, Ahmed M. Gharib, Mary Walter, Amber Courville, Gail Hall, Kong Y. Chen, Nora D. Volkow, George Kunos, Marilyn A. Huestis, and Monica C. Skarulis. "Metabolic Effects of Chronic Cannabis Smoking." *Diabetes Care* (2013). doi:10.2337/dc12-2303.

Neumeister, A., M. D. Normandin, R. H. Pietrzak, D. Piomelli, M. Q. Zheng, A. Gujarro-Anton, M. N. Potenza, C. R. Bailey, S. F. Lin, S. Najafzadeh, J. Ropchan, S. Henry, S. Corsi-Travali, R. E. Carson, and Y. Huang. "Elevated Brain Cannabinoid CB_1 Receptor Availability in Post-Traumatic Stress Disorder: A Positron Emission Tomography Study." *Molecular Psychiatry* 18 (September 2013): 1034–40. doi:10.1038/mp.2013.61.

Olson, Dave. "Hemp Culture in Japan." *Journal of the International Hemp Association* 4, no. 2 (June 1997): 40–50.

O'Shaughnessy, William Brooke. "On the preparations of the Indian hemp, or gunjah (*Cannabis indica*); Their effects on the animal system in health, and their utility in the treatment of tetanus and other convulsive diseases." *Transactions of the Medical and Physical Society of Bengal* (1838): 71–102, 421, 461.

Pace, Nicholas, Henry Clay Frick, Kenneth Sutin, William Manger, George Hyman, and Gabriel Nahas. "The Medical Use of Marihuana and THC in Perspective." In *Marihuana and Medicine*, 76–80. New York: Humana Press, 1999.

Pacher, Pál. "Towards the Use of Non-Psychoactive Cannabinoids for Prostate Cancer." *British Journal of Pharmacology* 168, no. 1 (2013): 76–78.

Pacher, Pál, Sándor Bátkai, and George Kunos. "The Endocannabinoid System as an Emerging Target of Pharmacotherapy." *Pharmacological Reviews* 58, no. 3

(2006): 389–462.
Pacher, Pál, Joseph S. Beckman, and Lucas Liaudet. "Nitric Oxide and Peroxynitrite in Health and Disease." *Physiological Reviews* 87, no. 1 (2007): 315–424.
Parker, Linda A., Erin M. Rock, and Cheryl L. Limebeer. "Regulation of Nausea and Vomiting by Cannabinoids." *British Journal of Pharmacology* 163, no. 7 (2011): 1411–22.
Passie, Torsten, H. M. Emrich, M. Karst, S. D. Brandt, and J. H. Halpern. "Mitigation of Post-Traumatic Stress Symptoms by Cannabis Resin: A Review of the Clinical and Neurobiological Evidence." *Drug Testing and Analysis* 4, nos. 7–8 (2012): 649–59.
Penner, Elizabeth A., Hannah Buettner, and Murray A. Mittleman. "The Impact of Marijuana Use on Glucose, Insulin, and Insulin Resistance among US Adults." *American Journal of Medicine* 126, no. 7 (July 2013): 583–89. doi:10.1016/j.amjmed.2013.03.002.
Pertwee, R. G. "The Diverse CB_1 and CB_2 Receptor Pharmacology of Three Plant Cannabinoids: Delta 9-Tetrahydrocannabinol, Cannabidiol and Delta 9-Tetrahydrocannabivarin." *British Journal of Pharmacology* 153, no. 2 (2008): 199–215.
Phillips, L. J., C. Curry, A. R. Yung, H. P. Yuen, S. Adlard, and P. D. McGorry. "Cannabis Use Is Not Associated with the Development of Psychosis in an 'Ultra' High-Risk Group." *Australian and New Zealand Journal of Psychiatry* 36, no. 6 (2002): 800–6.
Pletcher, Mark J., Eric Vittinghoff, Ravi Kalhan, Joshua Richmann, Monika Safford, Stephen Sidney, Feng Lin, and Stefan Kertesz. "Association Between Marijuana Exposure and Pulmonary Function over 20 years." *Journal of the American Medical Association* 307, no. 2 (2012): 173–81.
Portenoy, Russell K., E. D. Ganae-Motan, S. Allende, R. Yanagihara, L. Shaiova, S. Weinstein, R. McQuade, S. Wright, and M. T. Fallon. "Nabiximols for Opioid-Treated Cancer Patients with Poorly-Controlled Chronic Pain: A Randomized, Placebo-Controlled, Graded-Dose Trial." *Journal of Pain* 13, no. 5 (2012): 438–49.
Potter, David. "Growth and Morphology of Medicinal Cannabis." In *The Medicinal Uses of Cannabis and Cannabinoids*, edited by Geoffrey W. Guy, Brian A. Whittle, and Philip J.
———. "The Propagation, Characterisation and Optimisation of Cannabis *Sativa L* as a Phytopharmaceutical. Diss., King's College London, 2009.
Reinarman, Craig, H. Nunberg, F. Lanthier, and T. Heddleston. "Who Are Medical Marijuana Patients? Population Characteristics from Nine California Assessment Clinics." *Journal of Psychoactive Drugs* 43, no. 2 (2011): 128–35.
Report of the Indian Hemp Drugs Commission, 1893–94, 7 vols. Simla, India: Government Central Printing House, 1894.
Richardson, Jim, and Arik Woods. *Sinsemilla: Marijuana Flowers*. Berkeley: And/Or Press, 1976.
Robson, P. J., G. W. Guy, and V. Di Marzo. "Cannabinoids and Schizophrenia: Therapeutic Prospects." *Current Pharmaceutical Design* (2013).
Rosenthal, Franz. *The Herb: Hashish versus Medieval Muslim Society*. Leiden: Brill, 1971.
Russo, Ethan B. "Cannabis Treatments in Obstetrics and Gynecology: A Historical Review." *Journal of Cannabis Therapeutics* 2, nos. 3–4 (2002): 5–35.
———. "Clinical Endocannabinoid Deficiency (CECD): Can This Concept Explain Therapeutic Benefits of Cannabis in Migraine, Fibromyalgia, Irritable Bowel Syndrome and Other Treatment-Resistant Conditions?" *Neuroendocrinology Letters* 25, nos. 1–2 (2004): 31–3.
———. "Clinical Endocannabinoid Deficiency (CECD)." *Neuroendocrinology Letters* 29, no. 2 (2008): 192–200.
———. "Hemp for Headache: An In-Depth Historical and Scientific Review of Cannabis in Migraine Treatment." *Journal of Cannabis Therapeutics* 1, no. 2 (2001): 21–92.
———. "History of Cannabis and Its Preparations in Saga, Science, and Sobriquet." *Chemistry and Biodiversity* 4, no. 8 (2007): 1614–48.
———. "Taming THC: Potential Cannabis Synergy and Phytocannabinoid-Terpenoid Entourage Effects." *British Journal of Pharmacology* 163, no. 7 (2011): 1344–64.
Russo, Ethan B., and Geoffrey W. Guy. "A Tale of Two Cannabinoids: The Therapeutic Rationale for Combining Tetrahydrocannabinol and Cannabidiol." *Medical Hypotheses* 66, no. 2 (2006): 234–46.
Russo, Ethan B., and Andrea G. Hohmann. "Role of Cannabinoids in Pain Management." In *Comprehensive Treatment of Chronic Pain by Medical, Interventional, and Integrative Approaches*, edited by Timothy R. Deer, Michael S. Leong, Asokumar Buvanendran, Vitaly Gordin, Philip S. Kim, Sunil J. Panchal, and Albert L. Ray, 181–97. New York: Springer, 2013.
Russo, Ethan B., A. Burnett, B. Hall, and K. K. Parker. "Agonistic Properties of Cannabidiol at 5-HT1a Receptors." *Neurochemical Research* 30, no. 8 (2005): 1037–43.
Russo, Ethan B., Geoffrey W. Guy, and Philip J. Robson. "Cannabis, Pain, and Sleep: Lessons from

Therapeutic Clinical Trials of Sativex®, a Cannabis-Based Medicine." *Chemistry and Biodiversity* 4, no. 8 (2007): 1729–43.

Sallan, Stephen E., Norman E. Zinberg, and Emil Frei III. "Antiemetic Effect of Delta-9-Tetrahydro-cannabinol in Patients Receiving Cancer Chemotherapy." *New England Journal of Medicine* 293, no. 16 (1975): 795–97.

Sarfaraz, Sami, Vaqar M. Adhami, Deeba N. Syed, Farrukh Afaq, and Hasan Mukhtar. "Cannabinoids for Cancer Treatment: Progress and Promise." *Cancer research* 68, no. 2 (2008): 339-342.

Selye, Hans. "A Syndrome Produced by Diverse Nocuous Agents." *Nature*; *Nature* (1936): 32. doi:10.1038/138032a0

Sharma, G. K. "Ethnobotany and Its Significance for Cannabis Studies in the Himalayas." *Journal of Psychoactive Drugs* 9, no. 4 (1977): 337–39.

Shohami, E., A. Cohen-Yeshurun, L. Magid, M. Algali, and R. Mechoulam. "Endocannabinoids and Traumatic Brain Injury." *British Journal of Pharmacology* 163 (2011): 1402–10.

Simonetto, Douglas A., Amy S. Oxentenko, Margot L. Herman, and Jason H. Szostek. "Cannabinoid Hyperemesis: A Case Series of 98 Patients." *Mayo Clinic Proceedings* 87, no. 2 (2012).

Tam, Joseph, J. Liu, B. Mukhopadhyay, R. Cinar, G. Godlewski, and G. Kunos. "Endocannabinoids in Liver Disease" *Hepatology* 53, no. 1 (2011): 346–55.

Tashkin, Donald P. "Effects of Marijuana Smoking on the Lung." *Annals of the American Thoracic Society* 10, no. 3 (2013): 239–47.

Tashkin, Donald P., B. J. Shapiro, Y. E. Lee, and C. E. Harper. "Effects of Smoked Marijuana in Experimentally Induced Asthma." *American Review of Respiratory Disease* 112, no. 3 (1975): 377–86.

Tashkin, Donald P., G. C. Baldwin, T. Sarafian, S. Dubnett, and M. D. Roth. "Respiratory and Immunologic Consequences of Marijuana Smoking." *The Journal of Clinical Pharmacology* 42, no. 11 supplement (2002): 71S–81S.

Tetrault, Jeanette M., K. Crothers, B. A. Moore, R. Mehra, J. Concato, and D. A. Fiellin. "Effects of Marijuana Smoking on Pulmonary Function and Respiratory Complications: A Systematic Review." *Archives of Internal Medicine* 167, no. 3 (2007): 221.

Tomida, Ileana, A. Azuara-Blanco, H. House, M. Flint, R. G. Pertwee, and P. J. Robson. "Effect of Sublingual Application of Cannabinoids on Intraocular Pressure: A Pilot Study." *Journal of Glaucoma* 15, no. 5 (2006): 349–53.

Tubaro, Aurelia, A. Giangaspero, S. Sosa, R. Negri, G. Grassi, S. Casano, R. Della Loggia, and G. Appendino. "Comparative Topical Anti-Inflammatory Activity of Cannabinoids and Cannabivarins." *Fitoterapia* 81, no. 7 (2010): 816–19.

Wade, D. T., P. Makela, P. Robson, H. House, and C. Bateman. "Do Cannabis-Based Medicinal Extracts Have General or Specific Effects on Symptoms in Multiple Sclerosis? A Double-Blind, Randomized, Placebo-Controlled Study on 160 Patients." *Multiple Sclerosis Journal* 10 (2004): 434–41.

Wallace, Mark, G. Schulteis, J. H. Atkinson, T. Wolfson, D. Lazzaretto, H. Bentley, B. Gouaux, I. Abramson. "Dose-Dependent Effects of Smoked Cannabis on Capsaicin-Induced Pain and Hyperalgesia in Healthy Volunteers." *Anesthesiology* 107, no. 5 (2007): 785–96.

Ware, Mark A., M. A. Fitzcharles, L. Joseph, and Y. Shir. "The Effects of Nabilone on Sleep in Fibromyalgia: Results of a Randomized Controlled Trial." *Anesthesia and Analgesia* 110, no. 2 (2010): 604–10.

Ware, Mark A., T. Wang, S. Shapiro, A. Robinson, T. Ducruet, T. Huynh, A. Gamsa, G. J. Bennett, and J. P. Collet. "Smoked Cannabis for Chronic Neuropathic Pain: A Randomized Controlled Trial." *Canadian Medical Association Journal* 182, no. 14 (2010): E694–E701.

Weil, Andrew T., Norman E. Zinberg, and Judith M. Nelsen. "Clinical and psychological effects of marijuana in man." *Substance Use & Misuse* 4.3 (1969): 427-451.

Weil, Andrew. *The Natural Mind*.(Revised Edition). Jonathan Cape, London (1986).

Werner, Clint. *Marijuana: Gateway to Health: How Cannabis Protects Us from Cancer and Alzheimer's Disease*. San Francisco: Dachstar Press, 2011.

Werner, Clinton A. "Medical Marijuana and the AIDS Crisis." *Journal of Cannabis Therapeutics* 1, nos. 3–4 (2001): 17–33.

Zinberg, Norman E., and Andrew T. Weil. "A comparison of marijuana users and non-users." *Nature* (1970).

Zuardi, A. W., J. E. Hallak, S. M. Dursun, S. L. Morais, R. F. Sanches, R. E. Musty, and J. A. Crippa, "Cannabidiol Monotherapy for Treatment-Resistant Schizophrenia." *Journal of Psychopharmacology* 20, no. 5 (2006): 683–86.

Zuardi, A. W., S. L. Morais, F. S. Guimarães, and R. Mechoulam. "Antipsychotic Effect of Cannabidiol," *Journal of Clinical Psychiatry* 56, no. 10 (1995): 485–86.

GLOSSARY

2-AG (2-arachidonoylglycerol)—an endocannabinoid abundant within the central nervous system

7-hydroxy-CBD—the metabolite produced by liver metabolism of CBD

11-hydroxy-THC—the metabolite produced by liver metabolism of THC

abscission layer—the layer from which the gland head of the cannabis trichome can detach from its stalk

anandamide—*N*-arachidonoylethanolamine or AEA is an endogenous cannabinoid that regulates feeding and suckling behavior, along with baseline pain levels and sleep patterns

anthocyanin—plant pigment responsible for the color of purple cannabis

Ayurvedic—the traditional Indian medical system originating over 3,000 years ago

bagseed—seeds found in dried cannabis flowers

beta-caryophyllene—a spicy terpene produced by some cannabis varieties

bhang—a traditional Indian drink of cannabis, spices, and fermented milk

bioavailability—the portion of a cannabis dose that can be absorbed

BLD—broad-leafleted-drug (BLD) cannabis that is THC-predominant with wide leaflets, commonly referred to as "*indica*"

blood/brain barrier—a barrier consisting of cells that prevent bacteria and large or water-loving molecules from crossing into the central nervous system

blunt—a cannabis cigarette rolled in a cigar wrapper

bract—a leaflike floral structure surrounding the flowers and seed of the female cannabis plant

bubble hash—high-grade cannabis resin, typically extracted using ice water, which bubbles when flame is applied

Cannabaceae—small family of flowering plants including cannabis, hops, and hackberries

cannabichromene (CBC)—a cannabinoid found in cannabis that may be anti-inflammatory

cannabidiol (CBD)—non-psychoactive cannabinoid with broad medical applications; the second most common cannabinoid produced by the cannabis plant

cannabidiolic acid (CBDA)—the acidic form of CBD that is naturally produced by the cannabis plant

cannabidivarin (CBDVA)—CBDV is the propyl variant of CBD, and possesses a shorter molecular side chain than CBD; commonly found in some Nepalese and Indian varieties

cannabigerol (CBG)—non-psychoactive cannabinoid that serves as the precursor used by the plant's enzymes to produce THC and CBD

cannabinoids—compounds that activate cannabinoid receptors, including endocannabinoids produced by humans and animals, phytocannabinoids produced by cannabis and a few other plants, and synthetic cannabinoids

cannabinol (CBN)—the weakly psychoactive breakdown product of THC; not produced by the cannabis plant

cannabis hyperemesis syndrome—an uncommon condition affecting a small population of cannabis users characterized by nausea, vomiting, and abdominal pain that can be alleviated by abstinence from cannabis

capitate-stalked glandular trichomes—specialized plant hairs found on the floral bracts of the female cannabis plant. These trichomes are characterized by a stalk topped with a glandular head that swells with secretion of cannabinoid and terpene essential oils.

CB_1 receptor—a cannabinoid receptor located primarily in the central nervous system that is activated by cannabinoids

CB_2 receptor—a cannabinoid receptor that is expressed in the peripheral tissues of the immune system, the gastrointestinal system, the peripheral nervous system, and to a lesser degree in the central nervous system

charas—name given to cannabis resin or hashish in India, Nepal, and Pakistan

chemotype—a term for a plant type, including cannabis, that produces a distinct combination of chemical compounds

chromatography—the separation of a mixture by passing it through a medium in which the components move at different rates

cloning (or cutting)—a technique for propagating cannabis in which a piece of the mother plant is removed and placed in a grow medium, where it produces new roots and becomes a new plant

cola or collie—the top flower cluster of a female cannabis plant

cookie casualty—slang term for an oral cannabis overdose

couchlock—slang term for sedation without sleep brought on by high-THC cannabis
cultivar—a plant variety produced in cultivation through selective breeding
cutting—see *cloning*
decarboxylation—in cannabis, the process of converting acidic cannabinoids produced by the plant into their more bioavailable neutral form by removing a carboxyl group (consisting of one carbon, two oxygen, and a hydrogen atom) from the cannabinoid molecule, typically by the application of heat
dispensary—term used in the United States to refer to storefronts providing medical cannabis products
edibles—food products that have been infused with cannabis or cannabis extractions
endocannabinoid system—a system of neuromodulator chemicals and their receptors throughout the body involved in the regulation of appetite, pain, mood, and memory
entourage effect—the synergistic pharmacological effects that emerge through cannabinoid and terpene interaction
first-pass effect—a phenomenon in which the concentration of a drug is greatly reduced through the process of metabolism before it reaches systemic circulation. When cannabis is swallowed it is subjected to extensive first-pass effects by liver metabolism.
flowering time—the period required for cannabis flowers to develop and fully ripen
full melt—high-quality cannabis resin or hashish that readily melts when flame is applied; mistakenly believed to be an indicator of resin quality
ganja—Indian term for seedless female cannabis flower clusters, also known as *sinsemilla*
genotype—specific characteristic of a plant, the expression of which is controlled by genes
Golden Triangle—the drug-producing mountainous region of Myanmar, Thailand, and Laos in Southeast Asia
hashish—cannabis resin
hash oil—solvent extraction of cannabis
headspace—the gas space above the sample in a chromatography vial. Volatile constituents diffuse into their gas phase, forming the headspace gas. Headspace analysis is therefore the analysis of those volatile components.
hemp—low-THC content cannabis used for producing fiber. Hemp often produces CBD rather than THC.
***High Times* Cannabis Cup**—a competition sponsored by *High Times* magazine, held annually in Amsterdam, in which attendees judge herbal cannabis and hashish submitted by coffee shops and seed companies
hubble bubble—a large Afghani water pipe for smoking hashish
hydrophobic—repelling or failing to mix with water
hydroponics—the practice of growing plants without soil, typically in a medium consisting of sand, clay pellets, or gravel with liquid nutrient solutions
indica—a term commonly used to refer to broad-leafleted cannabis varieties
joint—a cannabis cigarette
kif—trichomes collected by sifting or tumbling dried cannabis
kush—a term broadly applied to high-potency varieties of cannabis, some of which originated in the Hindu Kush mountains of Central Asia
landrace—a variety of cannabis which has adapted to the local conditions without minimal intervention
leaflet—a leaflike part of a compound leaf, not borne by a branch or stem
limonene—a terpene possessing an orange aroma produced by some cannabis varieties
linalool—a terpene possessing a spicy, floral aroma produced by some cannabis varieties
lipophilic—literally "fat friendly," used to designate compounds such as cannabinoids that dissolve readily in fats, oils, lipids, and nonpolar solvents such as hexane
menstruum—a solvent used in extracting compounds from plants such as cannabis when preparing tinctures
metabolism—the biochemical modification of drugs by the body, usually by the actions of specialized enzymes
metabolite—the product that remains after a drug is broken down (metabolized) by the body
micro-dosing—a technique for employing the minimum effective dose of a cannabis medicine that delivers the desired outcome or level of effect
mother plant—a cannabis plant kept in a vegetative state (not allowed to flower) so that cuttings or clones may be taken to produce more plants identical to the mother
myrcene—a terpene produced by many plants, including cannabis, hops, and wild thyme, which is pharmacologically sedative and associated with the "*indica*" effect
nail—titanium or quartz fitting used in a specialized pipe ("dabbing rig") to vaporize hash oil. The nail is heated with a gas torch, then a dab of oil is applied, instantly vaporizing it for inhalation.
NLD—narrow-leafleted-drug (NLD) cannabis is THC-predominant with narrow leaflets, commonly called *sativa*
nontoxic cultivation—cultivation that eschews the use of all toxic pesticides and nutrients
ocimene—a terpene with a fruity, floral aroma occasionally found in cannabis
oromucosal delivery—administration that is intended for the oral cavity, especially the buccal mucosa that lines the mouth

pharmacodynamics—what a body does to a drug
pharmacokinetics—what a drug does to a body
phenotype—the distinct characteristics of an individual plant resulting from the interaction of the plant's genotype with the environment in which it is raised
phytocannabinoid—term for the cannabinoids produced by the cannabis plant and a few other plant species
pinene—a terpene with a pine smell produced by cannabis and many other plants, including conifers
plant growth regulator (PGR)—Synthetic plant hormones regulate plant growth, some of which may be harmful to humans
plant tissue culture—a method of growing plant cells, tissues, or organs under sterile conditions on a nutrient culture medium. Plant tissue culture is widely used to produce clones of plants, and recently has been used to produce cannabis.
poddar—an Indian field worker trained to identify and cull male plants from ganja fields
polm—hashish produced by sifting dried flowers through screens to capture the resin-filled trichome gland heads, then pressing the gland heads
postural/orthostatic hypotension—a form of low blood pressure that occurs when you stand up from sitting or lying down, and can be aggravated by cannabis use, especially among naive users. Orthostatic hypotension produces dizziness, lightheadedness, and can even result in unconsciousness.
psychoactivity—the measure of how cannabis and other drugs affect the mind, mood, or other mental states
purple cannabis—cannabis that possesses a genetic tendency to produce anthocyanin when cold stressed, which turns the leaves purple
receptor downregulation—the decrease in the number of receptors available to a cannabinoid molecule, which reduces the sensitivity to cannabinoid effects and underlies the buildup of tolerance
red oil—an early cannabis solvent extraction process developed in the 1940s that produced a clear, red oil
resin—the sticky exudation of the cannabis plant produced by its trichomes
resin head—the oil- and resin-filled gland head of a female cannabis plant's capitate-stalked glandular trichome
sativa—commonly used to describe narrow-leafleted cannabis varieties with stimulating psychoactivity
scissor hash—the resin that accumulates on manicuring tools used to remove extraneous leaf material in the preparation of dried cannabis
seed bank—a company that produce drug cannabis seed for cultivation
single drug/single target—the current system for developing prescription drugs that emphasizes the deployment of a single medicinal agent to target a specific tissue or system within the body
sinsemilla—Spanish for "without seed," referring to seedless, unpollinated female cannabis flowers
spliff—a large cannabis cigarette
sublingual—beneath the tongue
terpene—see *terpenoids*
terpenoids—volatile hydrocarbons found in the essential oils produced by many plants, including cannabis
terpinolene—a terpene found in a few cannabis varieties, as well as cardamom and marjoram
tetrahydrocannabinol (THC) or delta-9-tetrahydrocannabinol—the principal cannabinoid of the cannabis plant, responsible for much cannabis' psychoactivity
THCA (tetrahydrocannabinolic acid)—the acidic form of THC; the form of THC that is produced by the cannabis plant
THCV (tetrahydrocannabivarin)—a variant of tetrahydrocannabinol (THC) having a propyl (3-carbon) side chain. It has antagonistic effects on cannabinoid receptors, therefore it often exhibits effects contrary to THC, e.g., retarding appetite.
tincture—an ethyl alcohol extraction of a plant
tolerance—a reaction to dose (for cannabis or another drug) in which the effects are progressively reduced, requiring an increase in dose in order to achieve the desired effect
trichome—on cannabis, three types of specialized epidermal hairs: capitate-stalked glandular trichomes, capitate-sessile trichomes, and bulbous trichomes
TRPV1 (*transient receptor potential vanilloid receptor*)—the receptor responsible for initiating inflammatory response and pain
Veganics—a method of cannabis cultivation developed by Kyle Kushman that only employs vegan nutrients
water hash—cannabis resin, extracted using ice water and screens to capture resin heads
water leaves—the small leaves that surround the cannabis flower clusters

INDEX

Author Acknowledgments

I am fortunate to have enjoyed the support of many, many people, without whom this book could not have been written:

Amy Robertson, Richard Metzger, Tara McGinley, Mark Lewis, Brian Becker, Chris Holmes, and Sander Greenland gave freely of their brilliance, while providing extraordinary assistance, friendship, and encouragement; Shawn for his peerless vision; Gary, Jim, Don, Aundre, Ed, Matt, Laura, and Ramon for making a dream come true; Andrew Weil for his genius and kindness; Winslow Bouhier provided inspiration and support; My friends and colleagues at LAPCG, Abatin, CBCB, and Cornerstone.

Special thanks to my beloved son, Preston, and his mother, Martha; My parents and siblings: James, Bel, Mort, Marga Lee, Mark, Jeff, and Julie.

Ethan Russo, Mark Merlin, and Rob Clarke, John McPartland, Arno Hazekamp, Karl Hillig, and David Watson for their profound understanding of the plant and its uses.

My dearest friends (in order of appearance): David, Geoff, Robin, Chris, Michal, Ron Cobb and Robin Love, David and Teri Smith, Coco Conn, A.J. Peralta, Brian Callier, Greg Cummings, Peter Giblin, Steve Nalepa, Jonathan Watson and Karis Jagger, Nika Solomon, Mark Dippe, Bobby Tran, Carlos De La Torre, Marcos Lutyens, Freya Bardell and Brian Howe, Oliver Hess, Jeremy Morelli, and Jeff Hayden, who have taught me far more than I have learned.

Marc Geiger, Otis Jackson Jr., J Rocc, Steven Ellison, Daddy Kev, and Willie Bensussen provided the music by which I started this book. Paul and his fine man, John, provided music and inspiration by which I finished.

Fred Gardner and Martin Lee, Kymron DeCesare and Donald Land, Josh Wurzer and Alec Dixon, David Lampach and Addison DeMoura, Jeff Raber, DJ Short, Chimera and Todd McCormick.

I have been fortunate to interact with some excellent professionals who inspired me and helped this book immeasurably: Valerie Corral, Mike Corral, Liz McDuffie, Dr. Allan Frankel, Dale Gieringer, Dr. Donald Abrams, Dr. Maxine Barish-Wreden, Dr. Igor Grant, Dr. Larry Bedard, Roy Upton, Dr. Daniel Harder, Dr. Mark Ware, and my esteemed friends, Dr. Roger Barnes and Dr. Nick Berry. And a heartfelt thanks to the late Michael Crichton, for his eternal inspiration.

This book demanded an incredible amount of work from steady and experienced hands. Laura Ward, Will Steeds, Anna Southgate, and Magda Nakassis shaped every aspect of this book, generously providing their expertise and guidance throughout.

Thanks to J. P. Leventhal and Becky Koh at Black Dog & Leventhal for their extraordinary support and enthusiasm.

My deepest appreciation to all the patients that have shared their lives with me.

What is good in this book came from others, while the errors are mine alone.

Elephant Book Company would like to thank Mick Farren and Richard Metzger (latter of the Dangerous Minds blog), for their help at the earliest stages of this project. Mick (who, very sadly, died on stage during a comeback gig in London in the fall of 2013) suggested we talk to Richard. Richard very helpfully put us in touch with Michael Backes.

Picture Credits: Page 13: Jomon era cave painting near Shimonoseki, Japan—Dave Olson collection.